COMMUNICATING PROCESS ARCHITECTURES 2004

Concurrent Systems Engineering Series

Series Editors: M.R. Jane, J. Hulskamp, P.H. Welch, D. Stiles and T.L. Kunii

Volume 62

Previously published in this series:

ISSN 1383-7575

Communicating Process Architectures 2004

WoTUG-27

Edited by

Ian R. East
Oxford Brookes University, United Kingdom

Jeremy Martin
Oxagen Ltd., United Kingdom

Peter H. Welch
University of Kent, United Kingdom

David Duce
Oxford Brookes University, United Kingdom

and

Mark Green
Oxford Brookes University, United Kingdom

Proceedings of the 27th WoTUG Technical Meeting,
5–8 September 2004, Oxford Brookes University,
United Kingdom

IOS
Press

Amsterdam • Berlin • Oxford • Tokyo • Washington, DC

ISBN 1 58603 458 8
Library of Congress Control Number: 2004110872

Publisher
IOS Press
Nieuwe Hemweg 6B
1013 BG Amsterdam
The Netherlands
fax: +31 20 620 3419
e-mail: order@iospress.nl

Distributor in the UK and Ireland
IOS Press/Lavis Marketing
73 Lime Walk
Headington
Oxford OX3 7AD
England
fax: +44 1865 750079

Distributor in the USA and Canada
IOS Press, Inc.
4502 Rachael Manor Drive
Fairfax, VA 22032
USA
fax: +1 703 323 3668
e-mail: iosbooks@iospress.com

Contents

Preface

Communicating Process Architecture (CPA) describes an approach to system development that is *process*-oriented. It makes no great distinction between hardware and software. It has a major root in the theory of *Communicating Sequential Processes* (CSP) of C.A.R. Hoare, which celebrates its 25-year jubilee this year. However, the underlying theory is not limited to CSP. The importance of mobility of both channel and process within a network sees integration with ideas from the π-calculus. Other formalisms are also exploited, such as BSP and MPI. The focus is on sound methods for the engineering of significant concurrent systems, including those that are distributed (across the Internet or within a single chip) and/or software-scheduled on a single execution unit.

The series of CPA conferences, of which this is the twenty-seventh, has its origin in the technical meetings of the occam User Group, which later became WoTUG, and which now represents a shared interest reflected in the annual conference it sponsors. The ideas and methods that underpin occam and the transputer remain valid and important, especially when the latter may no longer be directly visible. Concurrency is demanded in commercial systems more than ever, yet has grown no easier to engineer. CPA embodies much that has been learned over the last two decades and offers a coherent solution.

Traditionally, at CPA, the emphasis has been on theory *and* practice – developing and applying tools based upon CSP and related theories to build high-integrity systems of significant size. In particular, interest focuses on achieving *scalability* and *security* against error. The development of Java, C, and C++, libraries to facilitate secure concurrent programming using 'mainstream' languages has allowed CPA to continue and proliferate. This work continues in support of the engineering of distributed applications.

Recently, there has been greater reference to theory and its more direct application to programming systems and languages. It is particularly reassuring this year to see the formal CSP community so well represented and we welcome keynote talks by Bill Roscoe and Michael Goldsmith, who have made such important contributions.

Session papers this year provide a healthy mixture of the academic and commercial, software and hardware, application and infrastructure. This reflects the nature of the discipline. CSP is applied to verify (FPGA) hardware descriptions, through model checking, as much as it is applied to verify software ones. Examples are also reported here for refining system architecture, distributed and otherwise, direct from specification. Programming abstraction and infrastructure is extended to include mobile channels and processes. At the academic end of the spectrum, there are valiant efforts to account for multiple views of a computation and to extend formal abstraction to include prioritisation. At the commercial end, parallel processing is finding new markets, such as telecom applications with picoChip™. We look forward to the continuing development of this single community of theoreticians and practitioners!

In a field where it is usual to find theory divorced from practice, we hope the delegate and reader will find Computing united here with a common theme.

Ian East, Mark Green and David Duce *(Oxford Brookes University)*
Jeremy Martin *(Oxagen Ltd)*
Peter Welch *(University of Kent)*

Programme Committee

Prof. Peter Welch, University of Kent, UK (Chair)

Prof. Hamid Arabnia, University of Georgia, USA

Prof. Peter Clayton, Rhodes University, South Africa

Prof. Jon Kerridge, Napier University, UK

Prof. Brian O'Neill, Nottingham Trent University, UK

Prof. Chris Nevison, Colgate University, New York, USA

Prof. Patrick Nixon, University of Strathclyde, UK

Prof. Nan Schaller, Rochester Institute of Technology, New York, USA

Prof. Dyke Stiles, Utah State University, USA

Prof. Rod Tosten, Gettysburg University, USA

Prof. Paul Tynman, Rochester Institute of Technology, New York, USA

Prof. Jim Woodcock, University of Kent, UK

Dr. Alastair Allen, Aberdeen University, UK

Dr. Fred Barnes, University of Kent, UK

Dr. Richard Beton, Roke Manor Research Ltd, UK

Dr. Marcel Boosten, Philips Medical Systems, Ltd, The Netherlands

Dr. Jan Broenink, University of Twente, The Netherlands

Dr. Alan Chalmers, University of Bristol, UK

Dr. Barry Cook, 4Links Ltd., UK

Ruth Ivimey-Cook, Creative Business Systems Ltd, UK

Dr. Ian East, Oxford Brookes University, UK

Dr. Mark Green, Oxford Brookes University, UK

Gerald Hilderink, University of Twente, The Netherlands

Christopher Jones, British Aerospace, UK

Dr. Tom Lake, InterGlossa, UK

Dr. Adrian Lawrence, Loughborough University, UK

Dr. Jeremy Martin, Oxagen Ltd., UK

Dr. Stephen Maudsley, Esgem Ltd, UK

Dr. Majid Mirmehdi, University of Bristol, UK

Dr. Henk Muller, University of Bristol, UK

Dr. Dennis Nicole, University of Southampton, UK

Dr. Matt Baekgaard Pedersen, Univeristy of Nevada, Las Vegas

Dr. Roger Peel, University of Surrey, UK

Herman Roebbers, Philips TASS, The Netherlands

Dr. Marc Smith, Colby College, Maine, USA

Johan Sunter, Philips TASS, The Netherlands

Oyvind Teig, Autronica Fire and Security, Norway

Dr. Stephen Turner, Nanyang Technological University, Singapore

Dr. Brian Vinter, University of Southern Denmark

Peter Visser, University of Twente, The Netherlands

Dr. Paul Walker, 4Links Ltd, UK

Communicating Process Architectures – 2004
Ian East, Jeremy Martin, Peter Welch, David Duce, and Mark Green (Eds.)
IOS Press, 2004

1

Finitary Refinement Checks for Infinitary Specifications

A.W. ROSCOE

Oxford University Computing Laboratory, Wolfson Building, Parks Road, Oxford OX1 3QD, UK

Abstract. We see how refinement against a variety of infinite-state CSP specifications can be translated into finitary refinement checks. Methods used include turning a process into its own specification inductively, and we recall Wolper's discovery that data independence can be used for this purpose.

1 Introduction

Thanks to the refinement checker FDR[1] [1], the question of what predicates on CSP models are decidable via a refinement check is practically as well as intellectually important. By this I mean: what predicates of a process P are equivalent to the question

$$F(P) \sqsubseteq G(P) \qquad (\dagger)$$

for CSP-definable functions F and G? In [7] I gave fairly complete characterisations of the unexpectedly wide range of predicates that can be represented like this. In particular, for the failures/divergences model over a finite alphabet, the metric/topological closed subsets are precisely the predicates that can be represented by metric-continuous F and G.

However, as observed in [7] this answer is of little practical use since the CSP contexts F and G it generates are, in general, infinitary – indeed, usually, they are in a strong sense infinitely large pieces of syntax. Nevertheless, experience and recent work [5] has shown that many useful and subtle properties can be expressed in practical ways.

In the present paper I will begin to study what can be done within the terms of what is practically possible on FDR. Namely, we will restrict ourselves to F and G which, when applied to a finite-state process P, have $F(P)$ and $G(P)$ finite state also. Note that this definition of a *finitary* function is grounded in the operational semantics of CSP, since that is where the notion of a 'finite state process' naturally rests.

By and large I will concentrate more on providing a range of useful recipes for representing predicates rather than full characterisations, simply because at present I have more of the former than the latter! Also the majority of this initial study will be devoted to discovering how to replace infinite-state fixed specification processes *Spec*, for simple checks *Spec* $\sqsubseteq P$, by finitary checks.

We will find that data independence plays an unexpectedly large role in this work.

In the next section we will study how to characterise a counter process, and in the following one we will extend this to the related specifications of bag, buffer and stack. We then discuss the potential for moving from our examples to general results.

---

[1]The references in this paper to FDR's capabilities are based on the tool in May 2004.

2   Counter Processes

Anyone who has studied CSP will have encountered infinite-state counter processes with events *up*, *down* and perhaps *iszero*, such as $Count_0$, $Count_0'$, *Zero* and *ZERO*, where

$$Count_0 = up \rightarrow Count_1$$

$$Count_{n+1} = up \rightarrow Count_{n+2}$$
$$\square \; down \rightarrow Count_n$$

$$Count_0' = up \rightarrow Count_1'$$
$$\square \; iszero \rightarrow Count_0'$$

$$Count_{n+1}' = up \rightarrow Count_{n+2}'$$
$$\square \; down \rightarrow Count_n'$$

$$Zero = up \rightarrow Pos; \; Zero$$
$$\square \; iszero \rightarrow Zero$$

$$Pos = up \rightarrow Pos; \; Pos$$
$$\square \; down \rightarrow SKIP$$

$$ZERO = up \rightarrow (ZERO \; ||| \; down \rightarrow STOP)$$

By analogy with the usual CSP specification of a buffer ([6], for example) we might reasonably specify a counter (of the first sort) to be a process which must accept *up* when it has value 0 and *down* when non-zero, and which never accepts more *down*s and *up*s. If (t, X) is a typical failure, this formalises to

(i) $t \in \{up, down^*\} \wedge t \downarrow down \leq t \downarrow up$

(ii) $t \downarrow up = t \downarrow down \implies up \notin X$

(iii) $t \downarrow up > t \downarrow down \implies down \notin X$

A counter of the second sort must accept *iszero* when zero and never when non-zero. (The value of a counter is defined to be the number of *up*s minus the number of *down*s.) This can be formalised by easy modifications to the above.

Satisfying this specification is equivalent to the process concerned refining $COUNT_0$ or $COUNT_0'$ as appropriate, where

$$COUNT_0 = up \rightarrow COUNT_1$$

$$COUNT_{n+1} = (STOP \sqcap up \rightarrow COUNT_{n+2})$$
$$\square \; down \rightarrow COUNT_n$$

$$COUNT_0' = up \rightarrow COUNT_1'$$
$$\square \; iszero \rightarrow COUNT_0'$$

$$COUNT_{n+1}' = (STOP \sqcap up \rightarrow COUNT_{n+2}')$$
$$\square \; down \rightarrow COUNT_n'$$

We therefore have a simple refinement check for both these predicates, but it is not finitary since the process on the left-hand side of the refinement is infinite state.[2] Note that there

---

[2] We note that, while the standard functionality of FDR is not able to deal with checks where the left-hand side is infinite state and the right-hand finite-state, it has long been known that this could be achieved by appropriate use of lazy normalisation, but it is suspected this would have a significant overhead in terms of running time.

are many finite-state processes that meet these specifications. For the time being we will concentrate on the first sort of counter (without *iszero*).

2.1 Approach 1: Two-sided Approximation

One solution to deciding whether a finite-state process is a counter using finite-state refinement checking is easily adapted from the approach set out in Chapter 5 of [6] for buffers. Define two series of processes:

- $COUNT^n$ is the most nondeterministic counter whose value never gets bigger than n. It behaves identically to $COUNT_0$ when its value is less than n, but when n it cannot accept an *up*.

- $WCOUNT^n$ is the most nondeterministic *weak* counter of size n: it may accept an *up* that takes its value over n but if so it becomes equal to the most chaotic process (**div** $\sqcap$ *Chaos* works in all standard models).

These specifications are in the relationship

$$\ldots \sqsubseteq WCOUNT^n \sqsubseteq WCOUNT^{n+1} \ldots \sqsubseteq COUNT_0 \sqsubseteq \ldots COUNT^{n+1} \sqsubseteq COUNT^n \ldots$$

It is then true that every finite state process which is a counter will refine one of the $COUNT^n$ and every finite-state process which is not a counter will fail to refine one of the $WCOUNT^n$.

Comparing a proposed counter against the specifications $WCOUNT^n$ and $COUNT^n$ for increasing values of n in turn therefore gives a decision procedure.

For obvious reasons, however, it would be nice to be able to resolve the issue in a small fixed number of checks.

2.2 Approach 2: Constructive Contexts

Recall that a CSP context $F(\cdot)$ is said to be *constructive*, or sometimes *guarded*, if for all processes P, Q and natural numbers n we have

$$P \downarrow n = Q \downarrow n \implies F(P) \downarrow (n+1) = F(Q) \downarrow (n+1)$$

where $P \downarrow n$ is the standard restriction to n steps of behaviour (see [6], for example). Recall also that every context built without hiding, where the process variable(s) only appear indirectly or directly guarded by some communication, is constructive.

Now suppose F is a constructive context which maps counters to counters, and that P is a process such that

$$F(P) \sqsubseteq P$$

If P were not itself a counter then there would be some shortest-length behaviour b which demonstrated this. Let the length of b be n in the sense that n is minimal such that $b \in Q \downarrow n$ if and only if $b \in Q$. n cannot be 0 since the only length 0 behaviour is the empty trace – which does not contradict being a counter – as both refusals and divergences on a trace of length k actually have length $k + 1$. It follows straightforwardly that there is a process C such that C is a counter and

$$C \downarrow (n-1) = P \downarrow (n-1)$$

(To construct C simply build a process which behaves identically to P for the first $n - 1$ steps and then behaves like $Count_r$ where the value of r is the excess of *ups* over *downs* in the preceding trace.) But then $F(C)$ is a counter with the property that $F(C) \downarrow n = F(P) \downarrow n$. Since P has behaviour b and $P \sqsupseteq F(P)$ it follows that $F(P)$ has it too. Since $b \in R \downarrow n \Leftrightarrow b \in R$, it follows that $b \in F(C)$ which contradicts the fact that $F(C)$ is a counter.[3]

Hence P is a counter. Obviously this argument applies to any specification, not just counters. We will see another example later.

$$
\begin{aligned}
CT_A(P) &= up \rightarrow (P \underset{\{up\}}{\|} D) \\
D &= down \rightarrow RUN(\{up\}) \\
&\quad \Box \ (STOP \sqcap up \rightarrow D)
\end{aligned}
$$

is a good simple context for proving counters. For example $CT_A(P) \sqsubseteq P$ holds whenever P is one of the $COUNT^n$ bounded nondeterministic counters, or the deterministic processes with the same traces which can always be taken up to value n.

There are, however, counter processes which do not satisfy this refinement relation, meaning that CT_A gives a sound but not complete rule for proving counters. As an example consider

$$ExpC = up \rightarrow down \rightarrow COUNT^2$$

This has the trace $\langle up, down, up, up \rangle$ but $CT_A(ExpC)$ does not, since the first pair of events must have come from the context itself, and $ExpC$ cannot initially perform a pair of ups.

Of course we can find a context that proves $ExpC$ by giving it the ability to handle a second up itself, but it seems very unlikely to the author that any single constructive context can handle all counters. The grounds for this are that in general a counter can suddenly develop the ability to accept an arbitrary extra number of ups after any particular trace, but when P has done this trace the $P(s)$ in $CT(P)$ has/have done a strictly shorter trace. He conjectures that this argument can be formalised into a proof of impossibility.

If we had adopted the second sort of counter specification (namely with $iszero$) then the context above can easily be adapted. Let

$$
\begin{aligned}
CT_B(P) &= up \rightarrow (P \underset{\{up,iszero\}}{\|} D') \\
&\quad \Box \ iszero \rightarrow CT_B(P) \\
\\
D' &= down \rightarrow RUN(\{up,izsero\}) \\
&\quad \Box \ (STOP \sqcap up \rightarrow D')
\end{aligned}
$$

Then this has the same properties with respect to the new specification. Note that D' prevents P from communicating $iszero$ until its own $down$ has occurred.

2.3 Pseudo-constructive Contexts

It is nevertheless possible to contract every nontrivial trace of a counter in a general and useful way. If t is a nonempty trace of a counter P then we can guarantee that it is also a trace of the process $P \ ||| \ UD$, where $UD = up \rightarrow down \rightarrow STOP$, in such a way that only a trace t' of P that is strictly shorter than t is used in the interleaving. To see this note that the last up in the trace followed by a $down$ if there is one following it might have come from UD however P has behaved.

---

[3]An alternative proof: as F is constructive it has a unique fixed point, which is the limit of the sequences $F^k(Q)$ for all processes Q in the standard metric space. If C is an arbitrary counter then so are all members of the sequence $F^k(C)$, and hence the limit. The limit of the sequence $F^k(P)$ is refined by P since $F(P) \sqsubseteq P$ and F is monotone. Since the two limits are the same it follows that P refines a counter, and so is a counter itself.

For the time being we will consider just the the traces of a possible counter process. There is of course a natural traces specification arising from the failures-divergences one:

$$t \downarrow up \geq t \downarrow down$$

and $t \in \{up, down\}^*$ for all traces t of the process we are considering. Call any process satisfying this a *trace counter*. However, while any counter satisfies this, failures-divergences counters actually satisfy stronger conditions on their sets of traces. For technical reasons that will soon be apparent, we will define a *strong trace counter* to be a process satisfying the above and which in addition, if t is a trace in which there are k less *down*s than *up*s, then $t^\frown \langle down \rangle^k$ is also a trace. (This is not a behavioural specification since it relates behaviours to each other, however every counter is a strong trace counter.)

Before turning to the failures aspects of counters we will try to capture the property of being a trace counter via a finitary refinement check.

If we could prove that

$$(P \, |||_C \, UD) \sqsubseteq_T P \qquad (\ddagger)$$

where $P \, |||_C \, UD$ consists of the empty trace together with all interleavings involving a non-empty trace of UD, then P is necessarily a trace-counter, as can easily be proved by induction on the length of trace. (We will see a similar induction in more detail below.)

Unfortunately $|||_C$ does not make sense as a CSP operator, and it is not implementable. In any implementation the first thing $P \, |||_C \, Q$ does has to come from Q, but it may need to have traces on which P performed the first action and Q didn't start till later!

We might term $P \, ||| \, UD$ a *pseudo-constructive* context: it is not constructive but in some way has to play the role of one for us.

It is in fact possible to achieve the desired effect by applying suitable transformations to both sides of ($\ddagger$). Specifically, we can identify the up that comes from UD by replacing UD on the left-hand side with

$$UD' = up' \rightarrow down \rightarrow STOP$$

Let $Counter'_L(P) = P \, ||| \, UD'$.

On the right-hand side of the refinement we can use a fairly standard double renaming trick to rename the last up to up':

$$
\begin{aligned}
Counter_R(P) &= P[\![up, up' / up, up]\!] \underset{\{up, up'\}}{\|} Reg \\
Reg &= up \rightarrow Reg \\
&\quad \square \, up' \rightarrow STOP
\end{aligned}
$$

The renamed up becomes the last one because all subsequent ones are banned. Note that the last one may not be renamed, but if any it is the last one, and for all traces of P with an up there is a corresponding one of $Counter_R(P)$ where the last one is renamed.

Now consider the refinement $Counter'_L(P) \sqsubseteq_T Counter_R(P)$. Since P's traces are all in $Counter'_L(P)$ the refinement can only fail if one of the traces of $Counter_R(P)$ with its final up renamed is not in $Counter'_L(P)$. If P is a strong trace counter then this cannot happen thanks to the argument above. The "strong" here is necessary because of examples like

$$up \rightarrow up \rightarrow down \rightarrow down \rightarrow STOP$$

(a trace counter but not a strong one) can fail to satisfy it because of varying patterns of *down*s: here, $\langle up, up', down, down \rangle \notin traces(Counter'_L(P))$ because $\langle up, down \rangle \notin traces(P)$.

It even turns out that the refinement might hold if P is not a trace counter: it holds for example when $P = down \rightarrow STOP$. This latter example is one which needs to be dealt with.

To deal with this problem we replace $Counter'_L(P)$ by $Counter_L(P)$ where

$$Counter_L(P) = Counter'_L(P) \underset{\Sigma}{\|} UpFirst$$

$$UpFirst = ?x : \{up, up'\} \rightarrow RUN(\{up, up', down\})$$

Now, if the refinement

$$Counter_L(P) \sqsubseteq Counter_R(P)$$

holds it follows that the first event of P is up. All traces of P of length 0 and 1 are legitimate counter traces. Suppose the same is true of all traces of length k or less and that t has length $k + 1$. Necessarily t has a last up, and the trace t' in which this is replaced by up' is a trace of $Counter_R(P)$. t' is therefore the interleaving of a trace t'' of P and either $\langle up' \rangle$ or $\langle up', down \rangle$. By induction $t'' \downarrow down \leq t'' \downarrow up$. It follows that the same is true of t.

It follows that $Counter_L(P) \sqsubseteq_T Counter_R(P)$ implies P is a trace-counter, and is implied by it being a strong trace counter.

If we move from the traces model to failures-divergences there is an obvious pathological case that passes the above refinement, namely **div**, the chaotic divergent process for which both $Counter_L$ and $Counter_R$ are strict. We can of course eliminate this possibility by a refinement check and it therefore makes sense to assume that P is known to be divergence-free.

In this case it is easier to create a refinement which establishes the correct failures specification if, noting that each counter is deadlock-free, we boost the divergence-freedom check to encompass deadlock-freedom (another one-state standard specification). Since the traces specification establishes that a trace counter with value 0 can only communicate up it follows that a deadlock-free trace counter cannot refuse up when 0. This is half of what we need, the other half being that it cannot refuse $down$ when non-zero.

If we were simply to check $Counter_L(P) \sqsubseteq Counter_R(P)$ in the failures or failures-divergences model, this would make assertions about what P has to do in both ups and $down$s. The former would, as it turns out, be too strong. If, however, we define

$$Counter_L^{\mathcal{N}}(P) = Counter_L(P) \underset{\{up\}}{\|} Chaos_{\{up\}}$$

we get exactly what is required (in addition to the deadlock and livelock freedom check). The proof just extends the trace version above, once we note that if P can refuse $down$ after a trace t with more ups than $down$s then $Counter_R(P)$ can do the same on t' where the last up has been replaced by up'. This is not permitted by the left-hand side since either the UD process offers $down$ or the trace s which the left-hand P has performed is shorter and has more ups than $down$s.

It is possible to deal with the failures requirement on ups in a similar case-specific way by allowing UD to refuse up' if and only if P has performed an earlier up. Reg needs to be altered also. The details are left to the reader.

Since of course any trace counter which satisfies the failures requirements of a counter is also a strong trace counter, instead of the not-quite characterisation of trace buffers we achieved earlier, we now have a precise characterisation: a process P is a counter if and only if it is deadlock and divergence free, and satisfies

$$Counter_L^{\mathcal{N}}(P) \sqsubseteq Counter_R(P)$$

Thus we have reduced the decision procedure about whether a general process is a counter to two finitary refinement checks. These can, if desired, by combined into a single one using the representation of conjunctions introduced in [7].

Notice how the interplay between traces and refusals in this natural specification allowed us to achieve a tighter result than we could with traces alone.

It is interesting to note that if the $Counter_{L/R}$ refinement were to fail on FDR, then the way that the refinement works inductively coupled with FDR finding the shortest counterexample will generally mean that the example behaviour it produces will be a direct counterexample to P being a counter. (The shorter behaviour against which it is judged will, one would expect, behave correctly.) This may not be true, however, since the shortest route to an offending behaviour on the RHS may have a longer trace than others thanks to the way FDR handles τs. The way to solve this difficulty, should one encounter it, is to apply some τ-eliminating compression such as *diamond* [9] to $Counter_R(P)$ before the refinement check. If this is done it is guaranteed that the counterexample behaviour will directly contradict the counter specification.

The method developed in this section relied on us being able to find a systematic way to transform every trace t of a process satisfying a specification into a shorter one t' which can be lifted back to t by the constructive action of an operator (even though the operator itself might not be constructive) which preserves the specification. What we are doing is using a process as its own specification inductively, so that each finite state process has its own custom-made finite state specification.

2.4 Approach 4: Watchdogs

In [2], we demonstrate how CSP behavioural specifications can be transformed to operate in parallel with the process being tested in such a way that if the specification fails then the parallel combination fails to refine a standard process which is independent of the problem. This form of specification is called a *watchdog* because it sits alongside the target process and 'woofs' when a mis-behaviour occurs. A typical watchdog for the counter specification is:

$$WatchC_0 = (STOP \sqcap down \to woof \to STOP)$$
$$\Box\ up \to WatchC_1$$

$$WatchC_{n+1} = (STOP \sqcap up \to WatchC_{n+2})$$
$$\Box\ down \to WatchC_n$$

Note how these are very similar to the $COUNT_n$ processes.

If $WatchC_0 \underset{\{up,down\}}{\|} P$ is run for a counter P, notice that the values of the two processes will always coincide, and that the combination will never *woof* or deadlock. On the other hand, any process with alphabet $\{up,down\}$ which fails the buffer specification will do one of these two things: an excess of *down*s will lead to a *woof*, and an illegal refusal of *up* (when 0) or *down* (when non-zero) will lead to deadlock.

One reason for our discussing watchdogs here is that, even though $WatchC_0$ is of course infinite state, if P is a finite-state counter then $WatchC_0 \underset{\{up,down\}}{\|} P$ is finite state (and can be run on FDR if care is taken to ensure the parallel combination is compiled at low level[4]: see

---

[4]For example, any $\checkmark$-free process P is compiled at low level if accessed as $low(P) = P; low(P)$. This is equivalent to P but contains a never-accessed recursion which forces low-level compilation. Since low-level compilation is slower and less space efficient than FDR's normal mode of running, it may be impractical to apply *low* to processes with large state spaces.

Appendix C of [6]). Notice however that if P is a finite-state process which is not a counter (such as $P = up \to P$, which is a trace counter) the parallel combination may be infinite state. Therefore this gives only a semi-decision procedure, and there are simple specifications where even this is not true.

Exactly the same applies to a counter with *iszero*. We quote the watchdog for this variant below. Note the way that, when one wants to test that a set of more than one elements are all available, each element has to be tested separately.

$$WatchC'_0 = (STOP \sqcap down \to woof \to STOP)$$
$$\square \, (up \to WatchC'_1$$
$$\sqcap \, iszero \to WatchC'_0)$$

$$WatchC'_{n+1} = (STOP \sqcap up \to WatchC_{n+2})$$
$$\square \, down \to WatchC_n$$
$$\square \, (STOP \sqcap iszero \to woof \to STOP)$$

Suppose C is a counter of this second sort. It is very easy to convert it into one if the first sort by $P \underset{\{iszero\}}{\parallel} STOP$. It is not nearly as easy to go the other way: if we have a context $C(P)$ which is operating on a counter of the first sort, the only clue that $C(P)$ has – by observing P – that P is in state 0 is that it refuses the event *down*. But there are no CSP operators which can introduce an extra event like *iszero* on the refusal of another: this would contradict monotonicity in trace sets. We conclude that the only way the context can know that it has to be able to say *iszero* is if it keeps a tally itself. The best way I can think of doing this is to put P in parallel with $Count'_0$: if P is a counter of the first sort then $P \underset{\{up,down\}}{\parallel} Count'_0$ is the corresponding counter of the second.

This method does, of course, have the same limitation as the watchdog, that it can only be guaranteed to produce a finite-state process if P is indeed a finite-state counter. (And is a failures/divergences counter, not just a trace counter.) Fortunately, of course, we have demonstrated in the previous section that it is possible to decide that question using finitary checks. So, as long as one is careful, infinite processes can be avoided for any finite-state P.

3 Processes with Data

Suppose that instead of having events *up*, *down* and perhaps *iszero*, we now have the channels *in*, *out*, and perhaps the event *isempty*. The channels communicate values in some type T that we want to store inside our process. In this section we will study three related specifications:

- A *bag* is a process which holds data it has input on *in*, outputting each item exactly once on *out*. It never refuses input when empty and is always willing to output when nonempty. If it has the *isempty* event, then this only happens when the bag is empty and cannot then be refused. A bag is not constrained as to which value to output if it has more than one (the items output are a permutation of those input).

- A *stack* is a bag which outputs on a strictly last-in first-out (LIFO) discipline. Of course the conventional names for the input and output channels of stacks are *push* and *pop*.

- A *buffer* is a bag which outputs on a strictly first-in first-out (FIFO) principle. Buffers have been extensively studied in CSP literature (generally without an *isempty* event).

Thus every stack and buffer is a bag, and the only process that is all three is *COPY* which can only hold a single item. Like counters, I will refer to first and second sort for ones that do and don't have *isempty*, and a trace bag (etc) will be one that just satisfies the trace constraints.

It is straightforward to adapt the counter failures divergences specification seen earlier into ones for each of these types of process. The buffer one can be found, for example, in chapter 5 of [6].

It is obvious that these three specifications are all close to that of a counter, and indeed the renaming

$$P[\![\, up, down, iszero \,/\, in.x, out.x, isempty \mid x \in T\,]\!] \qquad (\flat)$$

converts any bag into a counter. Of course my reason for using these specifications is that since we already know how to check if a finite-state process is a counter, then we can check the above transformation of any proposed bag is a counter as a large step on the way to verifying it. So all we have to do is concentrate on the data values that are passed around.

The most surprising discovery, however, is that under common conditions this transformation back to a counter is not necessary, because the introduction of data actually makes things easier as we shall see in the following section!

3.1 Data Independence

A process is said to be data independent in the type T when it makes sense for any type T. It can input and output members of T, and store them. For different purposes we can allow further operations, such as implicit and explicit equality tests, constants, relational and functional symbols, and arrays indexed by T. See for example [3]. Note that data independence is usually considered as a syntactic restriction on programs rather than a semantic one, though [4] gives a semantic characterisation. While there is no guarantee that a process that is intended to be a bag, stack or buffer is data independent, there is every reason to believe that such programs will often be so.

The first mention of data independence in the literature, Pierre Wolper's paper [10], took a version of data independence at its purest without any of the add-ons such as equality tests. One of the main examples in that paper includes a way of testing whether a data independent process is a buffer (though the concept of a buffer is not exactly the same as ours as it does not place the same failures obligations on the process). Wolper's method is finitary, and can readily be adapted into a finitary way of deciding whether a finite-state data independent process[5] is a buffer in our sense, which is conceptually simpler than the way we already have of testing a counter.

The idea underlying this is that, since data independent P's behaviour does not depend on which values have been input into it (except in exactly which values are output), we can put special 'marker' values into the input stream and by ensuring that these come out at exactly the right points be sure that the buffer is correct.

If a divergence-free data independent process failed to be a buffer, it would be for one of the following reasons:

(a) It loses an input x, meaning either that y input after x comes out before x, or it fails to perform any further output at some time even though non-empty.

(b) It re-orders two inputs: this will manifest itself in the same way as the first version of (a).

(c) It duplicates a value x: x is output twice when it has only been input once.

---

[5]This means finite state when the type T is finite.

(d) It refuses to input when empty: this will mean it is possible either to refuse an input initially, or after it has just output the last value x that it has input.

(e) It refuses to output when it has input some value x but not output it yet. (Note that, thanks to divergence-freedom, this includes the second aspect of (a).

We can always input specific values once only amongst a background of constant values to represent x and y in all these clauses. The crucial thing about data independence is that doing so will not change the control flow of the process: it would do the same on any other stream of inputs. Suppose all values input are 0 except for one 1 followed an arbitrary time later by one 2: the inputs are prefixes of members of the regular language $0^*10^*20^*$ (as used also by Wolper). Then the above clauses reduce to:

(b) 2 is never output before 1 (for if any two values were treated as in (a) above then we could arrange that the 1 and 2 are input at the same points in the input stream as x and y respectively).

(c) At most one 1 appears in the outputs.

(d) The process can refuse any input either initially or when the last input and output were both 1.

(e) The process can refuse to output when it has input the 1 but not yet output it. (Note that the output it must give is either a 0 or

(a) Is covered by the combination of (b) and (e) as discussed above.

All of these things reduce to a single failures-divergences refinement check of the process $P \parallel_{\{|in|\}} Reg$, where

$$
\begin{aligned}
Reg &= in.0 \rightarrow Reg \\
&\quad \Box\ in.1 \rightarrow Reg' \\[1em]
Reg' &= in.0 \rightarrow Reg' \\
&\quad \Box\ in.2 \rightarrow Reg'' \\[1em]
Reg'' &= in.0 \rightarrow Reg''
\end{aligned}
$$

against the specification $DIBspec_0$, defined in Figure 1.

There, $DIBspec_0$ is the initial state (which must accept inputs); $DIBspec_1$ is the state where only 0's have been transacted so far; $DIBspec_2$ is the state where the last input was 1 and there have been no other inputs since; $DIBspec_3$ is the state where a 1 has been input followed by some 0's; $DIBspec_4$ is the state where the buffer is meant to be empty as the 1 from state $DIBspec_2$ (i.e., the most recent input) has just been output; $DIBspec_5$ is a more general state where the 1 has come out but the 2 not yet gone in, and we are not sure whether the buffer is empty or not; $DIBspec_6$ is a state where both 1 and 2 are in the buffer; $DIBspec_7$ is a state where 2 is in the buffer; $DIBspec_8$ represents the states where both 1 and 2 have been and gone.

At the expense of making $DIBspec$ yet more elaborate (specifically, including a lot of extra events leading to **div** – for "don't care" – representing all the behaviours when the process does not follow the $0^*10^*20^*$ input pattern) this can be re-cast in the form $SPEC \sqsubseteq P$.

So data independence has removed the need for the self-referential refinement checking we encountered with counters in the last section. This is a rather remarkable fact. In essence

$$DIBspec_0 = in.0 \rightarrow DIBspec_1$$
$$\square \; in.1 \rightarrow DIBspec_2$$

$$DIBspec_1 = STOP \sqcap$$
$$(in.0 \rightarrow DIBspec_1$$
$$\square \; in.1 \rightarrow DIBspec_2$$
$$\square \; out.0 \rightarrow DIBspec_1)$$

$$DIBspec_2 = (STOP \sqcap$$
$$(in.0 \rightarrow DIBspec_3$$
$$\square \; in.2 \rightarrow DIBspec_6))$$
$$\square$$
$$(out.0 \rightarrow DIBspec_2$$
$$\sqcap \; out.1 \rightarrow DIBspec_4)$$

$$DIBspec_3 = (STOP \sqcap$$
$$(in.0 \rightarrow DIBspec_3$$
$$\square \; in.2 \rightarrow DIBspec_6))$$
$$\square$$
$$(out.0 \rightarrow DIBspec_3$$
$$\sqcap \; out.1 \rightarrow DIBspec_5)$$

$$DIBspec_4 = (in.0 \rightarrow DIBspec_5 \; \square \; in.2 \rightarrow DIBspec_7)$$

$$DIBspec_5 = STOP$$
$$\sqcap \; (in.0 \rightarrow DIBspec_5 \; \square \; in.2 \rightarrow DIBspec_7)$$
$$\sqcap \; out.0 \rightarrow DIBspec_5$$

$$DIBspec_6 = (out.0 \rightarrow DIBspec_6 \; \sqcap \; out.1 \rightarrow DIBspec_7)$$
$$\square \; (STOP \sqcap in.0 \rightarrow DIBspec_6)$$

$$DIBspec_7 = (out.0 \rightarrow DIBspec_7 \; \sqcap \; out.2 \rightarrow DIBspec_8)$$
$$\square \; (STOP \sqcap in.0 \rightarrow DIBspec_7)$$

$$DISspec_8 = Chaos_{\{in.0,out.0\}}$$

Figure 1: Specification for data independent buffer check

this is because we are able to get more of a handle on the number of pending outputs thanks to tagging them.

Those experienced in data independence will recognise that under the strong conditions we have assumed on our implementation, it is normally sufficient to check with T of size 2, whereas the above check uses one of size 3. The only property for which we have relied on 2 is establishing the absence of re-ordering. It is in fact possible to detect errors of this and the other forms by using the language $0^*(1 + 11)0^*$, thereby cutting the type to $\{0, 1\}$.

Subject to the remark in the next paragraph, it is easy to modify *DIBspec* to test $P \underset{\{|in|\}}{\|} Reg$ (with P data independent) for being a stack. Bags are easy because all one needs to do is to put a single 1 in amongst a stream of zeros and ensure (a) that 1 comes out no more than once and (b) that the bag cannot refuse to output while it contains the 1. Notice that 1 only coming out once implies (since all the output values were previously input somewhere) that the total number of outputs never exceeds that of inputs.

Neither the bag nor stack specifications described here address the question of forcing the processes to input when empty. This is because it is not possible for the specification to detect when the process is empty in a finite-state way, so it specially forces input. There is, however, a simple solution to this (also possible for buffers), namely modifying each specification state so it does not accept any deadlock.

3.2 Bags and Stacks without Data Independence

In this section we see what can be done without the assumption of data independence. The failures-divergences bag and stack specifications can be established with relatively minor modifications to the techniques used for counters. The first thing to remark is that there will be no problems with the refusal parts of the failure specification of a bag: for the *out.x* events the requirements are the same as for *down* events in counters. And for the requirement that a bag will input anything when empty all one has to do (in conjunction with proving it is trace-correct) is to show it refines:

$$IODF = (in?x \rightarrow IODF) \sqcap (\underset{x \in T}{\sqcap} out!x \rightarrow IODF)$$

In other words it can always either output, or accept all inputs.

Since a trace stack or trace buffer is respectively a stack or buffer if and only if it is a bag, we can therefore restrict ourselves to deciding whether a process is a bag, and whether it is a trace stack or buffer.

A little thought reveals that a bag is precisely a process P satisfying the strengthened deadlock freedom check above (also proving divergence freedom, of course), for which (a) the renaming given as ($\flat$) above satisfies the counter check

$$Counter_L^{\mathcal{N}}(P^{\flat}) \sqsubseteq Counter_R(P^{\flat}) \qquad (\sharp)$$

and (b) such that for each member x of T the process

$$(C_x(P) = P \setminus \{in.y, out.y \mid y \neq x\})[\![^{up,down}/_{in.x, out.x}]\!]$$

is a trace counter. Since any process satisfying this also has all the $C_x(P)$ strong trace counters, (b) is equivalent to $\sqcap\{C_x(P) \mid x \in T\}$ satisfying the trace refinement version of ($\sharp$).

The above check is less efficient than I would have liked since in essence it involves examining P's state space $n + 1$ times, where n is the size of T. To see why something like this seems to be necessary, and also to help our understanding of what can and cannot be done with pseudo-constructive contexts, I will now go over an earlier attempt at specifying bags that did not quite work.

It is reasonably obvious (and readily proved) that if B is a bag then so is $B \ ||| \ IO$, where $IO = in?x \rightarrow out!x \rightarrow STOP$. Clearly every nonempty trace of a bag starts with an event of the form $in.x$. It is tempting to believe that nonempty traces of B are also, analogously to counters, traces of $B \ ||| \ IO$ in which the last input of s is performed by IO (so that the interleaved copy of B performs a strictly shorter trace).

To see that this is not in general true let $B_K^?$ be a bag that uses a strict stack regime to output its pending values until its contents grow to size K for the first time, after which it for ever after outputs as though it were a buffer (including the outputs pending at the time). If $K = 3$ it will have the trace

$$\langle in.1, in.2, in.3, out.1, out.2, out.3 \rangle$$

but $\langle in.1, in.2, out.1, out.2 \rangle$ is not a trace, which it would have to be for the desired property to hold.

Let's define a *stable* bag to be one where, if $t^\frown\langle in.y, out.x_1, \ldots, out.x_n \rangle$ is a trace, then so is $t^\frown\langle out.y_1, \ldots, out.y_m \rangle$ where $m \in \{n - 1, n\}$ and the y_i are a subsequence of the x_i obtained by deleting (at most) $out.x$. (In the case where several x_i are equal to x all that is necessary is that there is one subsequence with this property.) In other words the order our process outputs values it had in it at the point where it performs the input $in.x$ was also possible before that input. Note that $B_3^?$ is not stable.

The following construction straightforwardly implies that any nonempty trace of B is one of $B \ ||| \ IO$ in which the last input was performed by IO.

So if we define

$$IO' \ = \ in'?x \rightarrow out!x \rightarrow STOP$$

$$InFirst \ = \ \begin{aligned} &in?x \rightarrow RUN_{\{|in,in',out|\}} \\ &\square \ in'?x \rightarrow RUN_{\{|in,in',out|\}} \end{aligned}$$

$$Bag_L(P) \ = \ (P \ ||| \ IO') \underset{\{in,in',out\}}{\Vert} InFirst$$

$$Reg \ = \ \begin{aligned} &in?x \rightarrow Reg \\ &\square \ in'?x \rightarrow STOP \end{aligned}$$

$$Bag_R(P) \ = \ P[\![\, in, in' \, / \, in, in]\!] \underset{\{|in,in'|\}}{\Vert} Reg$$

Then $Bag_L(P) \sqsubseteq_T Bag_R(P)$ if P is a stable strong traces bag and implies it is a stable traces bag. The proof of this is essentially the same as for counters.

The need for a condition such as stability in arises here because pseudo-constructive specifications, by their nature, have to reduce every nonempty trace of a process to a shorter one, so there cannot be any new sorts of behaviour suddenly appearing after a long trace. Note that, like our strong trace conditions, the stable bag condition is not a behavioural predicate.

It is easy to adapt the stable bag construction to characterise stacks. (Note that a stack is a stable bag.) What we know there is that as soon as the last input of a trace has gone in, the next input if any is tied to this input. So, whereas in $Bag_L(P)$ the output from IO' can occur any time after the input, we will now have to require that it is the next output. The easiest way to achieve this is to prime the output from IO, replacing it by

$$SIO = (in'?x \rightarrow out'x \rightarrow RUN_{\{|out|\}}) \ \square \ (out?x \rightarrow SIO)$$

and defining

$$Stack_L(P) = ((P \underset{\{|out|\}}{\|} SIO)[\![^{out}/_{out'}]\!]) \underset{\{in,in',out\}}{\|} InFirst$$

We can then set $Stack_R(P) = Bag_R(P)$, and have the expected result.

3.3 Buffers

I have been unable to find a similar and satisfactory construction to the above for buffers. The difficulty comes from the following:

- In looking for a pseudo-constructive context to characterise any of the sorts of specifications we have looked at, it is necessary to have the constructive action (i.e. the insertion of extra event(s)) towards the end of the trace. This is because the insertion towards the beginning of the trace (as was done in the section on constructive constructs above and which works equally well for buffers: see below) might change the LHS behaviour in a way that the pre- and post-insertion behaviours do not line up well enough for comparison.

- Given that we are inserting an input and perhaps output towards the end of a buffer trace, there seems (unlike with stacks) to be no straightforward way of placing the extra output in the right place.

So the best I have been able to do on previous models was to give a sound and incomplete rule, namely that P is a buffer if it satisfies

$$PB(P) \sqsubseteq P$$

where

$$PB(P) = in?x \to (P \underset{\{in,out\}}{\|} Z(x))[\![^{out}/_{out'}]\!]$$
$$Z(x) = (STOP \sqcap in?y \to Z(x))$$
$$\square\ out'!x \to RUN_{\{in,out\}}$$

This is not a complete rule because it cannot handle buffers which expand on the first output, for example

$$ExpB = in?x \to out!x \to B_2$$

where B_2 is a two-place buffer. Clearly this is essentially the same problem we found with counters when using the context CT_A.

Note the similarity of the PB-based rule to the rather more complex buffer laws $BL5$ and $BL5'$ from chapter 5 of [6] (originally proved in [8]) which apply to piped combinations rather than single processes.

The only way I have found to solve the problem of placing the last (rather than first) input into the correct place in the input stream borrows from the idea described earlier for turning a counter of the first sort into one of the second.

The first thing one has to do (to ensure that this exercise does not fail to terminate) is to check either that when renamed as in (♭) it is a counter. The left-hand side process is then constructed by running P in parallel with IO and the most nondeterministic buffer $BUFF'_{\langle\rangle}$ of the second sort. All the inputs of this process prior to IO's input are fed into $BUFF'$, but not that input or any subsequent one. Outputs of P prior to IO's output are synchronised with

$BUFF'$. IO's output is permitted once $BUFF'$ has become empty (which we can see thanks to the *isempty* event, which is synchronised with this output). Once this extra output has appeared then P is allowed to output freely again.

This generates a finite-state process which (with the extra input suitably renamed as usual) can be used to check the same right-hand side process we used for bags and stacks.

I feel, however, that this approach is clumsy and inelegant, and that it is less than appealing because of the way it uses an infinite state process in its definition. Fortunately, however, a different approach does give an elegant formulation.

Stacks and buffers share an interesting property that general bags do not have, namely, after any trace where an output is available, that output is completely determined by the trace. We can define a bag with this property to be *output deterministic*, noting that this certainly does not imply that the process itself is deterministic.

Lazić [3] developed a technique, reworked in [7], for establishing the determinism of a process via a finitary refinement check. Let P' be a copy of P renamed so that each event a in its alphabet A becomes $a' \in A'$, where this renaming is a bijection and $A \cap A' = \emptyset$, and let $Test = ?a : A \to a' \to Test$. Then P is deterministic if and only if

$$(P \,|||\, P') \underset{A \cup A'}{\|} Test$$

can never deadlock after an odd-length trace. This idea can be modified to produce a test for output determinism: let

$$TestOD \quad = \quad out?x \to out'?y \to (TestOD \Leftleft x = y \Rightright error \to STOP)$$
$$\Box \; in?x \to TestOD$$

and consider

$$(P \underset{\{|in|\}}{\|} P[\,^{out'}/\,_{out}]) \underset{\{|in,out,out'|\}}{\|} TestOD$$

This makes sure that the two copies of P have always done the same sequence of inputs and outputs, but if they do give different outputs at any time the event *error* appears. Evidently the combination refines $Chaos_{\{|in,out,out'|\}}$ precisely when P is output deterministic. So we can check if a process is an output deterministic bag via a few finitary refinement checks.

Recall that the CSP operator $P \gg Q$ connects the outputs of P to the inputs of Q and hides these internal communications. If P is a buffer then so is $CP = COPY \gg P$, where

$$COPY = in?x \to out!x \to COPY$$

is the simple one-place buffer (this is a consequence of BL1 in chapter 5 of [6]). CP is therefore output deterministic.

On the other hand, if P (known to be a bag) is not a buffer, then the only way this can happen is if it has a trace $s \langle out.x \rangle$ where x is the wrong value to be output (i.e. is not the next pending one). We can assume that this is a shortest such trace. Necessarily, after s (which is a buffer trace), there are at least two values pending since if there were only one the bag P would have to output the buffer-correct one. Now s is also a trace of CP, and this can happen in two ways:

- *Either COPY* transmits all its inputs directly to P so that in the final state P has performed the trace s;

- *or COPY* has retained the very last input *in.y* in s and not yet transmitted it to P. P can perform the trace s' which is s with its last input deleted since all outputs after this input are pending before that input occurs, and there is no shorter counterexample than $s \langle out.x \rangle$ to buffer behaviour. Note that, thanks to what we observed above, P is then (i.e., after s') in a state where it has a pending output.

In the first of these states CP can evidently output $out.x$ because P then can. In the second of the states it can, since P has performed a trace strictly shorter than s, output the correct $out.z$ based on FIFO in s. It follows that CP is not output deterministic.

An elegant decision procedure for P being a buffer is then to test if it is a stable bag (since all buffers are stable) and then to check that CP is output deterministic.

It is similarly possible to find out if a bag P is a stack by testing if a different context around P is output deterministic. This is left as an exercise to the reader.

4   The Problem of Generalisation

It is interesting to see what lessons we can learn from these examples and attempt to get some general results. For simplicity I will mainly consider trace specifications.

Any simple trace refinement is equivalent to the question of whether a given regular language (the traces of a finite-state process) is a subset of some set S of traces. Clearly the case in which the specification is also a finite-state process reduces to the question of whether one regular language is contained in another. However none of the cases we have been studying in this paper have S regular.

The traces of counters and stacks are prefix-closed context-free grammars, whereas the languages of buffers and bags are not. It seems very unlikely that prefix-closed subsets of any context-free language can be decided by a pseudo-constructive trace refinement (which is all we ought to be using to decide languages of traces, of course). We already had difficulties with, for example, weak counters (arbitrary prefix-closed subsets of the set of all counter traces), and consider for example the context-free language

$$a^*b^* \cup \{a^n b^n c \mid n \in \mathbb{N}\}$$

It seems very unlikely to me that a process's traces being contained within this is capturable by a finitary refinement using a pseudo-constructive context, bearing in mind that a trace of the form $a^n b^n c$ (which may, for arbitrarily large n, be the only such trace in our process) can be reduced meaningfully to another one of the same process. It can, however, be decided by a watchdog using the trick seen earlier which allows the inclusion of an infinite-state watchdog into a finite-state system.

We have already seen that the failures aspects of specifications can have significant effects: for example we were unable to characterise trace counters but were able to characterise failures-divergences one because of the interplay between refusals and traces. It almost seemed that the "naturalness" of our failures specifications, particularly the way they force a process to be reducible to zero/empty, played a big role in making them accessible.

There are obviously many different CSP contexts we could use which could play a pseudo-constructive role. In order to get any sorts of general characterisation of the specifications one could create using them we would have to understand the sorts of grammatical constructors they represent. This is something which needs to be investigated, but I have no idea if there is any sort of clean result here.

5   Conclusions and Future Work

We have seen how to characterise a number of related infinitary properties and seen a number of tricks for expressing them. While all the properties we aimed to characterise were behavioural specifications, we have found ourselves forced to use non behavioural approximations to them such as strong trace counters and stable bags.

While it is not too hard to see *why* data independence gave us extra power, the fact still seems rather wonderful and is certainly worthy of deeper investigation.

This work has brought extra insights into the nature of things like buffers and bags and potentially useful concepts such as stable bags and output determinism. I hope that by using these and the new specification techniques being developed I can shed more light on the important but difficult topic of *buffer tolerance* (see chapter 5 of [6] for example). It seems likely that the ideas like output determinism will be useful. Certainly it is a non-behavioural property which is of huge practical importance.

The ultimate goal is some sort of logical or mathematical characterisation of what properties are expressible as finitary refinement checks. The expressive power of CSP, coupled with the self-referential nature of the checks themselves (illustrated by our pseudo-constructive technique) make this a considerable challenge.

Acknowledgements

I would like to thank Gavin Lowe for his comments on an earlier draft of this paper.

References

[1] Formal Systems (Europe) Ltd., *Failures-Divergence Refinement*, User Manual, obtainable from www.fsel.com/documentation/fdr2/html/

[2] M.H. Goldsmith, N.Moffat, A.W. Roscoe, T. Whitworth and I. Zakiuddin, *Watchdog transformations for property-oriented model checking*, Proceedings of FME 2003.

[3] R.S. Lazić, *A semantic study of data-independence with applications to the mechanical verification of concurrent systems*, Oxford University D.Phil thesis, 1998.

[4] R.S. Lazić and D. Nowak, *A unifying approach to data-independence*, In Proceedings of the 11th International Conference on Concurrency Theory (CONCUR 2000), Lecture Notes in Computer Science. Springer-Verlag, August 2000.

[5] J.N. Reed, J. Sinclair and A.W. Roscoe, *Responsiveness of Interoperating Components*, To appear in FAC.

[6] A.W. Roscoe, *The theory and practice of concurrency*, Prentice Hall, 1998.

[7] A.W. Roscoe, *On the expressiveness of CSP refinement checking*, To appear in FAC (special issue related to AVOCS '03).

[8] A.W. Roscoe, *A mathematical theory of communicating processes* Oxford University D.Phil thesis, 1982.

[9] A.W. Roscoe, P.H.B. Gardiner, M.H. Goldsmith, J.R. Hulance, D.M. Jackson and J.B. Scattergood, *Hierarchical compression for model-checking CSP* or *how to check 10^{20} dining philosophers for deadlock*, Proceedings of the 1st TACAS, BRICS Notes Series NS-95-2, Department of Computer Science, University of Aarhus, 1995. (Also Springer LNCS 1019.)

[10] P. Wolper. Expressing interesting properties of programs in propositional temporal logic. In *Proceedings of the 13th PoPL* , pages 184–193, 1986.

Communicating Process Architectures 2004
Ian East, Jeremy Martin, Peter Welch, David Duce, and Mark Green (Eds.)
IOS Press, 2004

19

An Automatic Translation of CSP to Handel-C

Jonathan D. PHILLIPS

452½ East 700 North, Logan, UT 84321

jdphillips@cc.usu.edu

G. S. STILES

Utah State University, 4120 Old Main Hill, Logan, UT 84322-4120

dyke.stiles@ece.usu.edu

Abstract. We present tools that convert a subset of CSP into Handel-C code. Handel-C was derived from the original **occam** concurrency language, but has a syntax similar to the standard C programming language. It compiles to produce files to program an FPGA. We thus now have a process that can directly generate hardware from a verified high-level description. The CSP to Handel-C translator makes use of the Lex and Yacc programming tools. The Handel-C code produced is functional, but not necessarily optimized for all situations. The translator has been tested using several CSP scripts of varying complexity. The functionality of the resulting Handel-C programs has been verified with simulations, and two scripts were further checked with successful implementations on an FPGA.

1. Introduction

This paper describes tools to automate the conversion of a set of concurrent, interactive software processes into equivalent hardware. The tools are based on the development of an algorithm that automatically translates CSP [1] scripts into the Handel-C [2] language. A major benefit of creating specific hardware to implement software algorithms that are easily parallelized is a substantial increase in the throughput of the system; increased speed is vital in many real-time electronics applications, especially digital signal processing. CSP provides robust, reliable channels for inter-process communication, and CSP scripts can be checked to ensure absence of deadlock and – within certain limits – to verify correct implementation of formal specifications of the algorithms. Furthermore, automated translation of software into hardware, specifically in the case of large concurrent applications, can greatly reduce development time.

Communicating Sequential Processes, or CSP, is an algebra designed for describing and reasoning about synchronizations and communications between processes. Systems of processes that are described using CSP can be checked for non-determinism, freedom from deadlock and livelock, and correctness with respect to a formal specification through the use of the software tools FDR and ProBE [3]. The verified CSP script can then be used as a basis for implementing the algorithm in a high level language, or can be used as a guide to design hardware to perform the same task. In the case of this project, the verified CSP script is translated into Handel-C, which is then compiled to produce files for programming an FPGA device.

This automated verification and translation decreases the time generally spent on manually designing and testing an FPGA based on a CSP algorithm. Complicated systems with many processes and communicating channels can be easily implemented with minimal (or zero) errors in channel or process naming and channel synchronization.

The remainder of this paper is dedicated to the specifics of this project. The importance and relevance of this translation tool is discussed, and previous work along similar lines is reviewed. We will define the subset of CSP that was included and discuss the details of the translation tool, which is based on Lex and Yacc. The paper then presents examples of translations of simple and complex CSP scripts. The paper concludes with the successful simulations of the scripts using the Handel-C compiler and the results of two complete runs on an actual FPGAs.

2. Background

2.1 Project Significance

This project is an attempt to combine the mathematical strengths of CSP with the hardware-producing capabilities of Handel-C. Automating the translation of a CSP script into a Handel-C file minimizes the probability of human error. When complex systems of interacting processes are modelled in CSP, and then manually translated into a hardware or software programming language, it is easy for a human to confuse variable or channel names, improperly order processes, omit critical code synchronizations, and commit other syntactical or logical errors. Since CSP and Handel-C both have well-defined syntax and grammar rules, creating a compiler or translator to automate the conversion from one to the other immediately eliminates many errors that could otherwise occur during the translation process.

2.2 Previous Work

The area of hardware-software interaction has been addressed by several recent projects at Utah State University. John Campbell [6] developed and implemented algorithms for mapping regions of software into hardware based on dynamic behavior of the software. The mapping, based on profile information gathered in test executions of the software, configured hardware functions with high rates of communication in close proximity. He also investigated theoretical extensions of the algorithm for dynamic/run time caching of functionality to hardware.

Initial work on the automated conversion of CSP was done by Zhou and Stiles [7], where concurrent CSP scripts were translated into equivalent sequential scripts; this tool was developed in Mathematica©. The work most closely related to this paper is Raju, Rong, and Stiles [8], where CSP scripts were automatically translated into concurrency-capable, channel-oriented versions of Java and C (CTJ [9, 10], JCSP [11, 12], and CCSP [13]); the translation tools were Mathematica and C augmented with string-handling libraries.

Current research at the University of Surrey [14] is looking at the translation of occam directly into FPGA code. Preliminary results indicate that success has been obtained in modeling basic logic gates.

2.3 Project Details

The creation of an application-specific FPGA from a CSP specification involves several steps. The overall process is depicted in fig. 1. First, the CSP script must be verified for

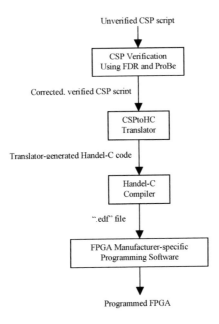

Unverified CSP script

CSP Verification
Using FDR and ProBe

Corrected. verified CSP script

CSPtoHC
Translator

Translator-generated Handel-C code

Handel-C
Compiler

".edf" file

FPGA Manufacturer-specific
Programming Software

Programmed FPGA

Figure 1: System overview.

correctness with respect to a specification, including absence of deadlock and livelock, using the ProBE and FDR tools. Once the CSP script is correct, it is passed to the CSPtoHC translator, which produces a Handel-C program based on the CSP design.

Handel-C is based on a subset of the traditional C programming language, with added features included to facilitate various facets of parallel hardware creation. Integers are the only data type that is allowed. Integers of any specific size can be declared, since unneeded bits would create inefficient hardware. A par construct allows for the parallel execution of instructions. The prialt construct behaves similarly to a switch or select statement, where the cases are triggered by data reception on an input channel. In addition to the traditional array construct, RAMs and ROMs can also be created, filled with data, and manipulated in similar fashion.

Handel-C programs can be simulated at the cycle level, using the Handel-C software, to observe how the hardware will respond. After simulation, the Handel-C compiler can produce an output file that can be fed into an FPGA-programming package, which ultimately results in a programmed FPGA that performs the functionality originally described in the CSP script.

This project concentrates mainly on the CSPtoHC translator. It is assumed that CSP scripts passed to the translator will have been verified for correctness previously, and thus the specifics of ProBE and FDR will not be discussed here. The Handel-C simulator will be employed extensively to demonstrate that the results match the desired output. An FPGA will be programmed with two of the more complex codes to show that the hardware does correspond as specified and to measure the performance.

The process of designing the CSPtoHC translator, which was done with the help of the Lex and Yacc utilities, will be described next. A brief overview on how to use the tool will also be provided.

3. The CSP to Handel-C Translator

3.1 CSP Subset Selection

CSP has considerable expressive power. However, a simple subset of CSP can be chosen that will serve to adequately model many real-world applications. Table I shows the subset that has been selected for translation in this compiler, and also lists the equivalent operation in Handel-C. (The CSP notation is expressed in the machine-readable version CSPM that is required by the tools).

Table 1: Handel-C Translation of CSPM Features

Feature	CSP	Handel-C
Comments	`-- ...`	`// ...`
	`{- ... -}`	`/* ... */`
Channel Declarations	`channel`	`chan, chanin, chanout`
Channel Operations	`in?x`	`in?x;`
	`out!x`	`out!x;`
Integer Declarations	`implied`	`int 8 x;`
External Choice	`[]`	`prialt {...}`
Synchronous Parallel	`[|{|...|}|]`	`par {...}`
Recursion	`P = ... → P`	`while(1) {...}`

CSP is an algebra concerned primarily with the interactions of multiple processes that communicate with each other via events. However, operations that are significant and internal to a process – such as complex mathematical expressions – may not be represented in CSP in an easy-to-translate form. Such operations are, however, of vital importance to the functionality of the FPGA, so a method has been developed for embedding arbitrary Handel-C statements in the CSP script as comments. For example:

```
{-MacroC calculation
      x = f(x);
      y = g(y);
EndMacroC-}
```

Assume that this CSP comment is associated with the following CSP script:

```
Ex = in?x -> in?y -> calculation -> out!x -> out!y -> Ex
```

The C statements included in the comment would be inserted in the Handel-C code anywhere that the term `calculation` was found. Thus a type of macro has been developed, where C code can be embedded as a comment in the CSP script and automatically inserted in the correct place in the Handel-C output file.

3.2 Lexical Analysis of CSP

The first step in creating any sort of a compiler-type program is to identify the tokens that are acceptable as input. The Lex utility makes the recognition of these tokens easy; the utility uses a list of tokens, along with a list of instructions on the actions that should take place when a specific token is found. For example, we present a piece of the translator's Lex file including the tokens "->" and "channel":

```
"->"            {return PREFIX;}                    /* PREFIX token */

channel         {                                   /* CHANNEL keyword */
                    var_dec = 1;
                    return CHANNEL;

                }
```

Note that in the case of the channel keyword, a variable is set for use in another part of the program before the token type is returned.

The complete list of tokens that the translator recognizes is very large and complex, with several tokens necessitating the call of various functions to set flags, store strings in memory, and perform a variety of other operations. In most cases, tokens are separated by white space, which is defined as any combination of spaces, tabs, and newline characters.

3.3 Grammatical Analysis of CSP

The lexical analysis breaks the input stream into tokens based on defined rules. This list of tokens is not very useful in itself, but when it is combined with a syntactical parser, it becomes invaluable. The Yacc utility is provided to help with the implementation of parsers. Code written using Yacc interacts with lexer code to produce a complete compiler.

Writing code using Yacc is similar to Lex. Once again, a list of allowable constructs is created. This time, however, combinations of tokens are represented. For example, here is part of the listing of possible combinations that the translator program will allow:

```
statement:  PROCESS '=' expression
         |  CHANNEL variable_list
         |  MACRO
         |  C_VAR
         |  COMMENT
         ;
```

This list signifies that a statement is one of five things: a process definition, a channel declaration, a macro, a C variable declaration, or a comment. These key words are provided to the Yacc program by the lexical analyzer described above.

As is the case with the lexer, the parser calls functions and set flags when specific constructs are recognized. If the lexer provides combinations of tokens that are not recognized as valid by the parser, a syntax error is generated.

The use of Lex and Yacc greatly improves the process of adding additional tokens or constructs to the translator. New features can be added simply by placing the appropriate tokens in the token list, and constructs in the construct list.

3.4 Code Design

The first step of the code design process is to determine which parts of CSP to accept. An appropriate subset has been selected, as shown in Table I. Next, a mapping of CSP to Handel-C was performed. Where there is a one-to-one correspondence between a CSP feature and a Handel-C feature, the translation process is simply a substitution of one character string for another.

The translation process is not always this simple, however. For example, the CSP "=" operator serves to assign an event or list of events to a process. In Handel-C, the events are listed sequentially, but the process name is meaningless as far as code execution is concerned. The list of events assigned to a specific process are stored in a linked list of processes, so that the individual processes can be combined properly when the inter-process interaction definitions are found later in the CSP script.

Another example of a complicated conversion involves the CSP synchronous parallel construct. A list of processes that would run in parallel in Handel-C requires the use of the `par` construct.

The translation of simple recursions required the creation of infinite `while` loops. A recursive process in CSP is written as:

```
GetVal = input?x -> GetVal
```

In Handel-C, this is represented as:

```
while(1)
{
        input?x;
}
```

This requires setting a flag in the process structure to indicate that the process in question is recursive. On another note, variables declared in Handel-C are visible to the entire function in question. Care should be taken in the CSP design to avoid the reuse of variable names, even in different processes, unless the intention is to allow these variables to be shared by the entire Handel-C program.

3.5 Using the CSPtoHC Translator

Consideration will now be given to the technique of using the `CSPtoHC` translator to produce Handel-C code. When a CSP script has been duly tested and proven reliable using the ProBE and FDR tools, the translator can be invoked to perform the conversion. The syntax expected by the `CSPtoHC` translator is as follows:

```
CSPtoHC <CSP filename> <Handel-C filename>
```

The CSP file must exist, or an error will occur and the program will exit. If the Handel-C file specified already exists, it cannot be overwritten, and an error will occur. If there are not exactly two files specified when the compiler is invoked, it will exit.

A typical `CSPtoHC` compiler session might appear as follows:

```
io% ./CSPtoHC Commstime.csp Commstime.hcc
Process PrefixInt0 found.
Process IdInt found.
Process Delta2Int found.
Process Consume found.
Process SuccessorInt found.
Process System found.
Translation successful -- File Commstime.hcc created.
```

Notice that `Commstime.csp` is the input file, and `Commstime.hcc` will be created as the output file. As the translation takes place, processes that have been identified are listed one by one. This process listing can be used as a means of checking to ensure that the compiler has actually found all the processes included in the CSP script. Once the translation succeeds, the user is alerted to this fact and notified that the output file has been created and is ready for use.

4. Testing The Translator

4.1 Simple Simulations

To test the functionality of the CSPtoHC translator, several simple programs were first employed to check the correctness of the different constructs. These simple CSP scripts and the Handel-C equivalent code are discussed in this section.

4.1.1 UpHandler

`UpHandler` is a very simple process that repeatedly reads in an integer on channel `input` and then exports the integer on channel `output`. The CSP script for this process is:

```
-- This is a test file for a simple process with recursion
channel input, output
UpHandler = input?x -> output!x -> UpHandler
```

The resulting Handel-C code appears as follows:

```
// This is a test file for a simple process with recursion
void main(void)
{
        chanin input;
        chanout output;
        int 8 UpHandler_flag, x;

        // UpHandler
        while(UpHandler_flag == 0)
        {
                input?x;
                output!x;
        }
}
```

There are several things to note about this translation. First, the CSPM comment is correctly translated into a C-style comment. The CSP channels are separated into input and output channels, and declared accordingly. The recursion is detected, and is properly represented through the use of the while loop. Observe that all `while` loops are given a loop flag, which is automatically initialized to zero in the C code, so that the programmer can manually insert a loop termination condition later on. (Alternatively the CSP programmer could insert an `if-the-else` clause in the CSP version, which would be correctly translated in Handel-C). The process name (UpHandler), is included in the Handel-C file as a comment. Semicolons have been inserted in the appropriate places. Tabs have been added to improve the readability of the code. Lastly, x is determined to be a variable, and is appropriately declared as an integer.

4.1.2 StopAndWait

The `StopAndWait` [15] protocol consists of two processes called `Send` and `Recv` that synchronize to establish a path of controlled data flow. In fig. 2, it can be seen that the `Send` process accepts data from an input channel, sends the data out on channel `mid`, and then waits for a response from channel `ack` before allowing further input. `Recv` reads data from channel `mid`, outputs it on channel `out`, and then sends an `ack` back to process `Send`.

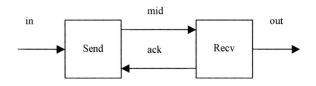

Figure 2: The `StopAndWait` protocol.

The CSP script that describes this system is:

```
-- Stop and Wait Protocol
channel in, mid, ack, out
Send = in?x -> mid!x -> ack?x -> Send
Recv = mid?y -> out!y -> ack!y -> Recv
System = (Send [|{| mid, ack |}|] Recv)
```

Executing the CSPtoHC compiler on this script produces the following Handel-C file:

```
// Stop and Wait Protocol
void main(void)
{
    chan ack, mid;
    chanin in;
    chanout out;
    int 8 Recv_flag, y, Send_flag, x;

    par    // System
    {
        // Send
        while(Send_flag == 0)
        {
            in?x;
            mid!x;
            ack?x;
        }

        // Recv
        while(Recv_flag == 0)
        {
            mid?y;
```

```
            out!y;
            ack!y;
        }
    }
}
```

The main feature is the use of the `par` construct, where `Send` and `Recv` are required to operate in synchronous parallel. The CSP channels are once again sorted as input, output, or bi-directional channels, based on the "?" and "!" tokens. One other factor of note is the length of the Handel-C program compared to the length of the original CSP script: the Handel-C program is about five times the length of the corresponding CSP script. Similar expansion of code was noted in Java and C translations of CSP [8].

4.1.3 ManyToOne

The last of the simple algorithms to be presented is the `ManyToOne` algorithm. This program acts as a simple multiplexer or switch. Four input channels are mapped to one output channel. The input channels are serviced by a first-in, first-out algorithm, where only one value at a time is output. Figure 3 shows how the channels interact.

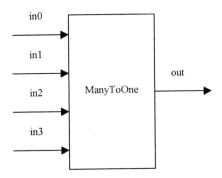

Figure 3: The `ManyToOne` algorithm.

The CSP description of this algorithm introduces the external choice operator:

```
-- This program maps four inputs to one output

channel in0, in1, in2, in3, out
MtoO = in0?x -> out!x -> MtoO
[] in1?y -> out!y -> MtoO
[] in2?z -> out!z -> MtoO
[] in3?w -> out!w -> MtoO
```

When this script is translated, the following Handel-C code is produced:

```
// This program maps four inputs to one output
void main(void)
{
    chanin in3, in2, in1, in0;
    chanout out;
    int 8 w, z, y, MToO_flag, x;

    // MToO
    while(MToO_flag == 0)
    {
        prialt
        {
            case in0?x:
            out!x;
            break;

            case in1?y:
            out!y;
            break;

            case in2?z:
            out!z;
            break;

            case in3?w:
            out!w;
            break;
        }
    }
}
```

This Handel-C program makes use of the `prialt` operator – Handel-C's implementation of CSP's external choice. Notice that there is a `prialt` case setup for each input channel, and once an input is read, that input value must be output before any other input channel can be serviced. Since all processes are part of the same C function, distinct variable names must be used in each case.

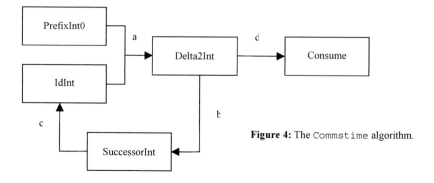

Figure 4: The Commstime algorithm.

4.2 Larger Programs

4.2.1 Commstime

The first example is Commstime, which is a commonly used timing benchmark [10]. The Commstime system is shown in fig. 4. The system starts with the number 0, and the number is circulated through the processes, being incremented by one each time it passes through the SuccessorInt process. Thus, the incrementing numbers are observed as they arrive at Consume, and the throughput of the system can be calculated.

The CSP script that corresponds to this figure is shown below. Notice the inclusion of a macro incw to define the addition operation present in the SuccessorInt process (in this case the simple arithmetic operation could be included in the channel output: c!(w+1)).

```
{-MacroC incw
w = w + 1;
EndMacroC-}

channel a, b, c, d, e

PrefixInt0 = a!0 -> Skip
IdInt = c?x -> a!x -> IdInt
Delta2Int = a?y -> d!y -> b!y -> Delta2Int
Consume = d?z -> e!z -> Consume
SuccessorInt = b?w -> incw -> c!w -> SuccessorInt
System = (SuccessorInt
        [|{| |}|] Consume
        [|{| |}|] Delta2Int
        [|{| |}|] IdInt
        [|{| |}|] PrefixInt0)
```

The equivalent Handel-C code:

```
void main(void)
{
        chan d, c, b, a;
        chanout e;
        int 8 SuccessorInt_flag, w, Consume_flag, z,
                Delta2Int_flag, y, IdInt_flag, x;

        par    // System
        {
                // PrefixInt0
                {
                        a!0;
                }

                // IdInt
                while(IdInt_flag == 0)
                {
                        c?x;
                        a!x;
                }

                // Delta2Int
                while(Delta2Int_flag == 0)
                {
                        a?y;
```

```
                        d!y;
                        b!y;
                }

                // Consume
                while(Consume_flag == 0)
                {
                        d?z;
                        e!z;
                }

                // SuccessorInt
                while(SuccessorInt_flag == 0)
                {
                        b?w;
                        w = w + 1;
                        c!w;
                }
        }
}
```

Upon analysis, it can be seen that there are four recursive processes and one non-recursive process that execute in parallel. Synchronization between processes is accomplished by using channels. The throughput of this system is easy to measure. Using the Handel-C simulator, the number of clock cycles it takes for the value output on channel e to increment can be observed (the current clock cycle is listed on the left of each line, and the value of each variable at that time is shown):

```
Compiled :     0 gates,     0 inverters,   11 latches,   84 others
Optimised :    0 gates,     0 inverters,   11 latches,   72 others
Expanded : 164 gates,     35 inverters,   58 latches,    8 others
Optimised :   76 gates,     13 inverters,   58 latches,    8 others

0:  w=0  z=0  y=0  x=0
1:  w=0  z=0  y=0  x=0
2:  w=0  z=0  y=0  x=0
2:  Ready to accept output from `e' ? (y/n) y
2:  Output from channel `e' = 0
3:  w=0  z=0  y=0  x=0
4:  w=1  z=0  y=0  x=0
5:  w=1  z=0  y=0  x=1
6:  w=1  z=0  y=1  x=1
7:  w=1  z=1  y=1  x=1
7:  Ready to accept output from `e' ? (y/n) y
7:  Output from channel `e' = 1
8:  w=1  z=1  y=1  x=1
9:  w=2  z=1  y=1  x=1
10:  w=2  z=1  y=1  x=2
11:  w=2  z=1  y=2  x=2
12:  w=2  z=2  y=2  x=2
12:  Ready to accept output from `e' ? (y/n) y
12:  Output from channel `e' = 2
```

Outputs are ready from channel e on clock cycles 2, 7, and 12. Thus, we can deduce that it takes five clock ticks for the system to loop one time. In addition to the current clock cycle, the simulator indicates the value held by each variable register on each clock cycle. Statistics are also given for the number of gates, inverters, latches, and other constructs that would be used if actual hardware was created. These numbers are helpful when determining the size of the FPGA that will be used to create the corresponding hardware.

4.2.2 Sieve of Eratosthenes

Another common benchmark program is the sieve of Eratosthenes, which was developed by the Greek mathematician Eratosthenes around 200 BC. This algorithm is an efficient method for calculating prime numbers, and lends itself well to pipelined parallelism. The diagram for a three-stage sieve is in fig. 5. This version passes all numbers through, attaching a tag (`primeout`) indicating whether the output is prime or non-prime.

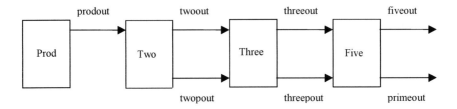

Figure 5: The sieve of Eratosthenes.

This model checks each input (`prodout`) to the pipe for multiples of two, three, and five, and thus will find all prime numbers up to five squared, or 25. Parallelism is possible, because each stage in the pipeline can be working on a different number at any given time. There are two channels for communication between most of the processes – one to pass the number being tested, and one to pass the status of that number as prime or non-prime. The CSP description of this system follows. A future version of the translator will allow if-then-else constructs in CSP, which would allow a much more efficient CSP script to be used for this algorithm.

```
-- An implementation of the Sieve of Eratosthenes that calculates
-- all prime numbers between 2 and 25.  This is done by marking
-- all numbers that are multiples of 2, 3, or 5 as non-prime (0).

--VarC int 8 i
--VarC int 8 j
--VarC int 8 k

{-MacroC incx
x++;
if(x > 25) x = 0;
EndMacroC-}

{-MacroC check2
g = 1;
for(i=4; i<=25; i=i+2)
{
   if(i == d) g = 0;
}
EndMacroC-}

{-MacroC check3
for(j=6; j<=25; j=j+3)
{
   if(j == e) h = 0;
}
EndMacroC-}

{-MacroC check5
```

```
for(k=10; k<=25; k=k+5)
{
  if(k == f) p = 0;
}
EndMacroC-}

channel prodout, twoout, threeout, fiveout, primeout
channel twopout, threepout

Prod = prodout!x -> incx ->  Prod
Two = prodout?d -> check2 -> twoout!d -> twopout!g -> Two
Three = twoout?e -> twopout?h -> check3 -> threeout!e ->
       threepout!h -> Three
Five = threeout?f -> threepout?p -> check5 -> fiveout!f ->
       primeout!p -> Five

Sieve = (Five || Three || Two || Prod)
```

When this CSP file is given to the CSPtoHC translator, the following output is obtained:

```
// An implementation of the Sieve of Eratosthenes that calculates
// all prime numbers between 2 and 25.  This is done by marking
// all numbers that are multiples of 2, 3, or 5 as non-prime (0).

void main(void)
{
        chan threepout, twopout, threeout, twoout, prodout;
        chanout primeout, fiveout;
        int 8 i;
        int 8 j;
        int 8 k;
        int 8 Five_flag, p, f, Three_flag, h, e, Two_flag, g, d,
            Prod_flag, x;
        par    // Sieve
        {
                // Prod
                while(Prod_flag == 0)
                {
                        prodout!x;
                        x++;
                        if(x > 25) x = 0;
                }

                // Two
                while(Two_flag == 0)
                {
                        prodout?d;
                        g = 1;
                        for(i=4; i<=25; i=i+2)
                        {
                                if(i == d) g = 0;
                        }
                        twoout!d;
                        twopout!g;
                }

                // Three
                while(Three_flag == 0)
                {
                        twoout?e;
                        twopout?h;
```

```
            for(j=6; j<=25; j=j+3)
            {
                    if(j == e) h = 0;
            }
            threeout!e;
            threepout!h;
    }

    // Five
    while(Five_flag == 0)
    {
            threeout?f;
            threepout?p;
            for(k=10; k<=25; k=k+5)
            {
                    if(k == f) p = 0;
            }
            fiveout!f;
            primeout!p;
    }
}
}
```

The Handel-C code contains four parallel processes that interact via channels to keep track of the current number, and whether or not that number is prime. Simulating this file yields the following hardware specifications:

```
Compiled :     0 gates,    0 inverters,   24 latches, 190 others
Optimised :     0 gates,    0 inverters,   21 latches, 161 others
Expanded : 476 gates, 179 inverters,  117 latches,  30 others
Optimised : 160 gates,   30 inverters,  110 latches,  30 others.
```

The simulator produces the following timing listing for the number 3 is prime:

```
65: i=26 j=6  k=30 p=1 f=2 h=1 e=3 d=4 x=4 g=1
66: i=26 j=9  k=30 p=1 f=2 h=1 e=3 d=4 x=5 g=1
67: i=4  j=12 k=30 p=1 f=2 h=1 e=3 d=4 x=5 g=1
68: i=4  j=15 k=30 p=1 f=2 h=1 e=3 d=4 x=5 g=0
69: i=6  j=18 k=30 p=1 f=2 h=1 e=3 d=4 x=5 g=0
70: i=8  j=21 k=30 p=1 f=2 h=1 e=3 d=4 x=5 g=0
71: i=10 j=24 k=30 p=1 f=2 h=1 e=3 d=4 x=5 g=0
72: i=12 j=27 k=30 p=1 f=2 h=1 e=3 d=4 x=5 g=0
73: i=14 j=27 k=30 p=1 f=3 h=1 e=3 d=4 x=5 g=0
74: i=16 j=27 k=30 p=1 f=3 h=1 e=3 d=4 x=5 g=0
75: i=18 j=27 k=10 p=1 f=3 h=1 e=3 d=4 x=5 g=0
76: i=20 j=27 k=15 p=1 f=3 h=1 e=3 d=4 x=5 g=0
77: i=22 j=27 k=20 p=1 f=3 h=1 e=3 d=4 x=5 g=0
78: i=24 j=27 k=25 p=1 f=3 h=1 e=3 d=4 x=5 g=0
79: i=26 j=27 k=30 p=1 f=3 h=1 e=3 d=4 x=5 g=0
79: Ready to accept output from `fiveout' ? (y/n) y
79: Output from channel `fiveout' = 3
80: i=26 j=27 k=30 p=1 f=3 h=1 e=4 d=4 x=5 g=0
80: Ready to accept output from `primeout' ? (y/n) y
80: Output from channel `primeout' = 1
```

It takes 15 clock cycles for the sieve to determine that 3 is a prime. Since this is a pipelined system, each of the three stage processes is working on a different number at any given time, and the speedup achieved would approach three times that of a non-pipelined version if the times for each stage were equal (in the future more efficient version).

4.3 Commstime in Hardware

We next produce actual hardware for two of these simulations, and then check that hardware to ensure that it does indeed match the CSP specification. The first program is the Commstime routine; it is more complicated than the simpler algorithms, and yet provides an easy-to-observe output – a continuously incrementing 8-bit number.

The hardware used in this test was a Celoxica RC200 development board [16]. The FPGA provided on this board is a Xilinx XC2V1000 [17], which includes 11,520 logic cells and 720 KB of RAM. This is ample room for the implementation of the Commstime algorithm.

The process of placing the Handel-C code on the FPGA is somewhat complicated. The CSPtoHC compiler translates CSP scripts into Handel-C code for the simulator. If an actual hardware build is required, the Handel-C file must be modified a little; a clock source must be defined, and any channels that communicate with external devices must be renamed and mapped to valid FPGA port pins. The beginning section of the modified Commstime Handel-C code is

```
#define PAL_TARGET_CLOCK_RATE 2000000
#include "pal_master.hch"

void main(void)
{
    chan d, c, b, a;
    int 8 e;

    interface bus_out() WriteData(int 8 DataOut = e) with
        {data = {"M3","P2","P1","N2","N1","M2","M1","R2"}};
```

Notice that a 2 MHz clock is defined, and the channel formally labeled output channel e is now a bus_out construct, mapped to eight I/O pins on the FPGA.

Once these modifications have been made, the Handel-C source code is opened in the Celoxica DK editor, where it can be compiled to an ".edif" file (among other options). The ".edif" file then needs to be fitted to a chip, where it is placed, routed, and tested, and a "bit" file is produced. Using the RC200 development board greatly simplifies this procedure, since the DK builder automatically performs the placement and routing routines, and produces an output file specifically configured for the RC200 board. The Celoxica FPU utility is then employed to program the FPGA.

Once the FPGA is programmed, the output can be observed by connecting a logic analyzer to the output pins of the FPGA. The results obtained are displayed in fig. 6 (remember that Commstime is a benchmark program used to observe the speed in which different processes connected by channels interact). The output of Commstime is an 8-bit number that continuously increments. The results obtained in fig. 6 confirm that this is indeed the case.

The least-significant bit, bit 0, changes every time the 8-bit number is incremented, which occurs every 2.5 microseconds. Going back to the earlier simulation of the Commstime algorithm, we predicted that each cycle would take 5 clock ticks. Since the FPGA is running at 2 MHz, that equates to a clock period of 500 ns. If the cycle truly takes 5 clock ticks, that would be 500 ns times 5, or 2.5 microseconds; thus, the simulator and the hardware agree precisely.

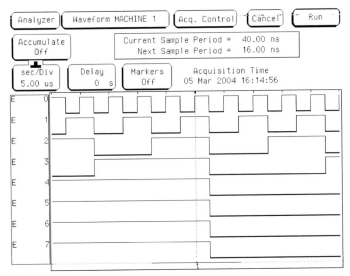

Figure 6: Commstime output from logic analyzer.

4.4 Sieve of Eratosthenes in Hardware

The second Handel-C program that was taken to the FPGA stage was the sieve of Eratosthenes. The same steps were taken to program the FPGA in this case as were in the Commstime example. The Handel-C code was modified to provide a clock source, and output signals were mapped to pins on the FPGA. The modified portion of the Handel-C source code is shown here:

```
// An implementation of the Sieve of Eratosthenes that calculates
// all prime numbers between 2 and 25.  This is done by marking
// all numbers that are multiples of 2, 3, or 5 (which is the
// square root of 25) as non-prime.

#define PAL_TARGET_CLOCK_RATE 2000000
#include "pal_master.hch"

void main(void)
{
        chan threepout, twopout, threeout, twoout, prodout;
        int 8 y, z;

        interface bus_out() WriteData(int 8 DataOut = y) with
                {data = {"M3","P2","P1","N2","N1","M2","M1","R2"}};
        interface bus_out() WritePrime(int 8 PrimeOut = z) with
                {data = {"T2","R4","R3","P3","P4","N4","N3","M4"}};
```

A logic analyzer was once again connected to the output pins of the programmed FPGA to observe the operations taking place. Figure 8 shows the resulting output. The top five data lines show the number being output from process Five, while the bottom line indicates whether that number is prime. Reading straight from the output, the numbers 0, 1, 2, 3, 5, 7, 11, 13, 17, 19, and 23 are marked as primes, all the others are not. It can be concluded that this implementation of a 3-stage sieve of Eratosthenes is correct. (Note that 0, not a prime, is marked as prime by the algorithm; added complexity could avoid this.)

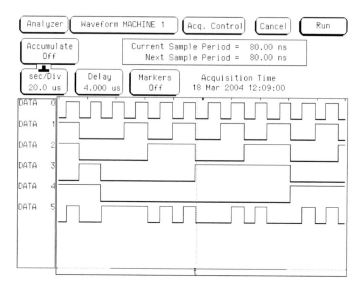

Figure 8: Sieve of Eratosthenes output from logic analyzer.

5. Summary and Conclusions

5.1 Successes

A translator has been constructed that correctly converts a useful subset of the CSP process description language into C code that can be implemented directly in FPGAs. Simulations and actual FPGA implementations verify that the hardware created does indeed match the original CSP specification.

5.2 Possible Improvements

There are many facets of CSP and Handel-C that have not been represented here. The most prominent is that of the introduction of discrete timing to a set of processes, which is critical for real-time systems.

A second improvement that could be provided is that of intra-process verification. CSP does an excellent job of modeling and verifying the external communications between processes, but using other tools, such as Promela [18], could improve the specification and verification of the internal operations.

A more user-friendly interface, possibly some sort of graphical user interface (GUI), could be developed to increase usefulness of the translator and provide more options and feedback. Options could also be added to compile the CSP script into simulation-style or release-style Handel-C.

Optimization of the Handel-C code is also possible. The Handel-C code produced by the compiler is functional, but there are many ways that the code could be rewritten to enhance and optimize its functionality. Optimization could occur at the CSP level, during the CSP to Handel-C conversion, or after the Handel-C has been translated.

5.3 Future Work

This project is just a small step in the field of studying the relationships and interactions between software and hardware. This project has significant room for improvement, including adding additional features of CSP to the allowable input and making the CSPtoHC translator more user-friendly.

Another area for future research would be comparing the efficiency of the generated Handel-C code with Handel-C code that was written by hand. A comparison of the efficiency of Handel-C with hardware languages such as VHDL, Verilog, or ABEL might prove interesting.

There is significant room for optimization in the Handel-C code. As mentioned previously, the focus during this project was to create Handel-C that was robust and functional, with efficiency being a lesser goal. Now that the functionality has been proven, more effort can be put towards making the code more efficient.

References

[1]   C.A.R. Hoare, "Communicating sequential processes," *CACM*, vol. 21(8), pp. 666-667, Aug. 1978.

[2]   Celoxica, "Handel-C Software-Compiled System Design." Available: http://www.celoxica.com/methodology/handelc.asp

[3]   Formal Systems (Europe) Ltd, "Formal Systems Software." Available: http://www.fsel.com/software.html

[4]   J. R. Levine, T. Mason, and D. Brown. Lex and Yacc. Sebastopol, CA: O'Reilly, 1992.

[5]   STMicroelectronics. "Welcome to ST." Available: http://www.st.com

[6]   J. Campbell, *"Efficient automatic mapping of hardware to software,"* PhD dissertation, Utah State University, Logan, UT. 2002.

[7]   W. Zhou and G. S. Stiles, "The automated serialization of concurrent CSP scripts using Mathematica," presented at the Communicating Process Architectures Conference, Enschede, the Netherlands, 2000.

[8]   V. Raju, L. Rong, and G. S. Stiles, "Automatic conversion of CSP to CTJ, JCSP, and CCSP," presented at the Communicating Process Architectures Conference, Enschede, the Netherlands, 2003.

[9]   G. Hilderink, J. Broenink, W. Vervoort, and A. Bakkers, "Communicating java threads," in *Proceedings of WoTUG 20: Parallel Programming and Java*, A. Bakkers, Ed. Amsterdam, the Netherlands: IOS Press, 1997, pp. 48-76.

[10] University of Twente, "CSP for Java." Available: http://www.rt.el.utwente.nl/

[11] P. H. Welch, "Process oriented design for Java: concurrency for all," in *Proceedings of the International Conference on Parallel and Distributed Processing Techniques and Applications*, H. R. Arabnia, Ed. Athens, GA: CSREA Press, 2000, pp. 51-57.

[12] University of Kent, "Communicating Sequential Processes for Java (JCSP)." Available: http://www.cs.ukc.ac.uk/projects/ofa/jcsp/

[13] Quickstone Technologies Ltd, "CCSP." Available: http://www.quickstone.com/xcsp/ccspnetworkedition/

[14] R. M. A. Peel and J. W. H. Feng, "Steps in the Verification of an Occam-to-FPGA Compiler". University of Surrey. Guildford, Surrey, U.K.

[15] S. Schneider. Concurrent and Real-Time Systems: The CSP Approach. Chichester, UK: Wiley, 1999.

[16] Celoxica, "Products: RC200 Development Board." Available: http://www.celoxica.com/products/boards/rc200.asp

[17] Xilinx, "Xilinx Products and Services." Available: http://www.xilinx.com/xlnx/xil_prodcat_product.jsp

[18] Promela, "Concise Promela Reference." Available: http://spinroot.com/spin/Man/Quick.html

Communicating Process Architectures 2004
Ian East, Jeremy Martin, Peter Welch, David Duce, and Mark Green (Eds.)
IOS Press, 2004

On Linear Time and Congruence in Channel-passing Calculi

Frédéric PESCHANSKI

University of Tokyo, Bunkyo-ku Hongo 7-3-1, 113-0033 Tokyo, Japan.
also with *LIP6, 8, rue du Capitaine Scott, 75015 Paris, France.*

Abstract. Process algebras such as CSP or the Pi-calculus are theories to reason about concurrent software. The Pi-calculus also introduces channel passing to address specific issues in mobility. Despite their similarity, the languages expose salient divergences at the formal level. CSP is built upon trace semantics while labeled transition systems and bisimulation are the privileged tools to discuss the Pi-calculus semantics. In this paper, we try to bring closer both approaches at the theoretical level by showing that proper trace semantics can be built upon the Pi-calculus. Moreover, by introducing locations, we obtain the same discriminative power for both the trace and bisimulation equivalences, in the particular case of early semantics. In a second part, we propose to develop the semantics of a slightly modified language directly in terms of traces. This language retains the full expressive power of the Pi-calculus and most notably supports channel passing. Interestingly, the resulting equivalence, obtained from late semantics, exhibits a nice congruence property over process expressions.

1 Introduction

CSP [1] and the Pi-calculus [2] are two well-developed theories to reason about concurrent software. Both approaches expose similar concepts, notably *interleaving semantics* and *synchronous communication*. They also diverge in some important areas. First of all, CSP is arguably richer and of higher-level than Pi. It provides various forms of parallel, choice and sequential constructs; it is also open to a rich set of datatypes. The Pi-calculus, on the other hand, only provides minimalistic forms of parallel and choice constructs; and it only supports the datatype of *names*. However, the Pi-calculus offers an interesting form of mobility through name/channel passing which is not present in CSP.

The divergence between the two language amplifies at the level of the underlying semantics. The Pi-calculus semantics are (generally) proposed through *labeled transition systems* whereas CSP mostly builds on top of *trace semantics*. It is our opinion that the latter, denoting set-based equivalences, are easier to deal with than the former, relying on more complex *bisimulation* equivalences. It is often stated, however, that *"Bisimulation equivalence discriminates more processes than trace semantics"* [3]. In this paper we show that mobile calculi close to the Pi-calculus can be analyzed *with full precision* using techniques similar to the ones developed within the CSP framework, namely *trace equivalence*. We hope that this preliminary step could help (re)conciliating the two approaches that have a lot in common. Strikingly enough, mobile channel types are now implemented in many CSP-based programming languages and implementations [4, 5, 6].

In section 2, we present a minimal language of concurrent sequential processes with a channel-passing form of mobility. The language is almost identical to the Pi-calculus. It can also be seen as a subset of CSP extended by channel passing. We further propose to characterize the operational semantics of this language, in two complementary ways. First, in section 3, we show that by inserting *locations* at well-chosen positions in terms (mostly

Table 1: A common syntax for mobile calculi

<expr> ::=	0	inert
	$\mid$ (*<expr>*)	precedence
	$\mid$ *<prefix>.<expr>*	sequence
	$\mid \nu(x)$ *<expr>*	restriction
	$\mid [x = y]$ *<expr>*	match
	$\mid [x \neq y]$ *<expr>*	mismatch
	$\mid$ *<expr>* $+$ *<expr>*	choice
	$\mid$ *<expr>* $\parallel$ *<expr>*	parallel
	$\mid *$*<expr>*	replication
<prefix> ::=	$c!y$	output
	$\mid c?(x)$	input
	$\mid \tau$	silent

around parallel and choice sub-terms), we can provide a linear-time form of Pi-calculus that retains all the features of its branching-time counterpart. We then prove that the LTS-based semantics can be equated to CSP-like trace semantics thus allowing reasoning based on both these complementary approaches. As a second contribution, developed in section 4, we take the counterpoint of developing CSP-like trace semantics directly, without having to construct a LTS first, on a slightly modified version of the language. Interestingly, this complementary development allows us to characterize a trace-based equivalence that enjoys a congruence property on process expressions which is not present in the "traditional" semantics for the Pi-calculus. A panorama of related work, a conclusion and a selection of references follow.

2   A Concurrent Language with Channel Passing

Several theories for concurrency have been developed during the past twenty years. Some of these theories, often designed as *process calculi* or *process algebras*, focus on *compositional semantics*. In such approaches, the behavior of high-level components are explained in terms of their lower-level sub-components and the way they interact. Successful members of this compositional family include the *Communicating Sequential Processes* (CSP) work introduced by Hoare [1], the *Calculus of Communicating Systems* (CCS) by Milner, further developed in its mobile counterpart the *Pi-calculus* [2], and the *Algebra of Communicating Processes* by Bergstra and Klop [7]. Empirically, one can say that all these languages allow to express the behavior of concurrent and sequential processes that can communicate with each other. In this section we give the minimalistic syntax of such a process calculus, which is almost identical to the Pi-calculus but with an additional – and intentional – CSP "feel".

In Table 1 we give the BNF syntax of the proposed language. Concurrent processes are expressed as terms separated by the parallel construct (noted here $\parallel$ as in the CSP). The following example is a canonical communication system:

$$c!e.0 \parallel c?(x).P(x)$$

Following the process algebra terminology, we can distinguish the *prefix* and the *continuation* of both processes. For example, the prefix of the left-side process is $c!e$ (for *emitting the value e on the channel c*) and its continuation is 0 (for *terminating the process*). The prefix of the right-side process is $c?(x)$ which denotes the reception of a value through the channel c. The value is bound to name x in the continuation $P(x)$. So the rewrite we expect from such a term may be informally noted as follows:

$$c!e.0 \parallel c?(x).P(x) \rightarrow 0 \parallel P(e)$$

The 0 (inert) process of the Pi-calculus indicates a process termination. Since there is no sequential composition operator, it is not possible to synchronize on termination as in CSP. That is why trailing 0's may generally be omitted in terms, which might seems unfamiliar for CSP experts. Note that synchronization on termination can be encoded in the Pi-calculus, for example by introducing dedicated *end* channels.

The Pi-calculus also provides channel mobility, which we can illustrate on the following example:

$$c!e.0 \parallel c?(x).x!f.0 \parallel e?(y).Q(y)$$

The value e we pass through the channel c from the left-side process to the one in the middle is bound to x in the destination, which is then used as a channel. The expected rewrites for the previous example are as follows:

$$c!e.0 \parallel c?(x).x!f.0 \parallel e?(y).Q(y) \rightarrow 0 \parallel e!f.0 \parallel e?(y).Q(y)$$
$$\rightarrow 0 \parallel 0 \parallel Q(f)$$

One may also employ *restriction* (ν construct) to encapsulate names/channels. Consider the following variant of the previous example:

$$\nu(e)(c!e.0) \parallel c?(x).x!f.0 \parallel e?(y).Q(y)$$

Here, the name e is restricted to the scope of the left process. This means that the name e in the right process, which is a free name, is different from the bound occurrence of e in the left process. The rewrite we expect is as follows:

$$\nu(e)(c!e.0) \parallel c?(x).x!f.0 \parallel e?(y).Q(y) \rightarrow \nu(e)\,(0 \parallel e!f.0) \parallel e?(y).Q(y)$$

The highlighted scope modification is called a *scope extrusion*, it will be discussed in the next section. The difference with the previous example is that no more rewrite is possible since we cannot extend further the scope of e to the right-side process without renaming either the restricted e (inside the ν) or the free one (outside). Unlike CSP, the proposed language does not provide a recursion operator. But such an operator can be encoded using *replication* ($*$ operator) and communication (see [2]). Moreover, only the datatype of *names* (sometimes considered as channels) is available. Names can solely be tested for (in)equality using the *match* $[x = y]$ and *mismatch* $[x \neq y]$ operators.

As such, the proposed language, which is equivalent to the Pi-calculus, can be seen as a severe restriction if compared to the CSP language. Except for communication prefixes and generalized forms of parallel and choice operators, most of CSP is not supported. However, channel passing itself gives almost all its expressiveness to the Pi-calculus, as largely exemplified in the literature (starting from [2]).

3   Linear-time Channel Passing

Bisimulation and *trace equivalences* are often opposed in the literature. Even in introductory textbooks (such as [3]), the former is generally considered as a *finer* equivalence (*i.e.* it discriminates more processes) than the latter.

Consider the following process expressions:

$$a!e.c!f + b!e.d!g \text{ and } a!e.c!f + a!e.d!g$$

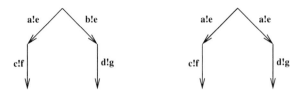

Figure 1: Branching vs linear-time tree structures

These expressions can be represented as tree structures (cf. figure 1). The left tree represents the behavior of the left process that can first perform either an output on a or an output on b, non-deterministically. If $a!e$ occurs, then $c!f$ follows, or if $b!e$ occurs, then $d!g$ follows. This *linear-time* behavior can be fully and naturally characterized with both trace and bisimulation equivalences. This is not true for the right-side process expression which exhibits *branching-time* semantics. In that case, the first action that can occur is always an output of a name e on a. Then, either $c!f$ or $d!g$ can follow. But the *choice* among which of these should occur is performed at the time $a!e$ occurs. Trace equivalence will equate such process to a less precise $a!e.(c!f + d!g)$. Intuitively, you cannot discriminate the "left" $a!e$ and the "right" $a!e$. Bisimulation equivalence, in contrast, properly discriminates here.

3.1   A Linearized Language with Locations

Trace equivalence can be extended with *stable failures* and *divergences* in order to obtain a more precise equivalence [1]. However, the resulting model does not integrate channel passing. In this paper, we thus propose a complementary approach which consists in changing slightly the language of section 2 so that trace semantics may be used even in the case of branching-time behaviors (such as the "splitting" action $a!e$ in our example).

Table 2: The syntax enriched with locations

$<expr>$ ::=	$[0]@l$	inert
	$\mid [(<expr>)]@l$	precedence
	$\mid [<prefix>.<expr>]@l$	sequence
	$\mid \nu(x)\,[<expr>]@l$	restriction
	$\mid [x = y]\,[<expr>]@l$	match
	$\mid [x \neq y]\,[<expr>]@l$	mismatch
	$\mid [<expr>]@l_1 + [\,<expr>]@l_2$	choice ($l_1 \neq l_2$)
	$\mid [<expr>]@l_1 \parallel [<expr>]@l_2$	parallel($l_1 \neq l_2$)
	$\mid [*<expr>]@l$	replication
$<prefix>$ ::=	$c!y$	output
	$\mid c?(x)$	input
	$\mid \tau$	silent

Our objective is to "linearize" the language and its semantics using *locations*. These are simple positional informations inserted into terms. The updated syntax is presented in Table 2. In this variant, a process P must be written $[P]@l$ which means intuitively that P "resides at" location l. Two processes P and Q, if composed in parallel, must reside at locations that are *different*. For instance, we write:

$$[P]@l_1 \parallel [Q]@l_2 \text{ with } l_1 \neq l_2$$

The only operation available on locations is to test their (in)equality, $l_1 = l_2$ or $l_1 \neq l_2$. It is important to note that locations are here abstract entities that do not only help at separating concurrent processes. In fact, locations must also be used to disambiguate choice alternatives. Suppose we decorate the branching trees with locations, as depicted on figure 2. In the localized syntax, the two processes may be written as follows:

$$[a!e.[c!f]@l_3]@l_1 + [b!e.[d!g]@l_4]@l_2 \text{ and } [a!e.[c!f]@l_3]@l_1 + [a!e.[d!g]@l_4]@l_2$$

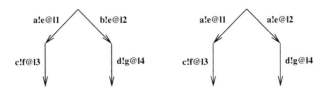

Figure 2: Linearized tree structures with locations

On the right-side of figure 2 we can see that locations solve the branching-time vs. linear-time issue. Now the choice of which among the "left" or "right" $a!e$ should occur is captured by the two distinct traces $a!e@l_1$ and $a!e@l_2$.

3.2   LTS-based Operational Semantics

We propose in this section the operational semantics of our channel-passing language using labeled transition systems. The presentation is brief since it is not the purpose of this paper to discuss precisely the LTS-based semantics, which are fully exposed in various documents (*e.g.* [8]). It is common to develop two levels in the semantics: *(i)* a *structural congruence* noted $\equiv$ (for now also noted $\equiv_{(2)}$) which equates "trivially" equivalent processes, and *(ii)* a set of *inference rules*, presented in the structural operational semantics style, from which the behavior of a process expression can be derived. We suppose the existence of two functions over processes $fn([P]@l)$ and $bn([P]@l)$ respectively denoting the *free names* and *bound names* of P. Names can be bound in either input prefix or restriction scopes. Note that locations are not considered as names and are thus "invisible" for these functions.

The structural congruence is defined by the axioms of Table 3. First, by rule (1), terms are alpha-convertible as in the lambda-calculus. Rules (2), (3) and (4) allow to simplify expressions by removing unnecessary locations. Parallel and choice operators expose common abelian monoid laws (commutativity, associativity and unit), as expressed by rules (5) to (10). Rules (11) and (12) are elimination rules for the match and mismatch operators. Rule (13) gives the semantics for replicated processes. Note that a fresh location must be introduced here. The most interesting rules are the last ones: they "implement" the combination of channel passing and restriction. For example, rule (14) states that a restricted name (a name in the scope of a ν) can see its scope *extruded* (if we read the equivalence from right-to-left) or conversely *intruded* within parallel constructs if there is no name conflict. More precisely, if read right-to-left, the rule states that a name x with restricted scope $[Q]@l_2$ can see its scope extruded to $[P]@l_1 \parallel [Q]@l_2$ if x is not a free name of P. The remaining rules (15) to (18) describe similar interactions with restricted names.

In the operational semantics defined in Table 4, the $(Struct)$ rule establishes the connection with the structural congruence. The (In), (Out) and (Tau) rules relate the prefixes of the languages to labels in the transition systems. The possible labels (or actions) are $a?u@l$ (input), $a!x@l$ (output), $a!\nu x@l$ (*bound output*) and $\tau@L$ (silent step, with possible multiple locations). Note that the labels are also localized, as suggested previously. We use the *early*

Table 3: Definition of structural congruence

(1) $[P]@l \equiv_{(2)} [Q]@l$ if P and Q are variants of alpha-conversion

(2) $[[P]@l_2]@l_1 \equiv_{(2)} [P]@l_2$
(3) $[[P]@l_2 \parallel [Q]@l_3]@l_1 \equiv_{(2)} [P]@l_2 \parallel [Q]@l_3$
(4) $[[P]@l_2 + [Q]@l_3]@l_1 \equiv_{(2)} [P]@l_2 + [Q]@l_3$

(5) $[P]@l_1 \parallel [Q]@l_2 \equiv_{(2)} [Q]@l_2 \parallel [P]@l_1$
(6) $([P]@l_1 \parallel [Q]@l_2) \parallel [R]@l_3 \equiv_{(2)} [P]@l_1 \parallel ([Q]@l_2 \parallel [R]@l_3)$
(7) $[P]@l_1 \parallel [0]@l_2 \equiv_{(2)} [P]@l_1$
(8) $[P]@l_1 + [Q]@l_2 \equiv_{(2)} [Q]@l_2 + [P]@l_1$
(9) $([P]@l_1 + [Q]@l_2) + [R]@l_3 \equiv_{(2)} [P]@l_1 + ([Q]@l_2 + [R]@l_3)$
(10) $[P]@l_1 + [0]@l_2 \equiv_{(2)} [P]@l_1$

(11) $[x = y][P]@l \equiv [P]@l$ if $x = y$, $[0]@l$ either
(12) $[x \neq y][P]@l \equiv [P]@l$ if $x \neq y$, $[0]@l$ either

(13) $[*P]@l_1 \equiv_{(2)} [*P]@l_1 \parallel [P]@l_2$ with $l_1 \neq l_2$

(14) $\nu(x)([P]@l_1 \parallel [Q]@l_2) \equiv [P]@l_1 \parallel \nu(x)[Q]@l_2$ if $x \notin fn(P)$
(15) $\nu(x)([P]@l_1 + [Q]@l_2) \equiv [P]@l_1 + \nu(x)[Q]@l_2$ if $x \notin fn(P)$
(16) $\nu(x)[u = v][P]@l \equiv [u = v]\nu(x)[P]@l$ if $x \neq u$ and $x \neq v$
(17) $\nu(x)[u \neq v][P]@l \equiv [u \neq v]\nu(x)[P]@l$ if $x \neq u$ and $x \neq v$
(18) $\nu(x)\nu(y)[P]@l \equiv \nu(y)\nu(x)[P]@l$

Table 4: Definition of transition rules

$$\frac{[P]@l \equiv [P']@l \quad [P]@l \xrightarrow{\alpha} [Q]@l' \quad [Q]@l' \equiv [Q']@l'}{[P']@l \xrightarrow{\alpha} [Q']@l'} \ (Struct)$$

$$\frac{[P]@l_1 \xrightarrow{\alpha} [P']@l_1'}{[P]@l_1 + [Q]@l_2 \xrightarrow{\alpha} [P']@l_1'} \ (Sum)$$

$$\frac{[P]@l_1 \xrightarrow{\alpha} [P']@l_1' \quad bn(\alpha) \cap fn(Q) = \emptyset}{[P]@l_1 \parallel [Q]@l_2 \xrightarrow{\alpha} [P']@l_1' \parallel [Q]@l_2} \ (Par)$$

$$\frac{}{[c!y.P]@l \xrightarrow{c!y@l} [P]@l} \ (Out) \quad \frac{}{[c?(x).P]@l \xrightarrow{c?u@l} [P]@l\{u/x\}} \ (In) \quad \frac{}{[\tau.P]@l \xrightarrow{\tau@l} [P]@l} \ (Tau)$$

$$\frac{[P]@l_1 \xrightarrow{a?u@l_1} [P']@l_1 \quad [Q]@l_2 \xrightarrow{a!u@l_2} [Q']@l_2}{[P]@l_1 \parallel [Q]@l_2 \xrightarrow{\tau@\{l_1,l_2\}} [P']@l_1 \parallel [Q']@l_2} \ (Com)$$

$$\frac{[P]@l_1 \xrightarrow{\alpha} [P']@l_1' \quad x \notin \alpha}{\nu(x)[P]@l \xrightarrow{\alpha} \nu(x)[P']@l_1'} \ (Res) \quad \frac{[P]@l_1 \xrightarrow{a!x@l_1} [P']@l_1 \quad a \neq x}{\nu(x)[P]@l \xrightarrow{a!\nu x@l_1} [P']@l_1} \ (Open)$$

semantics that perform substitutions directly through instantiations of the (In) inference rule. This rule relates a single input prefix $a?(x)$ to an infinite number of transitions/labels $a?u$ for every possible name u that can be received. The *late semantics* delay substitutions in instantiations of rule (Com). But in the early case, it only matches pairs of input and output actions to infer silent steps. The (Res) rule explains that restriction is preserved by transitions that do not refer to the restricted name. Finally, the $(Open)$ rule implements the communication of a restricted channel as a bound output action.

3.3 Behavioral Equivalences

The labeled transition systems defined previously denote a "natural" bisimulation equivalence that can be stated as follows:

Definition 1 *The (**strong early**) **bisimulation equivalence** of two processes $[P]@l$ and $[Q]@l$ is noted $[P]@l \sim [Q]@l$. This is the largest symmetric relation such that:*

$$\text{if } [P]@l \xrightarrow{\alpha} [P']@l', \text{ then } \exists Q' \text{ such as } [Q]@l \xrightarrow{\alpha} [Q']@l' \text{ and } [P']@l' \sim [Q']@l'$$

Intuitively, this relation equates the tree-like structure of process behaviors by ensuring that both equivalent terms covers the same possible transition paths. In comparison with more "traditional" definitions for *early bisimulation* (cf. [8]), our variant only differs by the introduction of locations. Only co-located process may be equated here.

As illustrated in [2] and many other works, such equivalence relations can be used in various ways to derive semantic laws about the language. However, the CSP community developed an arguably simpler equivalence in which processes are considered as equivalent if they expose the same traces, which is a natural equality on sets of sequences. Thanks to locations, we can reformulate the equivalence for the language proposed in section 2 in similar terms. We first need to define the notion of *trace*:

Definition 2 *The (LTS-based) **trace** of a process $[P]@l$, noted $tr([P]@l)$, is obtained inductively by the following rules:*

(i) $tr([0]@l) = \{\langle\rangle\}$
(ii) if $[P]@l \xrightarrow{\alpha} [P']@l'$ then $\langle\alpha\rangle.tr([P']@l') \subseteq tr([P]@l)$

*We also define the **trace prefixing** (. operator) on traces with the following rules:*

(i) $\langle\alpha\rangle.\{\langle\rangle\} = \langle\rangle.\{\langle\alpha\rangle\} = \{\langle\alpha\rangle\}$
(ii) $\langle\alpha\rangle.\{\langle\beta\rangle\} = \langle\alpha, \beta\rangle$
(iii) $\langle\alpha\rangle.A \cup B = \langle\alpha\rangle.A \cup \langle\alpha\rangle.B$

As discussed previously, the main issue with such connection between labeled transitions and traces is that one may not distinguish traces corresponding to different transitions sharing the same label. However, thanks to locations, we have the following important lemma:

Lemma 1 *(**Linear time**)*
if $[P]@l \xrightarrow{\alpha} [P']@l'$ and $[P]@l \xrightarrow{\beta} [P'']@l''$ with $[P']@l' \not\sim [P'']@l''$ then $\alpha \neq \beta$

The proof sketch for this lemma is as follows. First, only the choice and parallel operator can lead to multiple transitions for similar actions. This non-determinism stems from the interaction of the commutativity axiom for $+$ and $\|$, reflected in the semantics by the $(Struct)$ rule of Table 4, with the (Par), (Com) and (Sum) rules. We have to consider the cases of expression P corresponding to either $[Q]@l_1 \| [R]@l_2$ or $[S]@l_3 + [T]@l_4$. By definition of the localized syntax, we have $l_1 \neq l_2$ and $l_3 \neq l_4$. And from distinct locations we may only form distinct labels (*e.g.* $a?u@l_1 \neq a?u@l_2$) so that $\alpha \neq \beta$ □

We may now deduce an important reformulation for the equivalence of processes, under the form of the following theorem:

Theorem 1 *(Trace and bisimulation equivalences coincide)*
$[P]@l \sim [Q]@l \iff tr([P]@l) = tr([Q]@l)$

This theorem is a trivial consequence of lemma 1 on definitions 1 and 2   □

Note that this result does not translate to late semantics because of the more complex bisimulation equivalence they denote. However, we can formulate similar results on *observational* variants of the semantics, which consist in disabling the silent steps (the τ actions) when comparing processes. Given our two formulations for process equivalence, we have two ways to define such observational variant. In the Pi-calculus, *weak transitions* are introduced; they are noted $[P]@l \xRightarrow{\alpha} [P']@l'$. These transitions are transitive closures on τ steps around non-silent actions, which may be noted $[P]@l(\xrightarrow{\tau@L})^*[P_1]@l_1 \xrightarrow{\alpha} [P_2]@l_2(\xrightarrow{\tau@L'})^*[P']@l'$. From these weak semantics we can define a *weak (early) bisimulation equivalence*. But we can also propose an observational variant directly based on the trace-equivalence of theorem 1. We define a function otr of *observational traces* over processes as:

$$otr([P]@l) = \{S \in tr([P]@l) \mid \forall L, \tau@L \notin S\}$$

This is the set of traces $tr([P]@l)$ in which we filter out all silent steps. We could also provide a model closer to the CSP trace model by making otr closed over prefixes, which we note otr^* and define as follows:

$$\forall S.T \subseteq otr([P]@l),\ S \subseteq otr^*([P]@l)$$

We may finally introduce a *refinement operator* on processes, noted $\sqsubseteq$, as follows:

$$[P']@l \sqsubseteq [P]@l \iff otr^*([P']@l) \subseteq otr^*([P]@l)$$

Refinement techniques are largely exploited in trace-based semantics such as CSP. It is a very practical tool to reason in a top-down manner from specifications to actual implementations. Refinement is harder to define in terms of labeled transition systems [9]. This illustrates the advantage of the proposed model in which both semantics coincide.

4   Congruent Channel-passing

The equivalences defined in the previous sections raise important issues we propose to address now. First, there is some inconvenience in the fact that we defined trace equivalence upon LTS for process expressions. One has to build the transition system before being able to apply the trace model. Also, the equivalence relations of section 3 only coincide in early semantics, in which input prefixes denote impractical infinite branching. We would like to obtain similar results with late semantics. But more importantly, both the equivalences are *not preserved by input prefixes*. Consider the following example:

$$[d!e]@l_1 \parallel [c?(x)]@l_2 \sim [d!e.[c?(x)]@l_2]@l_1 + [c?(x).[d!e]@l_1]@l_2 \quad (1)$$

This corresponds to the *interleaving semantics* as implemented by the semantics proposed in the previous section. This equivalence is true for bisimulation equivalence (see [8]) and also for trace-equivalence since both match. However, we can also prove that:

$$[b?(d).([d!e]@l_1 \parallel [c?(x)]@l_2)]@l \not\sim [b?(d).([d!e.[c?(x)]@l_2]@l_1 + [c?(x).[d!e]@l_1]@l_2)]@l$$

Table 5: The revised syntax

\<expr\> ::=	$[0]@l$	inert
	$\mid [(\text{\textit{\<expr\>}})]@l$	precedence
	$\mid [\text{\textit{\<prefix\>}}.\text{\textit{\<expr\>}}]@l$	sequence
	$\mid [\text{\textit{\<expr\>}}]@l_1 + [\text{\textit{\<expr\>}}]@l_2$	choice ($l_1 \neq l_2$)
	$\mid [\text{\textit{\<expr\>}}]@l_1 \parallel [\text{\textit{\<expr\>}}]@l_2$	parallel ($l_1 \neq l_2$)
	$\mid [*\text{\textit{\<expr\>}}]@l$	replication

\<prefix\> ::=	$c!y$	output
	$\mid c?(x)$	input
	$\mid \tau$	silent
	$\mid \nu(c)$	restriction
	$\mid [x = y]$	match
	$\mid [x \neq y]$	mismatch

Here, the name d is bound through the input prefix $b?(d)$ and the equivalence is infirmed for the substitution $\{c/d\}$ (remember that input prefixes denote all the possible substitutions for d in early semantics). This tells that the equivalence relation is not a congruence on process expression. The proposed language is thus not truly compositional, at least with the proposed equivalences.

4.1   A Syntax with Substitutables and Fresh Occurrences

Let us consider again the issue raised by example (1) in the previous section. The problem is that we do not know in advance if the name d is susceptible to be captured by a binder (either an input prefix or a restriction) in some context. In the variant of the semantics we define in this section, if we write $d?(x)$ or $d!y$, then both the names d and y are *not substitutable* at all. In that case, the equivalence becomes trivially a congruence but by the same occasion, we lose the ability to communicate or restrict names and channels ! To circumvent this limitation, we modify the language syntax in two ways, as described on Table 5.

First, we remove the syntax rules for restriction and match/mismatch (in Table 2) and introduce dedicated prefixes. We do this because we need specific rules for these constructs. The second modification involves two new kinds of names that are defined as follows:

Definition 3 *The **substitutable** of a name x, noted λx, is a name that can be bound by either an input prefix $d?(x)$ (for any channel d) or a restriction $\nu(x)$. A **fresh occurrence** of x, noted νx (or νy provided that νy is fresh), is a name used for substitution of λx in a restriction scope $\nu(x)$. Moreover, νx must be a fresh name, different from any other name.*

In the new syntax, the prefix $d!x$ expresses an output on a channel d that cannot be received or restricted (*i.e.* it cannot be bound) in any context. More precisely, if the term appears in a context where the name d is bound, then d remains a free occurrence. On the other hand, in the prefix $\lambda d!x$, if d is bound (*e.g.* in either $c?(d).\lambda d!x$ or $\nu(d).\lambda d!x$), then λd may be accordingly substituted in the sub-term.

The *freshness property* of a fresh occurrence νx states in particular that distinct restrictions must result in substitutions by distinct *and unique* names. For example, two restrictions on the same name x, both noted $\nu(x)$, will lead to substitutions by different names, such as νx_1 and νx_2 with $\nu x_1 \neq \nu x_2$. A sufficient condition is to consider fresh occurrences as globally unique names (which is a reasonable assumption in practice).

Table 6: The trace semantics of the Pi-calculus with substitutables and fresh names

(1) $tr([P]@l) = tr([Q]@l)$ if $[P]@l \equiv_{(2)} [Q]@l$

(2) $tr([0]@l) = \langle\rangle$
(3) $tr([\tau.P]@l) = \langle\tau@l\rangle.tr([P]@l)$
(4) $tr([\xi?(x).P]@l) = \langle\xi?(x)@l\rangle.tr([P]@l)$
(5) $tr([\xi!\gamma.P]@l) = \langle\xi!\gamma@l\rangle.tr([P]@l)$
(6) $tr([\nu(x).P]@l) = tr([P]@l)\{\nu x/\lambda x\}$ with νx fresh
(7) $tr([[\xi = \gamma].P]@l) = tr([P]@l)$ if $\xi = \gamma$, $\langle\rangle$ either
(8) $tr([[\xi \neq \gamma].P]@l) = tr([P]@l)$ if $\xi \neq \gamma$, $\langle\rangle$ either

(9) $tr([P]@l_1 + [Q]@l_2) = tr([P]@l_1) \cup tr([Q]@l_2)$
(10) $tr([P]@l_1 \parallel [Q]@l_2) = tr([P]@l_1) \otimes tr([Q]@l_2)$

4.2   Revised Operational Semantics

We may now define the operational semantics for the extension of the language proposed in the previous section. We define these semantics *directly* in term of traces, through the function tr over processes as defined inductively on Table 6.

The first rule (1) relates the trace function tr to a structural congruence noted $\equiv_{(2)}$. This is the equivalence $\equiv$ (cf. Table 3) in which we remove all rules related to the "old" restriction and match/mismatch constructs (*i.e.* we remove the rules (11),(12), and (14) to (18) in Table 3). The rules (2) to (8) give the semantics of the language prefixes. The occurrences ξ and γ of names in these rules can represent either regular names x, substitutables λx, or fresh occurrences νx. This is to reduce the number of cases where the difference among name categories does not intervene. Of particular interest are rules (4) and (6) respectively for input prefix and restriction. In contrast to the LTS trace semantics given previously, the traces for input prefixes does not account for all (infinite) possible substitutions. The rule for restriction $\nu(x)$ involves the substitution of λx by a fresh occurrence νx. The substitution over process expressions trivially extends to traces, we thus have for any substitution σ, $(tr([P]@l))\sigma = tr(([P]@l)\sigma)$. We finally propose a rule for the choice operator, which is the union of traces for both the branches, and a rule for parallel which is obtained through *trace product and interleaving* defined as follows:

Definition 4 *The **trace product** of two process traces T_1 and T_2 is noted $T_1 \otimes T_2$. It produces the **trace interleaving**, noted $T_1 \oplus T_2$, in which communication steps are correctly substituted. It is defined inductively as follows:*
$T_1 \otimes \{\langle\rangle\} = T_1$ *and* $\{\langle\rangle\} \otimes T_2 = T_2$ *and* $\{\langle\rangle\} \otimes \{\langle\rangle\} = \{\langle\rangle\}$ *or*
$T = T_1 \otimes T_2$ *with* $\forall\langle\alpha\rangle.T_1' \subseteq T_1$ *and* $\forall\langle\beta\rangle.T_2' \subseteq T_2$ *then*
  (i) if $\alpha = c!\gamma@l_1$ *or* $\alpha = \lambda d!\gamma@l_1$ *and* $\beta = c?(x)@l_2$ *or* $\beta = \lambda e?(x)@l_2$
      then $\langle\tau@\{l_1,l_2\}\rangle. (T_1' \otimes T_2'\{\gamma/\lambda x\}) \cup (T_1 \oplus T_2) \subseteq T$
  (ii) if $\alpha = \nu c!\gamma@l_1$ *and* $\beta = \nu c?(x)@l_2$
      then $\langle\tau@\{l_1,l_2\}\rangle. (T_1' \otimes T_2'\{\gamma/\lambda x\}) \subseteq T$
  (iii) or $T_1 \oplus T_2 = \langle\alpha\rangle. (T_1' \otimes T_2) \cup \langle\beta\rangle. (T_1 \otimes T_2') \subseteq T$

The definition above is relatively complex since it mixes trace interleaving (case *(iii)*) and communications with substitution. Let us illustrate these semantics on some basic examples, starting with the canonical communication system written as follows:

$$[c!e]@l_1 \parallel [c?(x).P(\lambda x)]@l_2$$

Note that we now use a substitutable λx to denote the possible substitution of the bound name x. In contrast to the language and semantics of section 2, the plain name x cannot be substituted anymore. The semantics of the previous example are traces defined as follows:

$$\mathcal{T} = tr([c!e]@l_1 \parallel [c?(x).P(\lambda x)]@l_2) = tr([c!e]@l_1) \otimes tr([c?(x).P(\lambda x)]@l_2)$$

From the rules of Table 6 we have:

$$\left[\begin{array}{l} tr([c!e]@l_1) = \langle c!e@l_1 \rangle \\ tr([c?(x).P(\lambda x)]@l_2) = \langle c?(x)@l_2 \rangle.tr([P(\lambda x)]@l_2) \end{array} \right.$$

These traces can only be matched by case *(i)* in the definition of $\otimes$, from which we infer:

$$\mathcal{T} = \langle \tau@\{l_1,l_2\} \rangle.(\{\langle\rangle\} \otimes tr([P(\lambda x)]@l_2)\{e/\lambda x\})$$
$$\cup \{\langle c!e@l_1 \rangle\} \oplus (\langle c?(x)@l_2 \rangle.tr([P(\lambda x)]@l_2))$$

This may be simplified by applying the interleaving operator $\oplus$ as follows:

$$\mathcal{T} = \langle \tau@\{l_1,l_2\} \rangle.(\{\langle\rangle\} \otimes tr([P(\lambda x)]@l_2)\{e/\lambda x\})$$
$$\cup \langle c!e@l_1, c?(x)@l_2 \rangle.tr([P(\lambda x)]@l_2) \cup \langle c?(x)@l_2, c!e@l_1 \rangle.tr([P(\lambda x)]@l_2)$$

Finally, we end up with the following semantics:

$$\mathcal{T} = \langle \tau@\{l_1,l_2\} \rangle.tr([P(e)]@l_2)$$
$$\cup \langle c!e@l_1, c?(x)@l_2 \rangle.tr([P(\lambda x)]@l_2)$$
$$\cup \langle c?(x)@l_2, c!e@l_1 \rangle.tr([P(\lambda x)]@l_2)$$

Intuitively, the meaning of the program is that either the communication depicted occurs or we take into account the fact that someone else could resolve the communication on channel c through composition. Consider now the variant with a restriction on c as follows:

$$[\nu(c).\,([\lambda c!e]@l_1 \parallel [\lambda c?(x).(\lambda x)]@l_2)]@l$$

We use the substitutable λc because c itself cannot be restricted since it cannot be substituted. From rule (6) of Table 6, we derive the trace semantics $\mathcal{T}$ of this example as follows:

$$\mathcal{T} = tr([\lambda c!e]@l_1 \parallel [\lambda c?(x).P(\lambda x)]@l_2)\{\nu c/\lambda c\} \text{ with } \nu c \text{ fresh}$$
$$= tr([\nu c!e]@l_1 \parallel [\nu c?(x).P(\lambda x)]@l_2)$$

We are now in the case *(ii)* of the definition for the trace product, from which we obtain:

$$\mathcal{T} = \langle \tau@\{l_1,l_2\} \rangle.(\{\langle\rangle\} \otimes tr([P(\lambda x)]@l_2)\{e/\lambda x\})$$

And finally: $\mathcal{T} = \langle \tau@\{l_1,l_2\} \rangle.tr([P(e)]@l_2)$

We finally illustrate channel passing using the following example:

$$[c!e]@l_1 \parallel [c?(x).\lambda x!f]@l_2 \parallel [e?(y).P(\lambda y)]@l_3$$

The associativity of $\parallel$ allows us to treat the left or right composition in any order. Moreover, there are many possible executions in which the two communications we are interested in do not occur. We will thus only give the sub-traces $\mathcal{T}'$ of this expression in which the communication occur. For the left-side process which is an instance of the first example with $P = \lambda x!f$, we are left with the sequence : $\langle \tau@\{l_1,l_2\}, e!f@l_2 \rangle$. We see here that the passed name e is used as a channel in a subsequent trace. When combined with the traces of the right-side process, we can deduce the trace $\langle \tau@\{l_1,l_2\}, \tau@\{l_2,l_3\} \rangle.tr([P(f)]@l_3)$.

4.3   Revised Trace-equivalence

As illustrated in the previous section, the proposed language, if not equivalent, retains the major features of the Pi-calculus such as channel-passing. Moreover, we integrate locations and as such preserve the results of section 3. Thereupon, we can deduce from the previous semantics, directly expressed as traces, a precise *trace equivalence* as follows:

Definition 5 *The **trace equivalence** of two processes $[P]@l$ and $[Q]@l$, which is noted $[P]@l \sim [Q]@l$, is defined as the equality of the implied traces:*
$[P]@l \sim [Q]@l \iff tr([P]@l) = tr([Q]@l)$

In comparison to the equivalence proposed in section 3, this revised version is based on late semantics. Moreover, we can state a very important lemma about the revised equivalence:

Lemma 2 *($\sim$ is preserved by input prefixes)*
if $[P]@l \sim [Q]@l$ then $\forall \xi, \forall \gamma,\ \xi?(\gamma).[P]@l \sim \xi?(\gamma).[Q]@l$

We have $[P]@l \sim [Q]@l \iff tr([P]@l) = tr([Q]@l)$ by definition of trace equivalence. From the semantics for input prefixes, as defined by rule (4) in Table 6, we also have $tr(\xi?(\gamma).[P]@l) = \langle \xi?(\gamma)@l \rangle.tr([P]@l)$, which trivially equates $\langle \xi?(\gamma)@l \rangle.tr([Q]@l)$ $\square$

Now we can move on to the generalization of the congruence property of the proposed trace equivalence. We first need to establish the following lemma:

Lemma 3 *($\otimes$ left-preserves equality)*
Let T_1, T_2 and T_3 be traces, we then have $T_1 = T_2 \implies T_1 \otimes T_3 = T_2 \otimes T_3$.

The proof sketch for this lemma is by structural induction on traces, following the scheme for the definition of $\otimes$ (cf. definition 4). For the base case, in which $T_1 = T_2 = \langle \rangle$, the lemma is trivially verified since we have by definition $\langle \rangle \otimes T_3 = T_3$. Now we are left with the three inductive cases *(i)*, *(ii)* and *(iii)* of definition 4. In each case, we only have to look at the left trace since we only prove the preservation of equality on the left side of the $\otimes$ operator (the right-side case is handled through commutativity of $\|$). In the inductive cases, we define $T_i = \bigcup_{\alpha, T_i'} \langle \alpha \rangle.T_i'$ ($i \in \{1, 2, 3\}$). By the hypothesis of induction, we have $\forall \mathcal{U},\ T_1' \otimes \mathcal{U} = T_2' \otimes \mathcal{U}$. So, in particular, $\forall \gamma, \lambda x,\ T_1' \otimes T_3'\{\gamma/\lambda x\} = T_2' \otimes T_3'\{\gamma/\lambda x\}$. Finally, equality on sets is trivially preserved by both the union and prefixing relations (and also by $\oplus$ which is a composition of union and prefixing) so that we have $\langle \tau@\{l_1, l_2\} \rangle.((T_1' \otimes T_3'\{\gamma/\lambda x\}) \cup (T_1 \oplus T_3)) = \langle \tau@\{l_1, l_2\} \rangle.((T_2' \otimes T_3'\{\gamma/\lambda x\}) \cup (T_2 \oplus T_3))$. This covers the three inductive cases and thus concludes the proof $\square$

Theorem 2 *($\sim$ is a congruence on processes)*
For all terms $\mathcal{E}$ in which $[P]@l$ appears, if $[P]@l \sim [Q]@l$, then $\mathcal{E} \sim \mathcal{E}\{[P]@l/[Q]@l\}$

The proof for this theorem is by structural induction on the language constructors. First, structural congruence is a congruence by definition. Moreover, we can generalize lemma 2 for input, output and silent prefixes. For such a prefix α and a process P, we have the same basic fact that $tr([\alpha.P]@l) = \langle \alpha@l \rangle.tr([P]@l)$. Match and mismatch may reduce to the empty trace, but this does not impact the congruence property. The restriction semantics also involve substitutions by fresh (and free) names. Let σ and σ' be two substitutions on the same domain. Through alpha-conversion, we have $tr([P]@l) = tr([Q]@l) \implies tr([P]@l)\sigma = tr([Q]@l)\sigma'$ which is enough to cover the congruence property of the restriction prefixes.

Now consider the case of the choice operator. Suppose two processes P and P' such as $[P]@l_1 \sim [P']@l_1$, which means $tr([P]@l_1) = tr([P']@l_1)$. The semantics of $[P]@l_1 + [Q]@l_2$ are $tr([P]@l_1 + [Q]@l_2) = tr([P]@l_1) \cup tr([Q]@l_2)$. From simple properties of set union, we have $tr([P]@l_1) \cup tr([Q]@l_2) = tr([P']@l_1) \cup tr([Q]@l_2)$ since $tr([P]@l_1) = tr([P']@l_1)$. So we have $[P]@l_1 + [Q]@l_2 \sim [P']@l_1 + [Q]@l_2$. We can follow a similar scheme to prove the congruence property for the parallel operator. But for this we have to prove that if $tr([P]@l_1) = tr([P'@l_1])$ then $tr([P]@l_1) \otimes tr([Q]@l_2) = tr([P']@l_1) \otimes tr([Q]@l_2)$. This is true by lemma 3. □

The simple but fundamental corollary of theorem 2 is that unlike most Pi-calculus variants, the language we propose in this paper is truly *compositional*. This removes the burden of reasoning based on contextual informations, unavoidable in most behavioral equivalences on Pi-calculus processes [8].

5 Related Work

To our knowledge, there exist few works that aim at bringing CSP and the Pi-calculus closer at the formal level. Yet, many CSP-based programming languages and implementations such as Kroc/Linux [4], Icarus [5] or JCSP Network Edition [6] introduce channel-passing extensions. These works do not discuss, though, the influence of the new constructs on the formal semantics of the language. We hope that our propositions could be used as foundations for such mobile variants.

Testing theories can be used to compare trace-based and bisimulation-based equivalences for both static and channel-passing calculi. It is usual to associate bisimulation and trace models with respectively *may* and *must testing equivalences* [10]. In this work, we show that for a particular language, a variant of the pi-calculus with explicit locations and early semantics, both definitions coincide. There also exist transition-based models for CSP, for example in [11]. But channel passing is not discussed.

Various process algebras and programming language semantics have been recast and compared in the *unifying theories of programming* by Hoare and Jifeng [12]. Given a single denotational tool, namely relations and associated operators, most programming language concepts can be expressed and compared in this unifying framework. In contrast, our work focuses on operational semantics and discusses slight extensions making the departing worlds of bisimulation and trace equivalence coincide. Interestingly enough, trace equivalence on its own seems sufficient to characterize the category of language proposed in the paper. In the light of Hoare and Jifeng's unification work, it is probable that more profound coincidences exist. The fact that channel-passing may be expressed in more denotational terms, however, remains an open (and intriguing) question.

In this paper, we define a trace model that is an extension of a subset of the traditional CSP semantics (as defined in [1]) without prefix closure. Moreover, we integrate the silent steps to model the generalized choice operator of the Pi-calculus. In order to adapt the very practical refinement techniques of CSP, we must exhibit the prefix closure of the traces in which silent steps are filtered out. It is thankfully very easy to derive such semantics, noted otr^* in the paper. Stable failures and divergences are important tools we have not yet taken into account in the proposed model. The reason is that we capture the branching-time semantics and thus provide a precise equivalence we would like to investigate furthermore.

Explicit locations are introduced for a variant of the CCS language in [13] to discuss fairness models. Locations in this work are much more precise than ours. An order relation is introduced whereas we only rely on (in)equality. We may also remark that in both approaches, the frontier between safety and liveness properties is not as strongly delimited as usual. Moreover, the expressive power of localized variants does not seem to suffer much from the addition of locations. While this is not needed for the results presented, we may relax the semantics by proposing a weakest form of equivalence in which processes need not to be co-located in order to be compared. An interesting weaker variant is to only maintain (in)equality of locations among traces. For example the trace $\{\langle \alpha @ l_1, \beta @ l_2 \rangle\}$ with $l_1 \neq l_2$ would be equivalent to $\{\langle \alpha @ l_3, \beta @ l_4 \rangle\}$ *iff* $l_3 \neq l_4$.

There are many discussions on the basic syntax for Pi-calculus terms, and there exist in fact many variants of the language. In this paper, most of the language constructors are prefixes. In [8], the fact that most constructs of the Pi-calculus can be expressed in purely operational ways is discussed. For example, the restriction operator can be seen as an action through dedicated open and close rules. But it is then difficult to produce normal forms of terms, which is an important step for most proofs on congruence properties. It is notable that normalization is less prominent when the semantics are expressed in terms of traces. In fact, we do not rely on any normal form in our proposition.

From all characterizations of Pi-calculus semantics, our proposition is probably closest to the *open bisimulation* by Sangiorgi [14]. This is to our knowledge the only fully compositional characterization of the Pi-calculus semantics. To achieve this, open bisimulation integrates the quantification over all substitutions in its definition. In our proposition, the quantification occurs directly in the semantics, because substitutable channels can always be used for communication. This leads to an arguably simpler characterization of behavioral equivalence. Moreover, the mismatch operator remains available whereas no simple definition of open bisimulation with mismatch is known [8].

6   Conclusion

In this paper, we tried to illustrate that there were not always such *well delimited* frontiers between process algebras that are often considered as intrinsically dissimilar, for example CSP on one side and the Pi-calculus on the other side. As a matter of fact, we think that the activity of bringing things closer, by opposition of exhibiting differences, should be also of primary importance.

The difference between linear-time/branching-time semantics, the may/must testing dichotomy, or even the lack of precision of trace equivalence if compared to bisimulation, all these disappear with the surprisingly simple adjunction of *locations*. This does not seem to involve unbearable loss in terms of expressive power; though this issue should be further investigated.

Likewise, the often accepted idea that a channel passing language retaining all the features of the Pi-calculus may not be fully compositional seems, at least, unsatisfactory. Our proposition, once again, only involves a thin extension, namely the *substitutable* names, in order to obtain the most expected congruence property. Additionally, locations and substitutables may be treated separately. A motivating future work would be to define a congruent form of Pi-calculus, characterized through labeled transition systems and bisimulation exclusively.

Our main motivation, however, is to bring closer the CSP semantics and the Pi-calculus language. And there is a lot more to investigate in that direction. First, we should provide higher-level abstractions, most notably a richer set of datatypes. Distribution and explicit manipulation of locations ought to be explored as well. Termination of process is also somewhat neglected by Pi-calculus experts. On the semantic side, further experiments with the CSP-like refinement model are needed. For now, the translation to the proposed channel-passing calculus has been but roughly sketched. Later on, we wish that the proposed model could be used as foundations for practical languages and tools for the development of mobile systems with an emphasis on safety and assisted verification.

References

[1] C. A. R. Hoare. *Communicating Sequential Processes*. Prentice Hall, 1985.

[2] Robin Milner. *Communicating and Mobile Systems: The π-Calculus*. Cambridge University Press, 1999.

[3] Wan Fokkink. *Introduction to Process Algebra*. EATCS. Springer, 2000.

[4] F.R.M.Barnes and P.H.Welch. Prioritised Dynamic Communicating and Mobile Processes. *IEE Proceedings-Software*, 150(2):121–136, April 2003.

[5] David May and Henk Muller. Copying, moving and borrowing semantics. In *Communicating Process Architectures (CPA'2001)*. IOS Press, 2001.

[6] Quickstone Technologies. JCSP Network Edition. `http://www.quickstone.com/xcsp/jcspnetworkedition`.

[7] J.A. Bergstra and J.W. Klop. Process algebra for synchronous communication. *Information and Control*, 60(1/3):109–137, 1984.

[8] Joachim Parrow. *Handbook of Process Algebra*, chapter An Introduction to the Pi-calculus, pages 479–543. Elsevier, 2001.

[9] C. J. Frige and J. J. Zic. A notion of (weak) refinement for CCS. In *Fourth Australasian Refinement Workshop (ARW'95)*, April 1995.

[10] Michele Boreale and Rocco De Nicola. Testing equivalence for mobile processes. *Inf. Comput.*, 120(2):279–303, 1995.

[11] A. W. Roscoe. *The Theory and Practice of Concurrency*. Prentice Hall, 1997.

[12] C. A. R. Hoare and He Jifeng. *Unification Theories of Programming*. Prentice Hall, 1998.

[13] Gerardo Costa and Colin Stirling. Weak and strong fairness in CCS. *Inf. Comput.*, 73(3):207–244, 1987.

[14] D. Sangiorgi. A theory of bisimulation for the π-calculus. *Acta Informatica*, 33:69–97, 1996.

Communicating Process Architectures 2004
Ian East, Jeremy Martin, Peter Welch, David Duce, and Mark Green (Eds.)
IOS Press, 2004

Prioritised Service Architecture

Ian EAST

Dept. for Computing, Oxford Brookes University, Oxford OX33 1HX, England.
ireast@brookes.ac.uk

Abstract. Previously, Martin [1] gave formal conditions under which a simple design
rule guarantees deadlock-freedom in a system with service (client-server) architecture.
Both conditions and design rule may be statically verfied. Here, they are re-arranged
to define *service protocol*, *service network* (system), and *service network component*,
which together form a model for system abstraction. Adding mutual exclusion of
service provision and dependency between service connections enriches abstraction
and is shown to afford compositionality. *Prioritised alternation* of service provision
further enriches abstraction while retaining deadlock-freedom and denying priority
conflict, given appropriate new design rules.

1 Abstraction and Design

This work is predicated on the belief that abstraction is *paramount* in the engineering of any
system. Abstraction must capture system behaviour and provide for reduction via design.
Compositionality is therefore an essential consequence of the definition of system and component. Every system must form a valid component (for composition) and every component
a valid system (for decomposition).

It is further held that *concurrency*, *priority*, and *alternation*, are essential forms of abstraction and their expression should be supported by a programming language. Concurrency is
typically neglected because it invites pathological behaviour, such as deadlock, and the possibility of interference. However, formal *design rules* can provide security against most,
possibly all, pathology [2, 3, 4]. Components, each using a different rule, may be composed
without loss of guarantee, for example, of deadlock-freedom [5].

Guaranteeing interference-freedom in compositional concurrent system abstraction remains a challenge [6] and is not addressed here.

Design rules should be applied, and verified, as design proceeds. They thus need to
form part of the model for system abstraction, to be incorporated within the language in
which design is expressed, and to be *statically verified*. None of this is new. Structured
Programming may be regarded as the abstraction of procedure, enforced by design rules
expressed as the syntax of a "high-level" programming language, such as Pascal. In return
for the loss of some personal freedom in the way an algorithm is expressed, considerable
security against error is gained.

occam extended this principle with the incorporation of "usage rules" – statically verified
design rules which deny, for example, aliasing and concurrent access to a variable.

Static verification affords *correctness by construction*. The alternative is "trial-and-error",
which is *not* engineering. With static verification, every valid program is *a priori* guaranteed
free of certain errors. Obtaining the same security by trial-and-error introduces unpredictable
delay and requires additional capability in the development team. Both cost and risk increase.

Honeysuckle [7] relies upon a development of the Brinch-Hansen master-slave (client-
server) protocol for all communication [8]. Peter Welch *et al.* first applied this to systems with

communicating process architecture, and provided a proof of deadlock-freedom [3]. Jeremy Martin later provided a formal foundation and proof using the failures model in CSP [1, 9].

Honeysuckle requires formal definitions that are compositional and which can be efficiently verified upon compilation. Its model for abstraction relies upon the notions of *service protocol* and *service network (component)* which will be adequately defined in the next section, giving rise to the notion of *service architecture*.

Honeysuckle also seeks to serve engineers of *reactive systems*, which respond to external events via pre-emption according to some prioritisation. Such needs are typically met at the hardware level by *prioritised vectored interrupts*. Normal control-flow may be interrupted by a signal, whereupon an interrupt service routine is executed. Behaviour may be said to *alternate* between processes. (This should not be confused with the ALT construct in occam. ALT might better abbreviate *alternative* and denotes a "one-off" selection.) Hoare described an alternation operator which relied upon an external signal, so that interruption was outside the control of either process, and which did not prioritise [10, #5.4]. The author has previously proposed a prioritising operator and programming construct. These are summarised in a companion paper which explores their semantics [11].

Section 3 extends the notion of service architecture to include prioritised alternation, thus introducing *prioritised service architecture*, showing how deadlock-freedom may be retained and priority conflict denied.

2   Service Architecture

2.1   Hierarchical Data-Flow

Brinch-Hansen introduced the idea of enforcing a hierarchical dependency between "masters" and "servants" in order to avoid deadlock between communicating processes [8]. He defined service as the receipt of a request, possibly followed by a reply, and began with a "basic assumption":

> A servant will always eventually receive a request, and (if required) send a reply, unless delayed indefinitely by one of its own servants.

A simple inductive proof is then given that deadlock can never occur.

Rather than label processes 'master' or 'servant' (or the more liberal 'client' or 'server'), an oriented arc drawn between the two should be labelled 'serves'. A system can be abstracted by a directed graph, where each node represents a process, and each arc represents service provision.

Design proceeds from higher to lower levels of abstraction. Thus some means must be found by which to guarantee the basic assumption. Brinch-Hansen lists four conditions, establishing a *protocol* between connected components.

While, as Brinch-Hansen points out, such a protocol may be implemented simply via stepwise refinement, there can be no guarantee that it is then always in force. Errors are possible. These might be detected by some additional verification tool. However, such a tool will not be easy to compose, and in any case affords only trial and error.

2.2   Service Protocol and Network

CSP affords a definition of service at a level of abstraction above data-flow. Furthermore, there is no need to be limited to a sequence of two communications. Provided all partners to service protocol are 'live' (never refuse *every* offer of communication) and *deterministic* (allow the environment first authority to resolve any choice between two communications), the failures model [12] provides an adequate language in which to express the necessary conditions.

If, after trace s, an environment offers a process P the set of events X, and it refuses to participate in any of them, X is termed a *refusal* of P/s (P 'after' s). The combination of trace and refusal is referred to as a *failure* of P. Each failure is a very useful characteristic of a process as it constitutes a relation between past and imminent behaviour.

$$failures(P) = \{(s, X) \mid s \in traces(P), X \in refusals\,(P/s)\} \tag{1}$$

There is an important difference in the use of the terms 'client' and 'server'. Here, they refer to *ports* owned and regulated by the (distinct) processes that consume and provide a service. One should think of each end of a service connected to an appropriate port.

Definition 1 (Service). A *service* is a finite chain of communications between two processes P (provider) and Q (consumer)

$$S = \langle c_1, c_2, \ldots, c_n \rangle \subseteq \alpha P \cap \alpha Q \tag{2}$$

such that:

S1 *Client Condition.*

Q, as consumer, may request service at any time, by requesting c_1, but must then request each subsequent communication c_i immediately after the last, and continue to do so until it is granted.

$$\forall (s, X) \in failures(Q).\ \forall i \in N^>.$$
$$\begin{aligned} s \downarrow c_1 = s \downarrow c_n &\Rightarrow \forall j \in N^<.\, c_j \in X, \\ s \downarrow c_i > s \downarrow c_{i+1} &\Rightarrow c_{i+1} \notin X \end{aligned} \tag{3}$$

S2 *Server Condition.*

P, as provider, may initially offer only c_1, and must eventually grant each subsequent communication until service completion.

$$\forall (s, X) \in failures(P).\ \forall i \in N^>.$$
$$\begin{aligned} s \downarrow c_1 = s \downarrow c_n &\Rightarrow \forall j \in N^<.\, c_j \in X, \\ s \downarrow c_i > s \downarrow c_{i+1} &\Rightarrow \forall j \in N.\, j \neq i+1 \Rightarrow c_j \in X, \\ &\quad \exists (s \frown t, X') \in failures(P).\, c_{i+1} \notin X' \end{aligned} \tag{4}$$

where $N^> = \{1 \ldots n - 1\}$, $N = \{1 \ldots n\}$, and $N^< = \{2 \ldots n\}$.

This definition suffices whether service is offered just once or continuously.

Service may be guaranteed to proceed, once initiated, and in strict sequence. Conflict-freedom is assured. No service may be simultaneously both available and in progress. Service is never 're-entrant', and is oriented, according to initiation *not* data-flow.

The applicable set of client ports – $clients(P)$ – and server ports – $servers(P)$ – may now be attributed to any process P. The interface between any pair of processes can then be recorded as follows:

$$interface(P, Q) = (clients(P) \cap servers(Q)) \cup (clients(Q) \cap servers(P)) \tag{5}$$

Each communication within a service must, at some stage, be qualified according to:

- orientation of data-flow

- whether value or object is passed

- type of value or object passed.

Note that an interface may now be expressed without reference to any *channel*. A service is a higher form of abstraction. Channels are needed only for the implementation of a service. At most two channels suffice (one in each direction of data flow).

Design may be restricted to systems comprising only processes which communicate entirely, and always, according to service protocol. A first attempt at a suitable definition, of both system and component, follows.

Definition 2 (Service Network (a)). A *service network* V is a set of concurrent processes such that:

S3 *Network Communication Condition*
Every communication forms part of some predefined service.

$$\forall P \in V. \ \forall c \neq \tau \ \in \alpha P. \ \exists S \in (servers(P) \cup clients(P)) \, . \, c \in S \qquad (6)$$

S4 *Network Composition Condition*
Every service provided/consumed by any component of V is either consumed/provided by another component or forms part of the system interface.

$$\forall P \in V. \qquad\qquad\qquad\qquad\qquad\qquad\qquad\qquad\qquad (7)$$
$$\forall S \in servers(P). \ (\exists Q \in V. \ S \in clients(Q)) \ \not\Leftrightarrow \ S \in servers(V),$$
$$\forall S \in clients(P). \ (\exists Q \in V. \ S \in servers(Q)) \ \not\Leftrightarrow \ S \in clients(V)$$

S5 *Network Client Condition (a)*
No component of V may ever refuse everything.

$$\forall P \in V. \ \forall (s, X) \in failures(P). \ X \neq \Sigma \qquad\qquad\qquad (8)$$

S6 *Network Server Condition (a)*
Every component of V must either offer all its services, be actively providing at least one, or offer none.

$$\forall P \in V. \ \forall (s, X) \in failures(P).$$
$$\forall S \in servers(P). \ c_1 \notin X$$
$$\vee \ \exists S \in servers(P). \ \exists i \in N^<. \ c_i \notin X \qquad\qquad (9)$$
$$\vee \ \forall S \in servers(P). \ c_1 \in X$$

As well as governing internal communication, S3 also implies that the *system* interface be composed entirely of services provided or consumed. Similarly, S4 implies that V itself has no 'loops' (connections between a client and server port within its interface), should it form a component of a larger system.

The above definition of a service network also defines a class of process, termed a *service network component*, or SNC. S5 ensures that no SNC may ever deadlock, livelock, or terminate.

S6 is entirely consistent with a SNC never offering *any* service. Such a component is termed *pure-client*. One that never *requests* any service is called *pure-server*. S6 prohibits a system/component offering just some of its services while none are in progress.

S5 has two additional consequences. Any pure-client SNC must, at all times, request or consume at least one service. This also holds for any component that is not pure-client, but which insists on withholding all its services (permitted by S6). Second, any SNC that requests services only in response to requests for those of its own must offer them all when not engaged in providing one. When so engaged, it may suspend the offer of any or all other services. This is simply the familiar "basic assumption" made by Brinch-Hansen. Whether a component is able to offer one service while providing another is left open.

System design is documented as a *service digraph*, which overlays the corresponding (undirected) communication graph. Each node represents a component process. Each arc represents a service provided, and is oriented from client to server.

It is quite a simple matter to compose systems whose service graph enjoys one or more directed circuits but which remain free of deadlock. Security must always be purchased with a certain loss of liberty. It is hereby proposed that circuit-free networks comprise a diversity sufficient to fulfil a worthwhile set of applicable specifications.

Conversely, given the above definition, it remains easy to contrive systems composed of valid SNCs which are not valid components themselves. Figure 1 depicts two such systems.

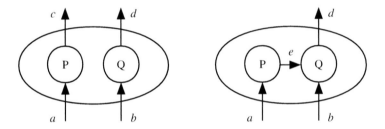

Figure 1: Service network components do not parallel-compose, under Definition 2.

On the LHS, services *a* and *b* are presumed dependent upon *c* and *d*, respectively. Following a request for *a*, the composite process is unable to satisfy any clause of S6. Once *P* requests *c*, it cannot immediately proceed with any service as provider. Neither can it offer all its services or deny them all.

On the RHS, *a* and *b* are presumed dependent upon *e* and *d*, respectively, but not *e* upon *d*. This time, following a request for *a*, S6 will be satisfied. *P* will withdraw *a*, and *Q* will withdraw *b*, when *e* is requested. However, following a request for *b*, *a* will remain on offer, while *b* suspends, pending completion of *d*. S6 is again denied.

It is the second clause of S6 that poses difficulty. Reliance upon it implies concurrency. To advance one service in progress, while offering others requires at least two processes. On the other hand, the set of SNCs, thus defined, does not close under the parallel operator. Two SNCs, composed in parallel, can together obtain states that breach the definition.

While a proof of deadlock-freedom is possible given Definition 2 and a simple design rule, it makes sense to seek compositionality first.

2.3 Composite Service Provision

With the rise in commercial importance of *component-based software development* [13], the need for precise and complete component specification is greater than ever. The ability to freely interchange components, without denying the system specification, depends upon *compositionality*, which can be traced back to the 19th century philosopher Gottlob Frege [14].

> The meaning of a sentence must remain unchanged when a part of the sentence is replaced by an expression having the same meaning.

With reference to engineering, 'sentence' refers to the design of a system, where a more practical definition is needed. The term 'component' is preferred over 'part'.

Definition 3 (Compositional).
In order to recursively decompose a system into components, we require:

- some indivisible components

- that compositions of components are themselves valid components

- that behaviour of any system is manifest in its interface, without reference to any internal structure. Any such interface shall be termed *adequate*.

Components whose definition complies with all the above conditions may be termed *compositional*.

Corollary. It is then possible to substitute any component with another, possessing the same interface, without affecting either design or compliance with specification.

Corollary. Since the above definition must clearly apply recursively, closure is required in the definition of system and component. Every system should form a valid component and every component a valid system.

Jeremy Martin began by defining an indivisible component [1]:

Definition 4 (Basic Process). A *basic process* (BP) P is one that:

S1–3 communicates solely via service protocol

S4 possesses an interface comprising precisely those services it either provides or consumes

S5 may never refuse everything

S7 offers either all the services it is committed to providing, or none (satisfying S6).

$$\forall (s, X) \in failures(P).$$
$$(\forall S \in servers(P).\ c_1 \notin X) \ \vee \ (\forall S \in servers(P).\ c_1 \in X) \qquad (10)$$

It is obvious that any BP qualifies as a valid SNC, as thus far defined. Therefore any system composed entirely of BPs will be inherently deadlock-free. Note that the ability has been lost to offer other services while one is in progress, and that any BP may be expressed using only sequence, repetition (or recursion), and selection.

Martin termed a parallel composition of BPs a *parallel-composite process* (PCP). While any BP is a PCP, the converse is false. It is was thus necessary to separately prove that parallel compositions of PCPs are both deadlock-free and themselves compose. Worse, the new proof rests on the absence of any directed circuit in a new service graph where each node depicts a PCP. This denies many systems that would lack a circuit when reduced to the original graph, comprising only BPs.

An alternative approach was later proposed by Martin and Welch [9], whereby a network of PCPs is "exploded" (converted to one of BPs) and then tested for circuit-freedom. This does not overcome the previous objection, and again reduces to trial-and-error, as the entire system must be re-assessed upon each refinement. (While a suitable programming environment might efficiently maintain an exploded description and rapidly add and test each refinement, such a description is *not* readily apparent to the designer, working at a (possibly much) higher level of abstraction.)

Clearly, a singular definition of system and component, together with a single design rule, is highly desirable, in order to permit secure recursive (de)composition.

2.4 Exclusion, Dependency, and Deadlock-Freedom

Services provided ("server connections", or just "servers") may be grouped into distinct *bunches*. Every server shall be a member of exactly one bunch.

$$\bigcup_i bunch_i(P) = servers(P), \quad \bigcap_i bunch_i(P) = \emptyset \tag{11}$$

$$\forall S \in servers(P) \; \exists i. \; S \in bunch_i(P) \tag{12}$$

Within any bunch, services are now declared mutually *exclusive*. From the moment the delivery of any service starts until completion, no other member of its bunch may be offered. We shall also ensure that no service need be delayed by the delivery of one from another bunch. For example, two clients must queue to receive services within a common bunch. However, they may be served *concurrently* if the services they request each belong to a different one.

Any *dependency* between server and client connections is noted, indicating that the provision of one service requires the consumption of another. In the interface to any given component, any pair of client and server connections are either dependent or independent. When independent, the server need not be delayed by the client.

$$dependencies(P) \hat{=} \{(S, C)\} . \; S \in servers(P), \; C \in clients(P) \tag{13}$$

Any dependency applicable to a server connection is shared by every member of its bunch.

Note that the dependency set of any process does not emerge from its definition but forms part of that definition. In other words, one *specifies* the servers, clients, bunching, and dependencies, in order to define a system or component. Design and implementation follow.

Dependency forms a relation between server and client connections, characteristic of a particular component or system. It is transitive and forms a strict partial order on the arcs of a service digraph.

Exclusion and dependency affords the decomposition of a process interface into *server interface components*, each comprising a server bunch together with the set of clients on which it depends. Since there is also a sense in which these clients also 'depend' upon the servers, and because it makes a useful distinction, we shall refer to them as 'dependent' clients.

$$SIC_i(P) \;=\; \{S \in servers(P) \mid S \in bunch_i(P)\} \;\cup\;$$
$$\{C \in clients(P) \mid (S, C) \in dependencies(P)\} \tag{14}$$

Other clients within an interface may be entirely *in*dependent. They pose no threat of deadlock since, by definition, they cannot compose to form a circuit of dependent services. Should they initiate a service, they remain bound by the service conditions (S1 and S2) and thus cannot give rise to conflict. It is useful to bunch any such ports together and refer to them as the *independent client component* of an interface.

Just as it was necessary to require the earlier form of service network (component) to be 'live' (never refuse all communication), a compositional service network must require all its server interface components to behave similarly.

Definition 5 (Service Network (b)). A *service network* V is a set of concurrent processes such that obey:

S3 *Network Communication Condition*

S4 *Network Composition Condition*

S8 *Network Client Condition (b):*
 No component of V may ever refuse everything within any server interface component:

$$\forall P \in V.\ \forall i.\ \neg \exists (s, X) \in failures(P).\ SIC_i(P) \subseteq X \qquad (15)$$

S9 *Network Server Condition (b):*
 Every component of V must either offer either all services provided or none, within each server bunch (interface component):

$$\forall P \in V.\ \forall i.\ \forall (s, X) \in failures(P).$$
$$(\forall S \in bunch_i(P).\ c_1 \notin X) \ \lor \ (\forall S \in bunch_i(P).\ c_1 \in X) \qquad (16)$$

The definition of SNC is now closed under parallel composition. Unlike S6, S9 does not retain a clause that implies concurrency. It is also no longer possible to compose two SNCs in parallel to form something that is not itself a valid component.

Each interface component may be implemented using a single BP. Parallel composition of BPs introduces new interface components, and *vice versa*. S8 merely mirrors S7, which requires each BP to be 'live', but it allows an interface to be constructed without foreknowledge of implementation.

A design rule may now be stated and proved to guarantee deadlock-freedom:

Design Rule 1 (Service Architecture Design Rule). *(SADR)*
 No circuit of dependent services is permitted in the service digraph.

Before we can offer a proof, a little more background is needed. For greater detail, refer either to the standard text [12] or Martin's thesis [1].

First, it is common to restrict interest to systems where communication occurs only between *pairs* of processes. Such systems are called *triple-disjoint*:

$$\forall \{i, j, k\}.i \neq j \neq k.\ \alpha P_i \cap \alpha P_j \cap \alpha P_k = \emptyset \qquad (17)$$

When a process finds itself ready to engage in at least one communication (shared event), it is said to make a *request*. If its partner is unready or unwilling to comply, the request is said to be *ungranted*.

$$P_i \longrightarrow \bullet P_j \ \Leftrightarrow \ (\alpha P_i \cap \alpha P_j \subseteq X_i \cup X_j) \qquad (18)$$

Each arc in a *snapshot digraph* represents an ungranted request. Any directed circuit manifest in a snapshot graph is termed a *cycle of ungranted requests* (CUR).

Conflict is said to occur between a pair of processes if both are ready to engage in a shared event but cannot agree on which one. Conflict-freedom implies the absence of any directed circuit of length two. Any circuit of length three or more is said to form a *proper cycle*, which is easily shown to be a necessary, but not sufficient, condition for deadlock.

A *system of interest* is one which is statically defined, connected, triple-disjoint, conflict-free, and composed of processes that are non-terminating and individually free of deadlock and divergence. None of these restrictions are severe in their consequences, and serve principally to simplify analysis.

The following theorem of Brookes and Roscoe can be used to prove deadlock-freedom in a wide range of systems, including service networks:

Theorem 1 (Fundamental Principle of Deadlock (FPD) [5]). *In any deadlock state of any system of interest, the snapshot digraph reveals at least one proper cycle of ungranted requests.*

Corollary. Any system of interest that never exhibits a proper cycle of ungranted requests is deadlock-free.

Corollary. Any system of interest whose communication graph contains no circuit is inherently deadlock-free.

There is no benefit here to separating the case of two processes in a "deadly embrace" from that of more than two. Conflict is a useful notion elsewhere, where local rules may be applied to pair-wise interaction. A generalization of the FPD [1, Theorem 1] may be applied instead that accounts directly for conflict-freedom, rather than treating it as a precondition. (It simply removes conflict-freedom from the definition of a system of interest.)

The following theorem may be proven by demonstrating that even when a CUR does occur, it is only temporary, and thus does indicate deadlock.

Theorem 2 (Service Network Theorem). *Any system whose service graph is free of any directed circuit of dependent services is free of deadlock.*

Proof. (adapted from that by Martin [1])

1. Assume a deadlock state exists. The FPD demands a CUR as a consequence.

2. Because there is no directed circuit of dependent services in the underlying service digraph, the CUR must contain a sub-path such that some process Q offers service to both its neighbours:

$$\exists P, Q, R \in V. \; \exists i, j \in N. \; P \xrightarrow{c_i} \bullet Q \xrightarrow{c_j} \bullet R \tag{19}$$

   P and R may represent the same process, which would then infer conflict.

3. The Client Condition (S1) allows R to refuse only the initiation of service, *i.e.* $j = 1$. (Whenever the orientations of ungranted request and service oppose, it is the service itself that is refused, *i.e.* its initial event.)

   Two possibilities must now be addressed separately: Either Q serves P and R via servers within a common bunch, or the two servers each lie in a separate bunch.

4. The Network Service Condition (S9) denies the possibility of a CUR passing through any single server bunch at Q. If $i = 1$ then c_i is granted. Q cannot offer service to R and not to P. If $i > 1$ then Q is denying P fresh service. It therefore cannot offer service to R.

5. Should the two servers at Q lie in separate bunches, a CUR through P, Q, and R is then possible. Another member of the bunch connected to P may be in progress, denying it service ($i = 1$). Should service be underway ($i > 1$), Q may be requesting or receiving a dependent service, and thus unable to immediately continue. Both situations

are temporary. The Server Condition (S2) guarantees that any service underway must eventually continue. The Network Client Condition (S8) ensures that any request for service will eventually be granted, provided there is no deadlock at a given server bunch (proven at previous step), and no "infinite overtaking" by other members (required in implementation).

There can thus be no CUR that corresponds to a deadlock state and therefore no deadlock.
□

It is worth adding that S8 and S9 prevent not only deadlock but also infinite overtaking (and thus indefinite postponement) as a result of any preference a process might otherwise have for one interface component over another. However, such "unfairness" is still possible *within* any server bunch. As with any form of selection, resolution must be sought in implementation, which in practice is not usually a problem.

Note also that Step 5 also guarantees that a circuit in the underlying service digraph linking *independent* services can cause no deadlock either.

2.5   Summary

In place of the conditions listed *ad hoc* by Martin [1], there is now clear and separate formal abstraction of service and service network. The channel has been removed from system abstraction, as has the restriction on service protocol to sequences of just one or two communications. The definition of service network has been rendered compositional under the parallel operator by the introduction of exclusion and dependency – both natural forms of abstraction.

It remains to add priority and alternation to complete the arsenal, without compromising security.

3   Prioritised Service Architecture

3.1   Prioritised Alternation

Many applications require systems that respond to events that occur in their environment according to some prioritisation. Such systems are said to exhibit *reactive* or *event-driven* behaviour. Processor architecture often provides for this with *prioritised vectored interrupts*. Some external mechanism provides both an interrupt signal and an interrupt vector. The signal causes interruption of normal (sequential) control flow. The vector identifies the interrupt service routine subsequently executed. Upon completion of that routine, control returns to the interrupted process. Resumption must typically await completion, even should the interrupt service routine become blocked. It is usually possible to prevent re-entrance to the routine prior to its completion. Performance of reactive systems is often measured according to *latency* (the delay between interrupt signal and commencement of service routine) rather than data or instruction throughput.

In his seminal book, Hoare discussed binary operators that capture both interruption and *alternation*, whereby some external signal causes behaviour of a system to switch between two processes [10, #5.4]. Upon change-over, the state of the interrupted process is preserved, allowing later resumption (interrupting its partner). This differs from the behaviour described earlier. First, the signal lies outside the alphabet of either process and must be repeated to cause resumption. Second, there is no prioritisation. Third, it is not immediately clear what happens should either component process terminate. An interrupt service routine sometimes *disables* further interruption. It may even disable interruption by other events.

A new operator has been proposed by the author, along with a corresponding programming construct, that is intended to reflect the behaviour of non-re-entrant prioritised vectored interruption, and better serve the abstraction of reactive systems [15]. A companion paper [11] seeks to clarify the semantics of such prioritised alternation (termed pri-alternation, for convenience). It also provides a complete description of operator and construct.

We are already well-equipped to abstract the behaviour of processes composed under pri-alternation, which can be seen as complementary to parallel composition. (The designer must choose whether to provide two services (or bunches) via two basic processes arranged in parallel or via the same processes in pri-alternation.) Communication with an interrupt service routine is easily abstracted as the conduct of a single service. The interrupt signal may be considered a request for that service – the first in its characteristic sequence. Response is captured by the remainder of that sequence. Finally, the behaviour of the interrupt service routine may be captured via a process that is typically cyclic about interruption and completion. The question of termination is addressed in the companion paper.

3.2 Cyclic Dependency

Pri-alternation may be easily added to a service digraph by the use of a second kind of directed arc, representing the possibility of interruption of one process (node) by another. A *prioritised service digraph* (PSD) can thus be drawn using one colour for each kind of arc — here, gray for interruption and black for service.

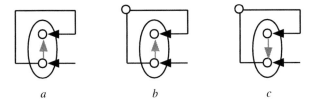

a　　　　　　　*b*　　　　　　　*c*

Figure 2: Three circuits within a prioritised service digraph (PSD).

With regard to deadlock in systems with PSA, consider the three circuits shown in Figure 2. Each diagram (*a*, *b*, and *c*) depicts two processes composed under prioritised alternation. In *a*, for example, a request for the service provided by the upper component will cause interruption of the lower one, as indicated by the gray arrow between them. The lower component will resume only when provision of that service has been completed.

Circuits of type *a* will clearly deadlock. Service cannot progress between two processes that alternate. If they alternate, they cannot be concurrent, and thus cannot synchronously communicate. Any attempt to connect services in this way will be denied by condition S4, which forbids loops, and by the SADR, which forbids circuits of any length.

Circuits of type *b* are permitted by the SADR and are inherently safe. Communication between upper and lower components of the alternation is mediated by the external process shown. It is free to gain a complete service from the upper component before proceeding to complete a service to the lower one. However, success depends upon the orientation of the gray arrow.

Those of type *c*, where the gray arrow is reversed, are still permitted by the SADR but are clearly unsafe. The upper component will *not* be at liberty to provide service to the external process. It must await completion by the lower one before it may resume. That will never occur.

To deny such eventualities, a new design rule is required for systems with *prioritised* service architecture.

Design Rule 2 (Prioritised Service Architecture Design Rule 1). *(PSA DR1)*
No directed circuit of dependent services and interruptions is permitted.

Note that this subsumes the earlier SADR, as a PSD subsumes a SD. PSA DR1 is thus the only design rule required, and the PSD is the only system design description required.

Prioritisation increases the scope for deadlock. As yet, deadlock-freedom cannot be guaranteed. PSA DR1 is a necessary but not a sufficient condition.

3.3   Priority Conflict

One other aim remains to be met — that prioritisation in one process should not conflict with that of another. Prioritisation here applies to services, not individual communications or processes, and forms part of the interface between processes. To be more precise, it is applied to server bunches, which are enumerated accordingly. The priority of each client connection is determined by the server bunch which, directly or indirectly, depends upon it.

Definition 6 (Priority Conflict). A *priority conflict* exists when the provision of some service is dependent upon the consumption of another of lower priority.

Inversion is one possible consequence, where an intended prioritisation is reversed as a result of parallel composition.

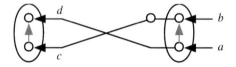

Figure 3: Priority inversion and potential deadlock in a PSD obeying PSA DR1.

Figure 3 shows how deadlock can arise from priority conflict even when PSA DR1 applies. Suppose a request for service *b* is made. The lower component of the right-hand alternation will be interrupted and service commenced. If it is dependent upon the service *c* then a request for that will be made, via the intervening node. All will be well unless the service *a* was already in progress and dependent upon *d*. If a request for *d* was made first at the left-hand alternation, deadlock will ensue.

Figure 3 also illustrates the futility of merely enforcing a local interface. No pair of processes can be found in direct conflict. More than a local connection rule is required.

The PSD has two dimensions – one representing interruption (gray), and one service (black). It will prove useful to require a normal form where all arcs are drawn oriented in common according to colour. For example, all gray arcs might be aligned vertically, with interruption proceeding upwards, and all black arcs aligned horizontally, with provision, say, on the left. Figure 3 is depicted in this fashion.

Design Rule 3 (Prioritised Service Architecture Design Rule 2). *(PSA DR2)*
When all arcs of the PSD are aligned according to colour, no pair of dependencies may cross.

This is clearly equivalent to a requirement that any prioritization of services, established via dependency, is consistent with that of the servers of any process to which they are connected. In other words, it must be possible to draw the PSD without any arcs of a given colour crossing. Freedom from priority conflict, and thus inversion, follows directly. (The proof is trivial but included for completeness.)

Theorem 3 (Prioritised Service Network Theorem 1).
Every system with PSA *that obeys* PSA DR1 *and* DR2 *is free of priority conflict.*

Proof. In the absence of a directed circuit in the SD (PSA DR1), it is possible to follow any dependency to its conclusion. Arcs along any dependency may be enumerated by back-tracking and decrementing the label each time an interruption is traversed in the corresponding PSD. The algorithm actually employed must take account of the fact that each arc may lie along multiple dependencies. For example, an existing label can be adopted and a correction applied back up the chain. It is thus possible to enumerate the global priority of every service.

It is therefore also possible to verify that the interface of each component is satisfied and thus that every system is free of priority conflict. □

PSA DR2 requires that the PSD can be *drawn* on a plane. One dimension corresponds to prioritisation (interruptability), the other to service dependency. It is proposed that this will also guarantee deadlock-freedom.

Theorem 4 (Service Network Theorem).
Every system with PSA *that obeys* PSA DR1 *and* DR2 *is free of deadlock.*

No proof is offered here of this theorem. This is because it would depend upon a formal definition of prioritised alternation — something which cannot be given using the failures model of CSP alone. (The formal definition of prioritised alternation is addressed in the companion paper [11].)

Formal conditions now govern whether any proposed system extension is admissible. It must be possible to incorporate the new subsystem within the existing (2-colour) PSD without dependency circuit or crossover. A suitable tool could verify this, still without the need to deploy mathematical skills in its application. The significance can be appreciated when it is remembered that around 98% of programmer activity is devoted to extending existing systems rather than constructing new ones.

As was noted earlier, performance of reactive systems frequently highlights latency rather than throughput. While physical time has not been introduced to the abstraction model presented here, in practice it remains possible to verify any latency requirement. A compiler will have knowledge of all aspects of the implementation of each pri-alternation. This can easily be extended to the timing parameters of the platform concerned. Thus verification of latency requirements could easily be accommodated within an appropriate programming environment.

4   Conclusion

Prioritised service architecture (PSA) is proposed for the abstraction of concurrent systems with a wide range of application, including those which are reactive (event-driven). It is suitable for the capture of both specification and design, where decomposition is safeguarded against deadlock and priority conflict by formal design rules. Direct implementation will be possible via the Honeysuckle programming language.

Figure 4 depicts a system with an interface comprising three components, each comprising a three-server bunch and a single dependent client. A prioritisation is also indicated. Provision of any service in bunch one will be pre-empted by a request for any in bunch two or three, for example.

PSA inherits the benefits of service architecture (SA). Not only are SA systems inherently deadlock-free, but they also are *compositional*; every component is a valid system, and every

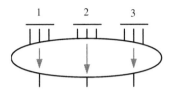

Figure 4: A prioritised service interface (PSI).

system a valid component. Components may be interchanged according only to their service interface.

Alternation provides a secure means by which to provide feedback within a system, avoiding the limitation to "process tree" structure inherent with client-server architecture defined according to data-flow. It also provides a simple, and natural, way to incorporate and express prioritisation.

Hybrid systems, where some components guarantee deadlock-freedom by enforcing other design rules, such as *cyclic order protocol* [4], can be achieved by exploiting the *Network Composition Theorem* of Brookes and Roscoe [5].

In addition to completing the definition of, and implementing, Honeysuckle, further work continues to address additional guarantees regarding pathological behaviour, and the issue of interference.

Acknowledgements

I am very grateful for many valuable and stimulating discussions with Jeremy Martin and Sabah Jassim.

References

[1] Jeremy M. R. Martin. *The Design and Construction of Deadlock-Free Concurrent Systems*. PhD thesis, University of Buckingham, Hunter Street, Buckingham, MK18 1EG, UK, 1996.

[2] A. W. Roscoe and N. Dathi. The pursuit of deadlock freedom. Technical Report PRG-57, Oxford University Computing Laboratory, 8-11, Keble Road, Oxford OX1 3QD, England, 1986.

[3] Peter H. Welch, G. Justo, and Colin Willcock. High-level paradigms for deadlock-free high performance systems. In R. Grebe et al., editor, *Transputer Applications and Systems '93*, pages 981–1004. IOS Press, 1993.

[4] Jeremy Martin, Ian East, and Sabah Jassim. Design rules for deadlock freedom. *Transputer Communications*, 2(3):121–133, 1994.

[5] S. D. Brookes and A. W. Roscoe. Deadlock analysis in networks of communicating processes. *Distributed Computing*, 4:209–230, 1991.

[6] C. B. Jones. Wanted: A compositional model for concurrency. In Annabelle McIver and Carroll Morgan, editors, *Programming Methodology*, Monographs in Computer Science, pages 1–15. Springer-Verlag, 2003.

[7] Ian R. East. The Honeysuckle programming language: An overview. *IEE Software*, 150(2):95–107, 2003.

[8] Per Brinch Hansen. *Operating System Principles*. Automatic Computation. Prentice Hall, 1973.

[9] Jeremy M. R. Martin and Peter H. Welch. A design strategy for deadlock-free concurrent systems. *Transputer Communications*, 3(3):1–18, 1997.

[10] C. A. R. Hoare. *Communicating Sequential Processes.* Series in Computer Science. Prentice Hall International, 1985.

[11] Ian R. East. Towards a semantics for prioritised alternation. In East and Martin et al., editors, *Communicating Process Architectures 2004*, Series in Concurrent Systems Engineering. IOS Press, 2004.

[12] A. W. Roscoe. *The Theory and Practice of Concurrency.* Series in Computer Science. Prentice-Hall, 1998.

[13] Clemens Szyperski. *Component Software: Beyond Object-Oriented Programming.* Component Software Series. Addison-Wesley, second edition, 2002.

[14] Gottlob Frege. Über sinn und bedeuting (on sense and reference). *Zeitschrift fr Philosophie und PhilosophischeKritik*, 100:25–50, 1892.

[15] Ian R. East. Programming prioritized alternation. In H. R. Arabnia, editor, *Parallel and Distributed Processing: Techniques and Applications 2002*, pages 531–537, Las Vegas, Nevada, USA, 2002. CSREA Press.

Communicating Process Architectures 2004   71
Ian East, Jeremy Martin, Peter Welch, David Duce, and Mark Green (Eds.)
IOS Press, 2004

Debugging and Verification of Parallel Systems — the *picoChip* Way!

Daniel TOWNER, Gajinder PANESAR, Andrew DULLER,
Alan GRAY and Will ROBBINS

picoChip Designs Ltd., Bath, UK

Abstract. This paper describes the methods that have been developed for debugging
and verifying systems using devices from the picoArray[TM] family. In order to increase
the computational ability of these devices the hardware debugging support has been
kept to a minimum and the methods and tools described take this into account. An
example of how some of these methods have been used to produce an 802.16 system
is given. The important features of the new PC102 device are outlined.

1 Introduction

The wireless communications field is experiencing a period of major expansion. This is
happening all over the world and is not dominated by any one region in particular. In a field
in which different standards are fixed for different regions of the world, where standards are
in a state of flux or even where no standards exist, it is very costly to enter the market with
a custom ASIC solution. What is required is a scalable programmable solution, which can
cater for most, if not all these areas. To this end picoChip created the picoArray[TM] and a rich
toolset.

The picoArray[TM] is a tiled processor architecture in which hundreds of processors are
connected together using a deterministic interconnect [1, 2]. The level of parallelism is relatively fine grained with each processor having a small amount of local memory. Each processor runs a single process in its own memory space and they use "signals" to synchronise
and communicate. Multiple picoArray[TM] devices may be connected together to form systems containing thousands of processors using on-chip peripherals which effectively extend
the on-chip bus structure.

In order to provide a commercially viable, massively parallel, scalable solution, picoChip
has had to re-think methods of debug and verification in the following areas:

scale: depending upon the target, systems solutions may require moderate or massive computational power. To address this, many picoArray[TM] devices may be connected together[1], creating systems containing thousands of processors.

reduced non-essential hardware: in order to produce a commercially viable chip, silicon
area is best used for computation. Specialised hardware for non-compute must be justified and the emphasis should be on system-wide rather than processor centric debug.
Therefore conventional processor support, such as register or memory trace mechanisms, are not as useful as they are in uni-processor systems. In the picoArray[TM], hardware support for debug has been kept to a minimum in order to allow more processors
to be fitted onto a single device.

---
[1]picoChip has boards with up to 16 devices.

environment: the picoArray™ devices are designed for use in embedded environments, where to keep costs to a minimum, there are relatively few inputs and outputs. In such an environment, the bandwidth available for debugging traffic is limited. picoChip provides relatively light weight access to the picoArray™ via a JTAG interface and the microprocessor interface.

communication and synchronisation: many parallel systems use special purpose libraries (e.g., Posix threads [3], Message Passing Interface [4]) or language support mechanisms (e.g., Java threads [5]) to handle communication and synchronisation of parallel processes. This is very difficult to justify in an embedded system where memory and system cost are areas of concern. The picoArray™ uses a deterministic interconnect fabric called the picoBus™. This behaves like a blocking, double-entry FIFO between processes, and is used for communication and synchronisation. No run-time arbitration of the picoBus™ is necessary, enabling the hardware to be made much simpler, and removing a possible source of bugs.

Conventional debuggers are usually designed for a single processor, and normally require a reasonable amount of hardware support. Even debuggers from vendors who claim to support multi-processor systems will require hardware support. More importantly however, conventional debuggers will not scale to systems consisting of hundreds or thousands of processors.

picoChip's approach to debug and verification has been to exploit the programming paradigm provided by the picoArray™ [1, 2] and to create a rich set of tools to aid system-wide debug and verification. Two main categories can be identified: language features and software tools.

The picoArray™ tools support an input language which is a combination of VHDL [6], ANSI/ISO C and assembly language. Individual processes are written in C and assembly, while structural VHDL is used to describe how processes are connected together using signals. Signals are strongly typed, and have specified bandwidths. They may be synchronous or asynchronous, point-to-point or point-to-multi-point. Processes are statically created by describing their number and type in the source files — no runtime creation of processes is possible. Thus, after a system has been compiled, the complete set of processes, and their connections is known, and the system will behave deterministically.

The most common software tool for debugging is the symbolic debugger, which allows the programmer's original source code to be displayed, along with the contents of source variables, on a per-process basis. The use of symbolic debugging is commonplace, so will not be considered further in this paper. The additional mechanisms that have been developed are as follows:

design browser: this allows both static and dynamic analysis of a user's design. The overall structure of a system can be graphically displayed in a number of ways. This allows the user to verify that the overall system has been connected in the way that was intended and to visualise and navigate through a complex design which may have been coded by many people. In addition, dynamic analysis can be performed and it can be used to visualise problems such as those associated with data throughput and deadlock.

simulation: the cycle accurate simulator allows all of the processor's internal state to be viewed, including aspects that the real hardware does not allow. Typically the user would start their development here and then migrate to hardware.

scripting: the debugger can be programmed using Tcl/Tk. This allows the user to build on top of the basic system provided by the standard debugger.

traces: track the contents of signals, variables, registers, and memory over time.

probes: a special type of process which can be inserted into a user's design during debugging, to enable complex real-time analysis.

traffic analysis: extract the states of the various communications and indicate the reasons for any stalling.

file I/O: stream data in to and out of a system, using files.

activity display: condensed graphical display of the state of many processes in a system.

The remainder of this paper is structured as follows. Section 2 contains an overview of the picoArray™ devices. We then describe how the debug and verification tools might be used over the lifetime of a design, from initial component to integrated system. We then describe each of the types of debug mechanism in more detail and finish with a conclusion.

2 The picoArray™ Concept

2.1 The picoArray™ Architecture

picoChip's latest device - PC102 is based around the picoArray™ tiled processor architecture in which over 300 processors (3-way VLIW, Harvard architecture with local memory), and 14 co-processors (Function Accelerator Units or FAU) are interconnected by a 32-bit picoBus and programmable switches.

The term Array Element (AE) is used to describe either processors or co-processors (i.e., there are 322 AEs in the array). There are three processor variants which share the same basic structure: Standard AE (STAN), Control AE (CTRL) and Memory AE (MEM). Memory configuration and the numbers of communications ports vary between AE types.

2.2 Inter-processor Communications

Within the picoArray™ core, AEs are organised in a two dimensional grid, and communicate over a network of 32-bit buses (the picoBus™) and programmable bus switches. AEs are connected to the picoBus™ by ports. The ports act as nodes on the picoBus™ and provide a simple interface to the bus based on "put" and "get" instructions in the instruction set.

The inter-processor communication protocol is based on a time division multiplexing (TDM) scheme, where data transfers between processor ports occur during time slots, scheduled automatically by the tools, and controlled using the bus switches. The bus switch programming and the scheduling of data transfers is fixed at compile time, and requires no run-time arbitration. Figure 1 shows an example in which the switches have been set to form two different signals between processors. Signals may be point-to-point, or point-to-multi-point. In the latter case, the data transfer will not take place until all the processor ports involved in the transfer are ready. The total internal data bandwidth for the signals is 3.3 Tera bits per second (322 processors x 2 buses x 32-bits x 160MHz clock).

The default signal transfer mode is synchronous; data is not transferred until both the sender and receiver ports are ready for the transfer. If either is ready before the other then the transfer will be retried during the next available time slot. If, during a *put* instruction no buffer space is available then the processor will sleep (hence reducing power consumption) until space becomes available. In the same way, if during a *get* instruction there is no data available in the buffers then the processor will also sleep. Using this protocol ensures that no data can be lost.

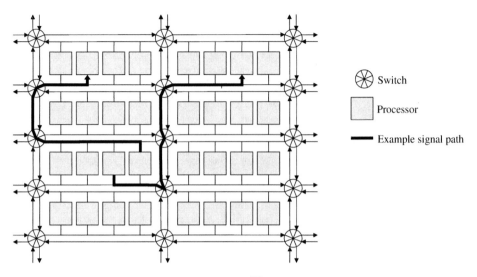

Figure 1: picoArray^{TM} Interconnect

There is also an asynchronous signal mode where transfer of data is not handshaken and in consequence data can be lost by being overwritten in the buffers without being read.

2.3   External Communications

The picoArray^{TM} has three methods of external communications. They are:

- Microprocessor Interface (MPI),

- Inter-picoArray^{TM} Interface (IPI),

- Asynchronous Data Interface (ADI).

These can all be connected to the picoBus^{TM} and can be accessed using signals. The MPI can be used to configure picoArray^{TM} devices and can be used by debugging tools for input and output of relatively low bandwidth (2.5 Giga bits per second) information.

The IPI is used to connect picoArray^{TM} devices together and can be viewed as a way of extending the picoBus^{TM} across devices.

The ADI is used for exchanging data with high bandwidth (5 Giga bits per second) external asynchronous data streams.

Each device has a single MPI and four interfaces which can be configured as either an IPI or an ADI.

3   A Method for Design and Debug

This section goes through a typical process that is used to create a picoArray^{TM} based application.

3.1 System Decomposition

Typically this is done by hierarchically breaking down the problem into components consisting of processes connected by signals. Experience has shown that components generally contain a few tens of processes, however the number of processes required does not have to be specified at this stage. The boundaries of these components will also have signals defined and will eventually be connected to other parts of the system. The user will use knowledge of the real-time system being developed to specify signal properties, such as maximum bandwidth and signal type. The properties can be checked during integration using signal assertions, which are described in section 3.3.

3.2 Component Coding

Two approaches can be taken, the choice being dictated by the complexity of the component.

For small components in which the division into AEs can be determined easily these AEs can be coded using C or ASM and connected using appropriate signals.

For larger components it may be preferable to initially produce a functional representation using C. This can be simulated even when the code size exceeds the memory for any AE and allows functional testing of this component prior to its division into individual AEs.

Whichever approach is used the code can be tested by creating test harnesses using FileIO to mimic the external components. The symbolic debugger and its attendant tools can be used to find bugs within the AEs.

The migration of the code to hardware is eased by the fact that the same FileIO test harnesses produced for simulation can be used for verification. This highlights a huge advantage of the picoChip approach since testing on hardware can be performed at a very early stage which means that components can be tested for minutes or hours of real time which would be impossible using simulation.

Other components can be written in parallel by other developers, or sequentially by the same developer.

3.3 Small Scale Integration

As components are completed they can be integrated. The strong typing, bandwidth allocation, and fixed process creation ensure that components developed by different people will fit together properly. Signal assertions can be written to encode properties (such as signal value or minimum throughput) of the signals, and these can be checked during integration using assertion probes.

If integration fails (components fail to communicate properly), then this is caused by problems between components, rather than within a component (since the component has been verified in isolation, it has static processes, fixed local signals, etc.). The suite of system-wide tools (probes, traces, activity display, etc.) can be used to identify the problem.

3.4 Large Scale Integration and Performance Testing

This phase of development can only really be done on the hardware. At this stage all of the FileIO will have been replaced by real components.

It is important to be able to monitor aspects of performance in real-time and this can be done using customised probes which monitor various signals and compare data throughput against predetermined limits. In addition it is possible to monitor the behaviour of the system when processing real-world data, and to inject data by using the microprocessor interface.

The results of the monitoring can be displayed using custom GUI's which the user can develop (an example of a custom GUI is shown in figure 5 in section 5).

3.5   Comparison with Traditional Techniques

The power of the overall approach described here is that once a component has been written and tested, it can be assumed to work from that point on. Other parallel systems can behave like this for individual components, but then fail to work during integration, or even worse, during customer use. Possible integration problems include:

- priority inversion (e.g., Mars Pathfinder [7]).

- rogue processes corrupting shared memory

- overflowing message queues

- scheduling failures (e.g., improperly bounded or excessively large critical sections).

- multi-processor bus contention causing non-deterministic communication delays

- incoherency of multi-processor caches

Some or all of these problems will afflict other types of parallel systems, from multi-threaded programs containing just two processes, through to large scale multi-processors. These problems are difficult to track down because they defy logical analysis, they behave non-deterministically and perhaps infrequently, or they disappear when debug code is inserted to find the problem. Even if the cause of the problem is found, it is often difficult to write verification to prevent the bug recurring, because of the need to verify the entire system, not just the component or interface which causes the problem. In the worst case, verification may not be possible because it is not apparent why a fix actually works!

The picoChip solution avoids these types of problem in integration. Individual components, which have been properly verified in isolation, will behave in the same way when integrated into a complete system. The system behaves deterministically, so if problems are found, they can be reproduced, isolated, fixed, and verified. The overall development of systems is more predictable (timescales, etc.), since development isn't held up by strange problems which can't be found until integration.

4   picoArray™ Debug and Analysis

4.1   Language Features

The language features aid verification and integration through three main features: strong type checking, fixed process creation, and bandwidth allocation.

Strong type checking is used to ensure that whenever data is communicated from one process to another, the data will be interpreted by both producer and consumer in the same way. Types are selected from a library of built-in types, or by the users defining their own types. Types used in communication are limited to 32-bits, which is the maximum size which may be transferred in a single communication over the picoBus™. At the structural level, processes will be defined with ports of specific types, and they will be connected with signals which must match the port types. Within a process, any data which is "put" or "get" from a port must be of the correct type. For processes written in C, this is achieved by synthesising the available types using C encoding rules (e.g., using typedef's, union's, and struct's), and

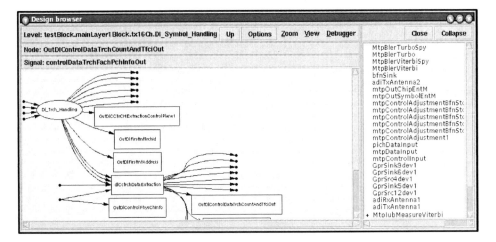

Figure 2: Design browser hierarchical display

hence tying into the C compiler's type system. Thus, end-to-end communication of data can only occur when all processes and signals agree on the type format. This makes integration of independently developed components easy since any discrepancies in type formats will be detected at compile time, when they are easily fixed.

The structural VHDL used to define a system requires the number of processes, and their interconnections to be fixed at compile time. During compilation, the tools will allocate each process to its own processor, and schedule the signals connecting the processes onto the picoBus™ interconnection fabric. Because of this compile-time scheduling, non-deterministic runtime effects such as process scheduling, or bus contention have been eliminated. This makes it easier to integrate systems. If problems are found, it also makes the reproduction of the problems, their debugging and the verification of their fixes easier.

In addition to specifying fixed signals connecting processes, the signals are also allocated bandwidth. This is achieved using a language notation which allows the frequency of communication over the signal to be specified. Processes requiring high signal bandwidths will use high frequencies (e.g., every 4 cycles), while processes requiring low bandwidth will use low frequencies (e.g., every 1024 cycles).

4.2 Design Browser

The design browser is a tool which allows the user's logical design to be viewed graphically and can be used both during simulation and when executing a design on hardware. The following different graphical views are possible:

- hierarchical,

- flat with a given scope,

- as the strongly connected components (SCC).

The hierarchical view mirrors the structural hierarchy that was created by the user and allows each level of this hierarchy to be explored. An example of this is shown in figure 2.

There are times when the user wishes to see more of a design than is permitted by the hierarchy display and the "flat" display provides this. If displayed from the root of the design the entire design is displayed at once. In addition by displaying from a scope other than

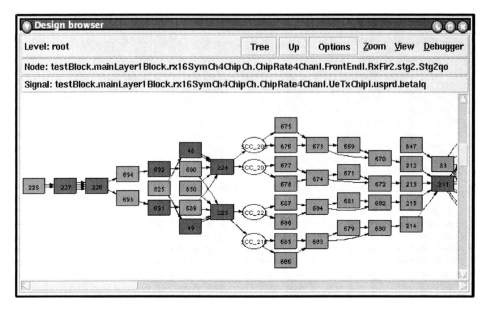

Figure 3: Design browser strongly connected component display

the root subtrees of the design can be viewed. The major difference between this and the hierarchy display is that from a given scope all of the leaf instances are displayed.

The final view comes from thinking of a design as a directed graph and then producing a single level of hierarchy by producing the strongly connected components (SCC). Each of the components can be viewed on their own. An example of this is shown in figure 3. The importance of the SCC view is that from the root level the graph becomes acyclic (directed acyclic graph, a DAG) and therefore this gives advantages when trying to debug a system which has deadlock, livelock or data throughput problems. This separates out the parts of the design that contain feedback from those that are simply pipeline processing.

In addition to these static features the design browser can provide dynamic information about the each instance in a design, for example whether it is processing or waiting for a communications operation. An example of this display is shown in figure 3 (in fact the boxes are coloured, green for processing, red for waiting on communications).

4.3   Simulation

The cycle accurate simulation system allows users to build, test and verify their entire design before moving to the hardware. The user is able to extract the state of the system (on a cycle-by-cycle basis) in order to check against the behaviour on hardware. Importantly, the same simulation system was used to provide a "golden reference" during the design and verification of the PC101 and PC102 chips.

The same source-level debugging interface exists on the hardware as on the simulator enabling the user to migrate from one environment to the another without making any changes to their design or their testbenches.

4.4   Scripting

While debugging large parallel systems, operations such as viewing the source code or variable values of individual processes become too low level; this is analogous to debugging a compiled process by inspecting its raw machine code and register values. For large parallel systems it is more convenient to be able to abstract the debugger to provide a higher, system-level interface. Such an interface allows the details of individual processes to be hidden, and replaced by system-specific displays instead. Clearly, it is impossible for picoChip to provide interfaces for every possible system, so instead the debugger can be programmed using Tcl/Tk [8]. This allows the users to create their own system-specific interfaces, built on top of the picoChip debugger. Figure 5 in section 5 shows an example of a WiMax system interface.

4.5   Traffic Analysis

Traffic analysis is used to monitor the state of the communications network. The AEs in a picoArray^{TM} use signals to communicate data (and hence synchronise), and traffic analysis can indicate to the user the states of the communication at any particular time. The relevant data is extracted from selected AEs or from all AEs in a design and either displayed immediately or stored to a file.

For each signal the maximum bandwidth of a signal has to be specified at design time but of particular interest to the user is the actual bandwidth used on a given signal. Using the traffic analysis data can provide information on the statistics of the bandwidth used and can help in the analysis of deadlock and livelock problems.

4.6   FileIO

When testing and debugging it is common to wish to use Unix files in order to inject data into a system or to record intermediate results. This is achieved by providing an AE template which interfaces to the picoBus in the usual way using signals but which is also "connected" to a Unix file. The advantage of this method is that the same user's code can be used whether the system is running as a simulation or on hardware. The FileIO AE has two different implementations, one for simulation and one for hardware. In a simulation the connection to the file is simple since the simulation simply consists of a piece of compiled C++. In hardware the data memory of the AE is used to buffer the data and when the AE requires it must request that the debugger either empty its memory (for an output FileIO) or fill its memory (for an input FileIO).

4.7   Traces

Traces allow specific types of data, such as register and memory contents, or signal values to be recorded during execution. The trace is stored as a sequence of tuples recording changes in value against the time at which that change occurred. This sequence can be saved to a file, and used by external programs such as gtkwave [9]. The tracing tool is used in a way that is similar to a hardware engineer using an oscilloscope to probe data paths in an electronic circuit. The trace allows a visual representation of the data to be shown with respect to time, which can make certain types of bug readily apparent. Tracing can also be used to perform code profiling, by tracing how the program counter changes over time, and post-processing the information to relate it to the original source code.

While many general purpose processors use special hardware to implement tracing (e.g., ARM Embedded Trace Macrocell [10]) the picoArray^{TM} devices do not. One reason for this is that traces can generate huge quantities of data (e.g., tracing the program counter for a single processor would generate 3.2×10^8 bytes/sec). While the picoArray^{TM} devices have impressive internal communications bandwidth, it would be impossible to transfer this much data off chip without affecting the system being debugged.

Two mechanisms are used to perform tracing. Signals are traced using probes, which are described in section 4.8. The probes mechanism allows signal traces to be performed while running a system at full hardware speed (160Mhz) but the dumping of data to a file means that this speed cannot be sustained. All other types of data (general/special purpose registers, and blocks of memory) are traced using software. The debugger tool repeatedly single-steps the debug system, recording traced values after each step. This can be slow. Typically, the debugged system will be traced off-line, and the results analysed using post-processing tools.

4.8   Probes

Probes are special purpose processes which the debugger inserts into the user's design by utilising unused processors. Probes can be connected to one or more signals, and can non-intrusively monitor all traffic which passes over the signals. They achieve this by using the bus interconnects ability to create 1-to-many connections. For example, suppose two processes in a system were connected by a 1-to-1 signal. If a probe is inserted during debugging to monitor that signal, the debug tools will change the 1-to-1 signal into a 1-to-many signal, with the probe acting as an extra destination. The original processes are unaffected by this change (both in terms of latency and bandwidth), but the probe is now able to monitor all communication over that signal.

Probes are implemented as processes, and so can run at full hardware speed. This enables probes to be used to debug systems in real-time. One use for probes is to allow real-time signal traces to be performed. Other uses include signal assertions, and on-chip analysis.

Signal assertion probes can be used to check that the data passing over a signal conforms to some compile-time specified property. For example, all signals in picoArray^{TM} devices have pre-allocated bandwidth. A signal assertion probe could be attached to a signal to record the bandwidth actually used, thus allowing signals with over-allocated bandwidth to be detected.

Probes can be used to perform on-chip analysis of signal data, rather than having to transport the data off-chip (e.g., using traces), for later analysis. For example, during the development of the picoChip base station, a probe was created which performed Bit-Error Rate (BER) computation on signals. These BER probes could be used to monitor the performance of the base station's Viterbi decoder's in real-time, under different system loads.

4.9   Activity Display

This is related to the trace facility but only looks at the type of activity being undertaken by an AE. This can be running, waiting on a communication or stalled on a memory pipeline fetch. This display allows the history of the activity of a number of AEs to be viewed.

5   A Design Example

picoChip is a member of the WiMax (802.16) Forum [11] and is actively working to produce a 802.16 compliant system. The current scope of the work is aimed at producing a system which can be used in either the base station or the consumer premises equipment (CPE) market. As part of this work, picoChip has developed the first part of this system solution - an 802.16 compliant PHY, whose functional decomposition can be seen in figure 4.

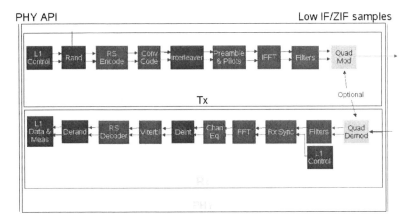

Figure 4: Functional decomposition of an 802.16 PHY

Using the PC101 device the system's team at picoChip have used most of the debugging aids to implement this PHY. This includes developing the individual blocks, executing the implementation on the simulator and creating testbenches in order to verify the correct (compliant) operation before moving onto integration.

It is the final integration of the whole PHY system, for both transmit and receive, that illustrates the key aspects of the debugging environment. The result of this is best shown in figure 5 where the systems group scripted an application specific GUI on top of the primitives provided by the toolkit and indeed the system debugging widgets. There are four areas of interest: three data output probes and one input probe.

The Data Constellation shows data captured by a probe at the output of the Channel Equaliser. This data is extracted in real-time and streamed (using DMA) out of the picoArray via the microprocessor interface.

The Channel Estimation shows the magnitude of preamble sub-carriers (consecutive preambles shown on plot) as captured by a probe at the output of the FFT.

The AWGN (additive white Gaussian noise) has been added to aid checking of the behaviour when there is noise in the channel. This injects data (noise) as input to the quad demodulation block.

The Viterbi BER display shows the Bit Error Rate at the output of the Viterbi, again in real-time, as captured by a probe.

Finally the RSSI (Received Signal Strength Indicator) display shows received signal statistics captured by a probe at the output of the ADI.

6   Conclusion

In order to address the target markets in wireless communications picoChip has created a family of code compatible devices (currently PC101 and PC102) using the picoArray[TM] concept that provides the large computation power required by these applications. To ensure the largest possible computational resource and recognising that system-wide debug is a major problem in multi-processor designs, a rethink of how to apply debugging was necessary. Therefore picoChip has shifted the debug burden from the hardware to the extensible software tools. The tools provide a way of debugging both single processors and more importantly the large multiprocessor systems possible on a picoArray[TM], or indeed an array of picoArray[TM] devices. Experience has shown that using these tools picoChip and its cus-

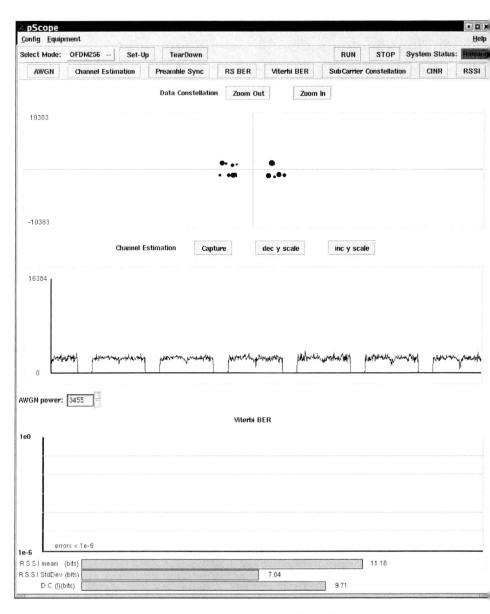

Figure 5: Diagnostics output from 802.16 PHY

tomers have been able to construct large working systems (currently up to 1000 processors) which have been put into our customers' products.

References

[1] Andrew Duller, Gajinder Panesar, and Daniel Towner. Parallel Processing — the picoChip way! In J.F. Broenink and G.H. Hilderink, editors, *Communicating Processing Architectures 2003*, pages 125–138, 2003.

[2] Peter Claydon. A Massively Parallel Array Processor. In *Embedded Processor Forum*, June 2003.

[3] David R. Butenhof. *Programming with POSIX Threads*. July 1997.

[4] Peter Pacheco. *Parallel Programming with MPI*. November 1996.

[5] Sun Microsystems Inc. Threads: Doing Two or More Tasks At Once. http://java.sun.com/docs/books/tutorial/essential/threads/.

[6] Peter Ashenden. The Designer's Guide to VHDL. Morgan Kaufmann, ISBN 1-55860-270-4, 1996.

[7] Mike Jones. What Really Happened on Mars? http://research.microsoft.com/~mbj/Mars_Pathfinder/, December 1997.

[8] John K. Ousterhout. *Tcl and the Tk Toolkit*. May 1994.

[9] The University of Manchester Advanced Processor Technologies Group. GTKWave Electronic Waveform Viewer. http://www.cs.man.ac.uk/apt/projects/tools/gtkwave/.

[10] Embedded Trace Macrocell. http://www.arm.com/products/solutions/ETM.html.

[11] Wimax forum. http://www.wimaxforum.org/home.

Communicating Process Architectures 2004
Ian East, Jeremy Martin, Peter Welch, David Duce, and Mark Green (Eds.)
IOS Press, 2004

Active Serial Port: A Component for JCSP.net Embedded Systems

Sarah CLAYTON and Jon KERRIDGE
School of Computing, Napier University, Edinburgh, Scotland

Abstract. The `javax.comm` package provides basic low-level access between Java programs and external input-output devices, in particular, serial devices. Such communications are handled using event listener technology similar to that used in the AWT package. Using the JCSP implementation of active AWT components as a model, we have constructed an active serial port (ASP), using `javax.comm`, that gives a channel interface that is more easily incorporated into a distributed JCSP.net collection of processes. The ASP has been tested in a real-time embedded system used to collect data from infrared detectors used to monitor the movement of pedestrians. The collected data is transferred across an Ethernet from the serial port process to the data manipulation processes. The performance of the JCSP.net based system has been compared with that supplied by the manufacturer of the detector and we conclude by showing how a complete monitoring system could be constructed in a scalable manner.

1. Introduction and Motivation

For some time research has been pursued to investigate the use of low-cost infrared detectors to monitor the path of pedestrians as they move through a space [1]. Of particular interest is the microscopic changes of direction people make as they interact with each other in a confined space. Such data is important when designers of spaces are considering the layout to ensure that movement is as efficient, pleasant and as free from conflict as possible.

The detectors we have investigated, manufactured by a British company IRISYS Ltd [2, 3], have a maximum field of view of 4m square and thus, to monitor a large area, a number of such detectors are required. Each detector generates a serial output data stream, which contains image data, counts of pedestrians crossing user defined datum lines and the instantaneous location of all the pedestrians in the field of view. The detector comprises a 16 by 16 pixel array and has an associated Digital Signal Processor, which undertakes image processing functions to fit an ellipse to each pedestrian that is then used to determine counts of pedestrians across datum lines and the sub-pixel location of each person.

The data output by the detector can be restricted to a subset of the available data. For the particular application we require only the location of each target in the field of view. The detector outputs serial data, with no flow control, equivalent to a frame rate of 30 frames per second. Each target in the field of view generates 34 bytes of data. Each frame of data requires a further 23 framing bytes. Thus the total data transfer for each frame of data comprises 23 + (n * 34) bytes where n is the number of people in the field of view of the detector. For normal spaces a suitable maximum value for the number of people, n, would be 10. Thus the total data transfer required for a single detector would be 10860 bytes per second. In more normal situations, we have rarely seen more than 6 people in the field of view at any one time, which gives a data rate of 6780 bytes per second. The serial communication port on the detector operates at 115k baud and thus the serial port should operate at about half its capacity.

2. Process Structure of the Data Collection System

Previous work undertaken by Kerridge had shown that it was possible to build a multi-process system using the *JCSP* Network Edition (*JCSP.net*) [4] that was capable of tracking the path of pedestrians as they move through a corridor, monitored by three detectors [5]. In this case, the data was read from files of data that had been captured by the detector manufacturer's software systems. The data was then read from the files at the equivalent of real-time using a *JCSP* CSTimer built into the system. This paper will not concern the design of that part of the system, except to confirm that we could deal with three detectors operating at an equivalent speed of 30 frames per second on an 850MHz processor. The system had been designed so that processes that accessed the detectors directly could replace the file reading processes. At the simplest level therefore the process architecture associated with a single detector is shown in Figure 1. This is broken down into two distinct parts. The first part, called the Detector Part, is concerned with receiving data from the detectors, parsing this into data objects that can then be transmitted over TCP/IP using *JCSP.net*. The second part is the Process Target Data (PTD) part. This receives the data sent across the Ethernet and then passes it on to the software that extract pedestrian trajectories from the data.

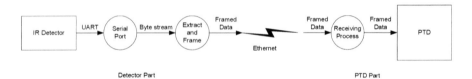

Figure 1: Initial System Design

The structure shown in Figure 1 assumes that there is a direct connection between each detector and the process that is going to analyse the target information. In practice, this would be a very limiting design, as each detector would need its own processor. Further, when a pedestrian leaves the field of view of a detector the path taken (as a series of [x,y] co-ordinates) has to be passed to an adjoining process where the pedestrian is likely to be observed next. For this to be efficient, it is better to have several Process Target Data processes in the same processor. If we have a large number of detectors it is also difficult to connect many serial ports to the same processor. In addition there is a limit to the length of a serial cable, which will limit the placement of the detectors and the processing system. A revised design was therefore proposed in which a relatively small number of detectors would be connected to a simple single board computer, which then used wireless technology to transfer packets of data to the processor dealing with the Process Target Data processes as shown in Figure 2.

The system comprises a number of Single Board Systems each connected to a number of detectors mounted physically close to the detectors. Data is read from the detector by means of the Active Serial Port process and a stream of data values are passed to the Extract and Frame process, which processes the data stream to extract the individual numbers that make up the data frame for each target (pedestrian) in the field of view of the detector. This data for each target is placed into a data frame object. The data frame from each of the detectors is packed into a single object for those detectors connected to the same single board system. It is this packed data that is sent across the network. Once the data has been received it is unpacked and each data frame is then communicated to the appropriate process that processes the target data from that detector.

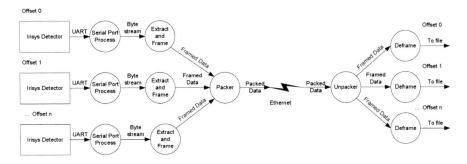

Figure 2: Overall System Design

3. Design and Implementation of Active Serial Port

The `javax.comm` API, released by Sun Microsystems and available as a download, provides Java with serial and parallel port functionality. Although this is often considered as an unfinished API by Java developers, it still provides all the necessary functionality for proper serial communications. In order to make the API portable across platforms, the API defines an abstract `SerialPort` class. This class is then subclassed and platform specific functionality is implemented in the subclassed object. For example on the Microsoft Windows platform, the class that implements the functionality is called `Win32SerialPort`. This concrete class then interacts with a Dynamic Link Library (DLL) file through the Java Native Interface (JNI). The applications programmer need have no knowledge of platform specific issues in managing serial communications, as these are provided through the concrete implementation of the abstract `SerialPort` class. Once a `SerialPort` object has been created, communications through the physical port are conducted through standard `InputStream` and `OutputStream` objects. These streams send and receive information as bytes, integers or arrays of bytes.

The `SerialPort` listener, the `SerialPortEventListener`, communicates 10 possible serial port events specified by the `SerialPortEvent` class.

According to Niemeyer and Knudsen [6]:

> *"Swing and AWT events are multicast; every event is associated with a single source but can be delivered to any number of receivers. When an event is fired, it is delivered individually to each listener on the list."*

This is not true of the classes in the `javax.comm` API. The `SerialPort` object is limited to only one listener, of one type, `SerialPortEventListener`. As Niemeyer and Knudsen [6] continue:

> *"If an event source can support only one event listener (unicast delivery), the add listener method can throw the `java.util.TooManyListenersException`."*

JCSP does not approve interaction between *processes* (i.e. *active* objects running in their own threads) other than through its various channel mechanisms (or other CSP-based synchronization primitives, such as multiway events). This is at odds with standard practices in OOP. In an *event-driven* context, the listener mechanism, or more strictly implicit invocation by the Java Event Thread, is the standard method for separate objects to respond to events. The architecture of Java is built entirely on these principles. Therefore, there is an architectural mismatch between the *process-oriented JCSP* and standard Java. This leaves the question of how to leverage the wealth of existing Java classes so that they can work as processes in a *JCSP* design. An answer is given by the *JCSP* AWT classes, provided with the *JCSP* API. These extend the Java AWT classes, allowing them to be run as processes, providing User Interface elements to *JCSP* applications. Insight into how the developers of *JCSP* overcame these problems was gained through decompilation of the *JCSP* AWT classes and from discussion with Welch [7]. The design patterns used have then been applied in the implementation of the serial port process.

To convert event-driven Java objects for use in *JCSP*, replace the listener and configure mechanisms with channel communications. For example, in *JCSP* AWT classes:

- the listener interface is implemented in a (hidden) event handler class, which communicates events through the *JCSP* AWT class' (published) output channel. This event handler class is added as a listener to the *JCSP* AWT class' superclass.
- a class based mechanism for configuring the *JCSP* AWT class at run time is provided via its (published) configure channel.

One of the concerns about *JCSP* was that, once a process had started, there was no obvious way of configuring that process; it would simply execute its `run()` method until it terminated. However, the designers of *JCSP* provided their *JCSP* AWT classes with inner interfaces called `Configure`: to configure, simply send them a `Configure`-implementing object along their configure channels.

The ActiveSerialPort (ASP) process cannot be implemented in quite the same way as the *JCSP* AWT [7] classes because `SerialPort` is an abstract class, thus it cannot be instantiated directly or derived from. It therefore has to be added to ASP as an attribute.

The need for the propagation of events in this context is far more straightforward than in a User Interface setting. Although the fact that `SerialPort` only supports one listener is often a matter of complaint among programmers using the `javax.comm` API, for our purposes there is no need for these events to be propagated beyond the ASP class itself. Therefore ASP implements the `SerialPortEventListener` interface itself, in addition to `CSProcess`, rather than this being delegated to a concrete event handler as in *JCSP* AWT. The UML class diagram for ASP is shown in figure 3.

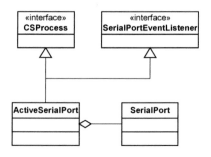

Figure 3: UML Diagram for ASP

The *JCSP* AWT classes, in general, had a single input channel and a single output channel. The situation in this case is more complicated however. In the final design, ASP has three channel interfaces: configure channel (`configure`), input channel (`input`) and an output channel (`output`). These are shown in the process diagram given in Figure 4.

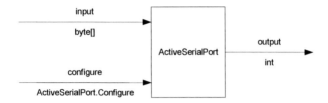

Figure 4: Process Diagram for ASP

The `configure` channel of an `ActiveSerialPort` is a `One2OneChannel` that expects an `ActiveSerialPort.Configure` object. It was decided early in the design process that configuration information and data input to ASP should be sent along separate channels. This is in line with the standard practice of separating control information and data. The design pattern, of specifying a `Configure` interface for the process, similar to that used in `jcsp.awt` classes, is implemented here. The `SerialPort` class requires a combination of settings that set flow control, baud rate, parity and stop bits. These need to be set up correctly for communication to proceed. It was decided, in order to avoid the returning of erroneous data from ASP, that no data should be sent from it until the object had been configured once.

On its own, ASP does not represent an API. Its workings as a process are summarized in Figure 4; it has a pure channel interface. However, as stated above, serial ports require a great deal of configuration information to work correctly. In addition to this, there are many separate notification options available to the programmer. Although in our application these are not used, the Irisys detectors employ a 'naïve' communications protocol with no flow control, the `java.comm` API lists some nine different notification events. These range from notify on ring indicator to notify on framing error, and encompass a number of events relevant to flow control. In order to make these available when using ASP, an `ASPConfigure` object was created, that inherits from `ActiveSerialPort.Configure`. This takes flow control, baud rate, parity, stop bit and notification information as parameters in its constructor. Once initialized, it can be communicated to the ASP's `configure` channel. As shown in the listing below, it is relatively simple to implement and to use.

```
public class ASPConfigure implements ActiveSerialPort.Configure
{

  int notify;
  int baud;
  int databits;
  int stopbits;
  int parity;

  public ASPConfigure(int baud, int databits, int stopbits, int parity)
  {
    this (baud, databits, stopbits, parity, 0);
  }
```

```
public ASPConfigure (int baud, int databits, int stopbits,
                     int parity, int notify)
{
  this.baud = baud;
  this.databits = databits;
  this.stopbits = stopbits;
  this.parity = parity;
  this.notify = notify;
}

public void configure (ActiveSerialPort s)
{
  s.setPortParameters (baud, databits, stopbits, parity);
  if (notify != 0)
    s.setNotify (notify);
}

}
```

The input channel of an `ActiveSerialPort` is also a `One2OneChannel` that expects data sent along it to be an array of bytes. `SerialPort`'s `OutputStream` can then write out that array of bytes to the port using one method call.

The output channel is `One2OneChannelInt`. The reason for using an `int` carrying channel requires some explanation, which will be given here. *JCSP* channels, other than the `int` channels, are typed so that only `Object`s may be sent along them. All Java classes, including arrays, are derived from `java.lang.Object`. However, as the serial port, potentially, produces an unlimited amount of new data, the manner in which this is returned requires some thought. According to Lindholm and Yellin [8]:

"There are three kinds or reference types: the class types, the interface types, and the array types. An object is a dynamically created class instance or an array. [...] An object is created in the Java heap, and is garbage collected after there are no more references to it. Objects are never reclaimed or freed by explicit Java language directives."

The `SerialPort`'s underlying `InputStream` is able to read data from the port either as an array of bytes, or one byte at a time. While it is possible to declare new arrays at each read, this can very quickly use up system resources. As stated above, the reclamation of these resources is not within the control of the Java programmer. It is governed entirely by the Java Virtual Machine's (JVM) garbage collector. The garbage collector is a low priority thread that from time to time is activated and searches the Java heap for objects that no longer have any references to them within scope. Object creation involves the allocation of resources on the heap, and the creation of a reference on the stack. In Java, objects are often referenced in more than one place. If, however, there are no references to the object within scope, the garbage collector reclaims these resources when it is run.

C++, in comparison, does not have this problem because class destructors can be specified, the `delete` keyword will invoke its operand's destructor to reclaim resources. However, this must be done explicitly, and any oversight in this regard leads to memory leaks, where orphaned objects stay on the heap without any reference to them on the stack. The aim of the Java garbage collector, a system that has been adopted for other languages such as C#, is to remove responsibility from the programmer for object deletion and resource reclamation.

A simple solution to this dilemma is to completely avoid object creation at the outset. This is particularly important in this situation. The target platform for this software is an embedded machine, with limited resources in terms of either processor time or memory. Venners [9] also states:

> "*Heap fragmentation occurs through the course of normal program execution. [...] On an embedded system with low memory, fragmentation could cause the virtual machine to 'run out of memory' unnecessarily.*"

The `One2OneChannelInt` interface provides an immediate solution to this problem. Unlike all other *JCSP* channels, the `Int` channels send only integer values. These are sent by value, not by reference. Primitive data types, such as `byte`, `int`, `float`, `double` and so forth, are created and allocated resources on the stack. These resources are automatically reclaimed when they pass out of scope. The heap is entirely unaffected.

Testing showed the software ran sufficiently quickly that, even when the serial port was running at 115200 baud, that there was no blocking when using simple integers rather than arrays of bytes to send data from ASP.

Only the input channels are dealt with entirely in ASP's `run()` method, as is consistent with *JCSP* programming principles. They form the guards in a `pri.select()` of an `Alternative` as shown in the following code snippet:

```
public void run ()
{

  Guard[] guards = {configure, input};
  final int CONFIGURE = 0;
  final int INPUT = 1;
  Alternative alt = new Alternative (guards);

  while (true)
  {
    switch (alt.priSelect())
    {
      case CONFIGURE:
        handleConfigure ();
        break;
      case INPUT:
        handleSerialWrite ();
        break;
    }
  }

}
```

The output channel is not handled directly in the `run()` method, however. It is only used when the `readFromSerial()` method is invoked, which only happens when the `DATA_AVAILABLE SerialPortEvent` is generated. The `SerialPort` object, running in the Java Event Thread, calls this method implicitly through the listener mechanism, whenever data is available. A criticism often levelled against Java's thread model, by Welch[10] and Hansen[11] amongst others is that threads can access an object's methods and data irrespective of whether or not it is ready to service that request. Objects become vulnerable to arbitrary requests at any time, irrespective of their state. For our purposes however, this makes ASP extremely efficient at reading from the serial port. The code is shown in the following snippets.

```
public void serialEvent (SerialPortEvent event)
{
  switch (event.getEventType ())
  {
    case SerialPortEvent.BI:
    case SerialPortEvent.OE:
    case SerialPortEvent.FE:
    case SerialPortEvent.PE:
    case SerialPortEvent.CD:
    case SerialPortEvent.CTS:
    case SerialPortEvent.DSR:
    case SerialPortEvent.RI:
    case SerialPortEvent.OUTPUT_BUFFER_EMPTY:
      break;
    case SerialPortEvent.DATA_AVAILABLE:
      readFromSerial ();
      break;
  }
}
```

The `readFromSerial()` method shows how the data is read from the serial stream into an integer variable and only written to the output channel if the `SerialPort` has been configured. The `output` channel is connected to the Extract and Frame process.

```
private void readFromSerial ()
{
  int i = 0;
  while (inputStream.available () > 0)
  {
    i = inputStream.read ();
    if (configured)
      output.write (i);
  }
}
```

4. Extract and Frame Process

The Extract and Frame process (EFP) is specific to this application but has a generally applicable process structure shown in Figure 5.

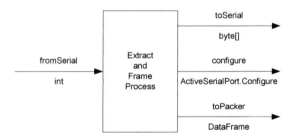

Figure 5: Process Diagram for Extract and Frame Process

EFP has one input channel, a `One2OneChannelInt`, that is unbuffered. It receives integers from ASP, as discussed in the previous section, that carry the bytes returned from the serial port.

EFP has three output channels that are all unbuffered `One2OneChannels`. They are:

- `toSerial`: this sends an array of bytes to be written to the serial port by ASP;
- `configure`: this sends an `ActiveSerialPort.Configure` object to the `ActiveSerialPort` process, which configures the ports settings;
- `toPacker`: this sends the parsed `DataFrame` object to the packer process.

The data sent by the sensor is limited to `shorts` and `floats`. The internal DSP uses the IEEE 754 Floating Point Format. Extracting the data values from the input byte stream was simply achieved by byte shifting to accommodate *endian* differences between Java and the DSP and, for floating point values, a call to the `Float.intBitsToFloat(int)` method to convert the resulting 32-bit pattern into a `float`. It was possible to do comparison testing of the data by capturing the byte stream passing through the serial port of a machine running Irisys' proprietary software using a serial port logging application. The bytes captured were then sent through the parser and the values returned were compared against the results given by the Irisys software. The results showed that these were entirely in agreement with each other and that the assumptions made about byte ordering and data formats were correct.

As discussed previously, this software is intended for use on an embedded machine, and therefore there is a need for reducing the amount of object creation to an absolute minimum. EFP sends `DataFrame` objects, containing an array of `TargetData` objects, through its output channel. The `TargetData` objects contain the parsed target data for each target (if any) in the parsed packet. Potentially, this could involve a great deal of object creation. As stated by Welch [10], *JCSP* channels (other than the `Int` channels) do not transmit *copies* of classes, they transmit *references* to the classes. Consequently, the sending and the receiving process can manipulate the same object at the same time and thus two processes can then, potentially, use that object's data and methods at the same time while running concurrently. This is known as *aliasing*, which is an endemic problem in Java, and in this situation would be a race hazard.

However, with careful thought and consideration, it can also be used to our advantage, and it is used in EFP to implement a *double buffer* between EFP and the `Pack` process. This is done as follows:

- an array of two `DataFrame` objects is declared and initialized in EFP;
- an index `counter` is also declared and initialized;
- before parsing, the active `DataFrame` is indexed from the array using the index counter;
- the active `DataFrame` is cleared of all data, as are its constituent `TargetData` objects;
- once the parsing is complete, the `DataFrame` is written out to the channel connecting EFP to the `Pack` process;
- the index `counter` is changed to either 0 or 1, depending on its value. The next parse then occurs using the other `DataFrame` object in the array.

To avoid aliasing race hazards downstream, we *copy* the received `DataFrame` in the `Pack` process. For this, we have chosen to use static functions that have the prototype:

```
SomeClass.copy (SomeClass src, SomeClass dest);
```

There are a certain number of advantages to using static functions in this way. Static functions are defined at the class rather than the instance level. They do not require the programmer to have a handle on the object to be called. Where data is being received through channel communication, as in this case, it removes the need to declare and initialise a reference pointer, and cast the input value to the correct type. This helps to make the code more readable, as the example shown below shows. We read from each sensor by means of a parallel read using JCSP's ProcessRead. The values obtained are copied into a local DataFrames vector and then added to the packedData object.

```
ProcessRead[] processReads = new ProcessRead[toPacker.length];

for (int i = 0; i < toPacker.length; i++)
  processReads[i] = new ProcessRead (toPacker[i].in());

CSProcess p = new Parallel (processReads);

while (running)
{
  p.run ();
  for (int i = 0; i < toPacker.length; i++)
  {
    DataFrame.copy((DataFrame) processReads[i].value, dataframes[i]);
    packedData.addFrame (dataframes[i]);
  }
  toNet.write (packedData);
}
```

This Pack process simply outputs the packed DataFrames saved in packedData over the Ethernet connection to an Unpack process in the main processing system, thence to be passed to the subsystem that processes target data.

Although effective, this does not represent a solution to the problem intrinsic to JCSP, in that two processes are *potentially* free to use references to the same object at the same time. For our design, that freedom is curtailed by the synchronisations forced by JCSP channel communications to make it safe. All EFP processes have two (DataFrame) buffers, which they use alternately. Having sent one to this Pack process, they work on their other buffer. When filled, they commit to send it to this process, but that blocks until this process takes them (p.run). That won't happen until this process has copied, packed, forwarded and finished with the first buffers from the EFPs, and looped around. In each cycle, Pack and the EPF processes work on different sets of DataFrame buffers – with the switch-over safely coordinated by the p.run communications.

5. Performance Evaluation of ASP

In order to test the software adequately, a number of outputs were added to the processes in the application. Figure 6 shows the outputs from each component.

The EFP process has two outputs: a binary output, which records every byte received from the ASP process, and a parsed data file, which records the result of the parsing operation. Pack records the metrics of three operations: parallel reading from all its channels, the time taken to copy the data into the PackedData object, and the time taken to write the PackedData object to the One2NetChannel. The Deframe process merely streams out to file all the data it receives.

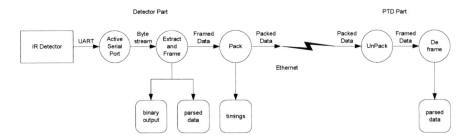

Figure 6: Test Outputs from the Software

If the system is working correctly, the parsed data output by the EFP process should be exactly the same as the data recorded by its analogous `Deframe` process. In this way, the correctness of the Ethernet channel communications can be tested. This does not test the parsing process itself, which was proved to be correct through comparison testing with Irisys' own software. For the sake of clarity, figure 6 shows only one set of ASP, EFP and `Deframe` processes. The intended system will have an arbitrary number of these running in parallel. As such, the tests defined in Table 1 all involve reading from between 3 to 4 serial ports.

Table 1: Allocation of Processes and Detectors to the Available Processors

	2 Ghz Athlon	**400Mhz Pentium**	**Detector 1**	**Detector 2**
Test 1	DetectorPart PTDPart	-	4 ports	-
Test 2	DetectorPart PTDPart	-	2 ports	2 ports
Test 3	DetectorPart	PTDPart	4 ports	-
Test 4	DetectorPart	PTDPart	2 ports	2 ports
Test 5	PTDPart	DetectorPart	3 ports	-
Test 6	PTDPart	DetectorPart	2 ports	1 port

The machines used for testing are a 2 Ghz Athlon with 1Gb RAM running Windows XP Pro and a 400MHz Pentium with 128Mb RAM running Windows 2000. Serial cable splitters were used, so that one detector could potentially be connected up to four serial ports. Although the Athlon could be upgraded to four serial ports, the Pentium could only be upgraded to three. This is reflected in Table 1, which gives an overview of the tests that were carried out. Two separate Irisys detectors of the same model were used. Splitting the signal from one detector to two or more ports has the effect of stressing the serial port and parsing processes, as they will all receive data at the same time. At the same time, this is also a good test of parallelism in action. Processing the outputs from two or more detectors is a good test of the efficacy of the `Pack` process, as this must handle inputs from three to four EFP processes in parallel. The binary output file, that recorded every input from the serial port process, permitted comparison between ports that received data from the same detector. Where parse errors occurred, it was possible to check the binary output and rule out errors in the parser itself.

Each test was run for two minutes. The metrics collected are presented here as average times, in milliseconds, for each packet to be parsed and each `PackedData` object to be written out to the Ethernet. The parsed data output file generated by each EFP process could be directly compared, byte for byte, with the file generated by its analogous `Deframe` process. In all of the tests, the files were exactly identical. The sharing of buffers between the EFP processes and the `Pack` process might allow for some data to be corrupted, if that sharing were not properly synchronised by the channel communication of their references. As all the output data files were identical, this shows that this never happened during any of the tests. Parse errors were only detected in the last test, where two detectors were connected to the slower 400Mhz Pentium. No other parse errors were reported.

Metrics were calculated for the parsing of each target in the byte stream, for each port. They were also calculated for the operations of the `Pack` process. Tables 2 and 3 shows the average time in milliseconds for each of the operations. There is a striking similarity in the network performance between the slower Pentium and the Athlon. However, as expected, the average parse operations were significantly slower.

Table 2: Average times for the Extract and Frame Process in milliseconds

	Port 1	Port 2	Port 3	Port 4
Test 1	29.217	29.217	29.213	29.213
Test 2	30.531	30.516	29.362	29.362
Test 3	31.947	31.947	31.947	31.947
Test 4	31.510	31.509	32.579	32.579
Test 5	34.693	34.707	34.696	-
Test 6	35.683	35.729	35.706	-

In Test 1 and Test 2, the time taken to read from all the channels in parallel was significantly higher than all the other tests. This is explained by the fact that, as these tests were conducted using the loopback address, network operations were only on average 3.77 milliseconds. Therefore, the process would have been waiting on input from its channels. As Table 3 shows, the times taken by the `Pack` process were overall very similar. From this we can conclude that the determining factor is the speed at which the detector sends its data, rather than the overhead of the network operation itself.

In Test 4 and Test 6, where two detectors were attached through serial cable splitters to each machine, the resulting time taken was exactly the same on the Athlon as the Pentium. This suggests that the difference between detector 1 and detector 2 sending their data accounts for the greater time taken in packing the data for transmission across the Ethernet.

Table 3: Average times for the `Pack` process in milliseconds

	Parallel read	Pack Data	Write to Ethernet	Total
Test 1	28.447	0.0339	3.841	32.322
Test 2	28.515	0.0376	3.718	32.271
Test 3	11.630	0.0294	20.679	32.338
Test 4	15.279	0.0870	19.785	35.151
Test 5	14.298	0.0711	19.663	34.032
Test 6	15.279	0.0870	19.785	35.151

6. Building a Scalable System

The test results given above demonstrate that a system with multiple detectors can be constructed and that the data can be transmitted over an Ethernet to a processing subsystem. The design is thus inherently scalable. The limit to scalability will in fact be determined by the number of people in the field of view of the detectors and the effect this has on the accuracy of the system in terms of the number of frames that will be lost and the effect this has on the performance of the system in tracking individuals from one detector's field of view to that of an adjacent one. Calculations suggest that if there are more than 10 people in the field of view then the time taken to transfer the data over the serial link is longer than the time available when the detector is working at 30 frames per second. From the evidence above, this would seem to be a more pressing limit to scalability than the performance of the underlying processing system.

The likely scenario would be a number of sensors connected, by wire, to an embedded system that undertakes initial data capture and immediate processing and then sends the data across a wireless network. The increasing availability of plug in wireless components that can be attached to the Ethernet port of such embedded Java based systems means that the size of the sensor layout is limited only by the coverage of the wireless network in the area to be monitored.

7. Conclusions and Further Work

The ASP described in this paper has been designed specifically for the infrared sensor application using PCs rather than embedded systems. For it to be used in a genuine embedded system some modifications would be needed because reporting errors on System.out is not feasible. However the modification is in fact quite simple. An additional output channel from ASP is introduced to the application process connected to it. This channel is used to send error values, which can then be interpreted by the application process. The package javax.comm defines most of the required error values and all that would be required are some additional error values pertaining to initialization and configuration.

This paper has demonstrated that it is possible to construct real-time systems using JCSP.net, which operate under constraints imposed by the devices that are connected to the system. Furthermore, the system is inherently scalable and with advances in modern embedded systems technology and the use of wireless network technologies the applicability of the approach is not limited to applications that rely on wired connections between components.

The next stage in the development is to use a number of sensors working together to monitor a larger area. This however, is not a problem for the input of the data from the sensors because we have demonstrated its feasibility. The challenge in the next phase is to track a person as they move from one field of view to that of another detector. We have achieved this in a corridor application, where the movements of pedestrians are confined, essentially to one direction [5]. When monitoring a rectangular area the complexity of processing increases and yet again we would expect to deploy parallel processing techniques to solve this problem

Acknowledgements

IRISYS Ltd, the manufacturers of the infrared detector, have given us access to confidential information concerning the internal operation of their detector, which we gratefully acknowledge. Sarah Clayton acknowledges the funding provided by the Student Awards Agency for Scotland, who paid her tuition fees for the undergraduate degree of which, the work reported in this paper formed her final year project. Discussions with colleagues, Alistair Armitage, David Binnie, Frank Greig and Tim Chamberlain are gratefully acknowledged. This research has been, in part, supported by a grant from the UK Department of Transport in the LINK programme Future Integrated Transport with the project PERMEATE (GR/N33706).

References

[1] A. Armitage, T.D. Binnie, J.M. Kerridge and L. Lei, "Measuring Pedestrian Trajectories with Low Cost Infrared Detectors: Preliminary Results", Pedestrian Evacuation and Dynamics – 2003, Galea, E.R. (ed), University of Greenwich, London, UK. 2003.

[2] M.V. Mansi, S.G. Porter, J.L. Galloway and N. Sumpter, "Very low cost infrared array based detection and imaging systems" (SPIE) Aerosense 2001, Orlando, Florida USA, 17-19 April 2001

[3] N. Stogdale, S. Hollock, N. Johnson and N. Sumpter (2003), "Array based infrared detection: an enabling technology for people counting, sensing, tracking and intelligent detection", SPIE, USE 3, 5071-94

[4] Quickstone Ltd. "An Introduction to the *JCSP* Network Edition". Retrieved November 20, 2003 from: http://www.quickstone.com/xcsp/jcspnetworkedition/ . 2003.

[5] J.M. Kerridge, A. Armitage, T.D. Binnie and L. Lei, "Monitoring the Movement of Pedestrians Using Low-cost Infrared Detectors: Initial Findings". 2004 Transportation Research Board, Washington, January 2004, paper 2185. 2004.

[6] P. Niemeyer and J. Knudsen, J. "Learning Java (2nd ed.)". Sebastopol: O'Reilly. 2002.

[7] P.H. Welch, private communication, January 2004, by email, concerning the structure of *JCSP* AWT components confirming a proposition sent to him.

[8] T. Lindholm and F. Yellin. "The Java Virtual Machine Specification". Reading: Addison-Wesley. 1997.

[9] B. Venners. "Inside the Java Virtual Machine". London: McGraw-Hill. 1998.

[10] P.H. Welch. "Process Oriented Design for Java: Concurrency for All". Retrieved, October 2003, from: http://www.cs.kent.ac.uk/projects/ofa/jcsp/jcsp.ppt . 2002.

[11] P. Brinch-Hansen. "Java's Insecure Parallelism", ACM SIGPLAN Notices, Volume 34, Issue 4, 1999, Pages: 38 – 45. 1999.

Communicating Process Architectures 2004
Ian East, Jeremy Martin, Peter Welch, David Duce, and Mark Green (Eds.)
IOS Press, 2004

The *Transterpreter*:
A Transputer Interpreter

Christian L. JACOBSEN

clj3@kent.ac.uk

Matthew C. JADUD

matthew.c@jadud.com

Computing Laboratory, University of Kent, Canterbury, CT2 7NF, UK

Abstract. This paper reports on the *Transterpreter*: a virtual machine for executing the Transputer instruction set. This interpreter is a small, portable, efficient and extensible run-time. It is intended to be easily ported to handheld computers, mobile phones, and other embedded contexts. In striving for this level of portability, occam programs compiled to Transputer byte-code can currently be run on desktop computers, handhelds, and even the LEGO Mindstorms robotics kit.

1 Introduction

occam [1] is an excellent language for reasoning about and writing programs dealing with concurrency and parallelism. Robots and other embedded systems are natural applications for occam, as are many programming problems which are often tackled with languages that have insufficient support for expressing concurrency [2]. We believe that writing programs for the LEGO Mindstorms [3], a small robotics platform produced by the LEGO Group, is a natural application of the occam programming language.

occam was originally the language of the Transputer, a microprocessor specifically designed for parallel processing. To encourage adoption of and development on the Transputer, Inmos Ltd. developed the Portakit, a portable occam interpreter [4]. In the spirit of the Portakit, we have written an interpreter that executes the Transputer instruction set. This interpreter, which we call the *Transterpreter*, can be easily built and executed on any platform with an ANSI-compliant C compiler. The Transterpreter currently runs on many operating systems and architectures, including Macintosh OS X (PowerPC), Linux (x86, MIPS), Windows (x86), and the LEGO Mindstorms (running the BrickOS [5] on a Renesas H8/300 series CPU).

In this paper, we begin by describing our pedagogic motivations for developing the Transterpreter. This is followed in section 3 by an exploration of related work regarding occam interpreters and the existing tool chains for compiling occam programs. In section 4 we discuss the architectural and design aspects of the Transterpreter that we believe to be interesting, some simple benchmarking results in 5, and close by briefly discussing future directions of our work.

2 Pedagogic Motivation

occam's syntax provides a concise way of expressing ideas about concurrency and parallelism, and we believe it to be an excellent language for teaching these ideas. However, students tend to perceive things differently: they tend to see occam as having little or no practical application in the world today. Our goal is to begin combating student misconceptions about occam by providing an enjoyable context to which students can relate. We believe occam on the LEGO Mindstorms will be an excellent starting point for students in their study of concurrency and parallelism.

2.1 The LEGO Mindstorms Robotics Kit

The LEGO Mindstorms Robotics Invention System is a commercial product from the LEGO Group that provides an inexpensive, re-configurable platform for exploring robotics [3]. It has three input ports (where touch, light, and other sensors can be attached), three output ports (for motors), and a two way infra-red port. This is used to download programs to the LEGO as well as enable line-of-sight communication between robots.

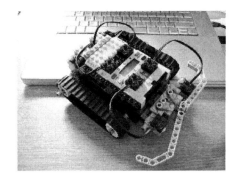

Figure 1: A treaded LEGO robot with two touch sensors

2.2 occam on the LEGO

When programming for the LEGO Mindstorms, students quickly face the difficulty of expressing ideas about concurrency in the procedural or object-oriented languages available. As an example, a robot which is intended to wander around the lab bench while communicating with other robots is difficult for novices to write in languages like C and Java.[1] Furthermore, libraries like JCSP [6] that provide explicit support for occam-style parallelism are too heavyweight (with respect to executable code size and run-time memory requirements, compounded by the already large requirements of the JVM interpreter) and therefore barely usable on machines the size of the LEGO.[2] Programmable robotics kits like the LEGO Mindstorms provide students with a real-world motivation for thinking about parallelism and concurrency; using occam to express those ideas seems like a natural choice in this domain.

We see the Mindstorms as an artefact with which students can begin to observe the abstract world of an executing program in a real and concrete way. A LEGO robot provides a focus for interactions between peers and the instructor, real-world learning situations, and an opportunity for students to have fun in the classroom [7]. To motivate students to think and program concurrently, we believe it is important to begin by creating a challenging and engaging environment for learning to take place in.

3 Related Work

To achieve our goal of running occam programs on the LEGO, we have implemented the Transterpreter, a virtual machine for executing Transputer byte-code. Our work is related to the interpretation of occam, the emulation of the Transputer, and occam compilers for modern architectures.

---

[1]Personal experience teaching with the LEGO in the classroom.
[2]Conversation with David Barnes regarding the use of JCSP on the LEGO Mindstorms, University of Kent.

3.1   Interpreters and Emulators

The Transterpreter is not the first interpreter of occam that has been written. The Inmos Portakit interpreted the occam1 programming language, and was first released in 1984. It was used to run occam programs before the Transputer was commercially available. The interpreters contained within the Portakit were written in several different languages, including Pascal, BCPL and occam1.

In the early 1990's, Julian Highfield authored a Transputer emulator in C for the Macintosh operating system running on the Motorola 68000 [8]; Highfield's software emulates a Transputer development board that one might have purchased from Inmos for doing Transputer development. The Transterpreter, unlike either of these approaches, is intended to be easily embedded in other applications and ported across multiple architectures.

3.2   Compilers

There are currently two tool chains available for compiling occam programs: the Kent Retargetable occam Compiler (KRoC) and the Southampton Portable occam Compiler (SPOC).

3.2.1   KRoC: The Kent Retargetable occam Compiler

KRoC uses a heavily modified version of the original Inmos occam compiler, and outputs byte-code in an extended version of the Transputer instruction set [9]. This byte-code has been augmented with new instructions to support dynamic memory, 32 levels of priority, mobile channels, and other constructs as introduced in F.R.M. Barnes's doctoral thesis [10]. This code is then further compiled to native code by a separate back-end translator, tranx86 [11].

Currently, KRoC only produces executable code for the Linux operating system running on the Intel x86 architecture. Although older back-end translators exist (targeting the SPARC and other processors), they are currently out of step with the most recent versions of KRoC and its extensions to the occam programming language [12].

3.2.2   SPOC: Southampton Portable occam Compiler

SPOC [13] predates KRoC, and is a completely separate tool chain; SPOC's implementation has nothing in common with KRoC. Whereas the KRoC tool chain produces native assembly as its output, SPOC is a high-level cross-compiler, converting occam programs into ANSI C. The resulting C programs can then be compiled to binary form on a number of different architectures using a standard ANSI C compiler.

3.2.3   Limitations of KRoC and SPOC

The latest version of KRoC does not currently produce native code for the three most common commercial operating systems in the world today: Windows, Macintosh OS X, and Sun/Solaris.[3] This is largely because of KRoC's reliance on a complex back-end to produce native executables from Transputer byte-code, as well as the need to port the CCSP run-time system to each new target platform [14]. Furthermore, the resulting executable programs must include this run-time, meaning that the size of the smallest executable program that can be produced is 70KB.

---

[3] As KRoC is open source, it can of course be made to target these in future versions.

While the C produced by SPOC can be compiled to a number of different platforms, it does not support the latest extensions[4] to occam provided by KRoC, such as mobility, and the size of the smallest possible executable on a 32-bit machine is 60KB. By comparison, the smallest Transterpreter executable on a 32-bit machine is 20K, which is three times smaller than the executables generated by either KRoC or SPOC.

3.3   The Transterpreter, a Portable Run-Time

In developing the Transterpreter, we have focused on addressing the limitations of the tools currently available for running and compiling occam programs. While the KRoC front-end is portable, its code generator must be modified for each new platform we might want to support. The Transterpreter is written in strict ANSI C, employing no libraries; as a result, the Transputer byte-code output by KRoC can interpreted on any platform with an ANSI-compliant C compiler. To ease the movement of the Transterpreter from one architecture to another, we have made use of the *autotools* suite to make building the Transterpreter on a new platform a simple, two-step process [15].

The choice to implement an interpreter of Transputer byte-code is in keeping with the current trend in modern programming language implementation. Sun's Java (JVM), Microsoft's C# (CLR), and Perl 6 (Parrot) all follow the same design: a compiler that targets a portable virtual machine. This design is particularly flexible from a language implementation perspective: as KRoC continues to explore new extensions to occam, the Transterpreter can easily be extended to support these new language constructs, which immediately become available on every architecture and operating system to which the virtual machine has been ported.

4   Design and Implementation

The Transterpreter replaces the current back-end of the KRoC tool chain (figure 2). KRoC generates byte-codes which are then transformed further by tranx86; using the Transterpreter, those byte-codes are instead processed by the linker (see 4.2) and fed to the Transterpreter, which interprets each instruction, simulating a real Transputer. Around the core interpreter is a portability wrapper that provides operating system dependent hooks for external channels (like kyb and scr), timers, the loading of byte-code, and graceful error handling.

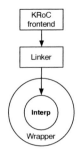

Figure 2: The structure of the Transterpreter

Both the linker and interpreter have been designed with growth and change in mind. The linker is implemented in a micro pass architecture that can be easily be extended to support new transformations of the byte-code. New instructions can be added to the core interpreter, and all operating system specific code has been pushed into a wrapper around the interpreter. When moving between similar (POSIX-compliant) operating systems, minimal changes are required in the wrapper; for more specialised applications, this wrapper may change more significantly.

4.1   One Machine, Two Interpreters

The C programming language can be compiled efficiently (with regards to the size and performance of resulting executable), but programming safely in C is difficult at best. To contend with this reality, we have written not one, but *two* interpreters.

---

[4] As SPOC is open source, this can also be remedied.

Our first interpreter is written in Scheme [16]. This "interpreted interpreter" gives us a running virtual Transputer in 1200 lines of a safe, high-level language. From a programmer's point of view, Scheme has a simple syntax, and by its nature we are protected from many of the tedious, dangerous aspects of programming—memory management, pointers—faced by developers working in C. Debugging our implementation of the Transputer's scheduler, for example, was made simple by the ability to easily interrupt and inspect everything about the state of the interpreter without resorting to tools like the GNU debugger.

4.1.1   External Channels and the Foreign Function Interface

Our virtual machine is not intended to replace a host OS; as a result, we have focused on making the ANSI C core portable by relying on the operating system and libraries compiled into the wrapper to provide as much external functionality as possible. Both external channels and the foreign function interface are arrays of pointers to procedures; these procedures are intended to be implemented in the wrapper by a developer porting the Transterpreter from one architecture to another [17, 18]. For example, the special input and output channels kyb and scr currently make use of the standard input and output ports on Linux and OS X via the general external channel mechanism. On the LEGO Mindstorms (running the BrickOS) we attach scr to its 5-character LCD; both the UNIX and LEGO solutions require a minimal amount of wrapper code. We can support an arbitrary number of external channels using this mechanism. In the context of the Mindstorms, motors, sensors, infra-red communications, and sound are all easily accessed via this external channel interface. Thinking more broadly about other platforms, we can imagine attaching to network sockets, graphical user interfaces, or a wide variety of hardware devices that are already programmatically accessible via C.

4.2   The Transterpreter Linker: a Stratified Architecture

In designing a linker that would take input from tools like KRoC and produce clean byte-code to execute on the Transterpreter, we stratified our design to accommodate future change. This design extends the UNIX notion of piping together two or more commands to transform data. We have carried this notion to a logical extreme in the implementation of our linker.

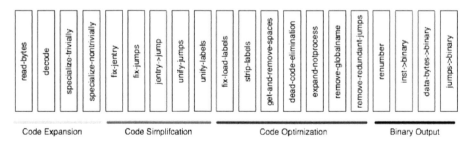

Figure 3: A twenty pass linker, clearly separating out semantic concerns in the linking process

A stratified architecture is appropriate to compilers and compiler-like software. We like to think of compilers and their supporting tools as having as many passes as necessary, where each pass does one thing and one thing only. tranx86, the native-code generating back-end of KRoC, has only four passes—input, translation, optimisation, and output. In each pass, tranx86 does many things to the instruction stream; as a result, dependancies between instructions add significantly to the complexity of the code [11]. By comparison, we isolate these complexities with separate micro passes, gaining conceptual clarity and sacrificing little in run-time efficiency on modern machines.

5 Performance

The Transterpreter was designed to be maintainable and portable; fast execution time was never a primary motivator in the design process. Despite this fact, the Transterpreter, as an interpreter of Transputer byte-code, compares favourably with existing occam implementations. First, we look at the number of source lines of code (SLoC) in KRoC and the Transterpreter as a simple metric related to maintenance. Second, we compare the execution of commstime [19], a common occam benchmark, across KRoC, SPOC, and the Transterpreter.

5.1 Source Lines of Code

Counting the number of lines of code in the linker, the interpreter core, and portability wrapper, there are only 3175 lines of code in the entire Transterpreter project.[5] The equivalent combination of tools in the KRoC tool chain would be the `tranx86` back-end and the CCSP run-time, totalling 29,012 lines of code. Porting the KRoC back-end to a new architecture means porting both of these tools, while porting the Transterpreter only requires modifying or rewriting the wrapper, which is seventy times smaller than the KRoC 1.3 back-end (Table 1).

Table 1: SLoC for occam implementations

Implementation	SLoC
Transterpreter wrapper	416
Transterpreter core	1257
Transterpreter linker	1502
CCSP v1.6	12,480
`tranx86` v0.9	16,532

5.2 Benchmarking

We have two sets of benchmarks: one set generated on an idle Sun v480 with 4GB of RAM and two 900MHz UltraSparc III processors, and one generated on an idle Dell Optiplex GX260 with 512MB of RAM and a 2.4GHz Pentium 4 processor. In all cases, we are comparing different occam compilers and run-times; as a result, the numbers reported are a representative indication of performance, and should not be construed otherwise.

We chose commstime as a simple benchmark that can be run on KRoC, SPOC, and the Transterpreter. It lets us compare two important features of an occam run-time: the time it takes for a context switch, and the time it takes to startup and shutdown a PAR.

5.2.1 SunOS/UltraSparc III

Table 2 shows the time required for context switches and the startup/shutdown time of a PAR in KRoC 1.0 [9], SPOC, and the Transterpreter on a Sun v480. With a sequential delta, SPOC runs 7 times slower than KRoC 1.0. The Transterpreter is 15 times slower than KRoC 1.0, which means it handles a context switch roughly twice as slowly as the SPOC run-time.

The Transterpreter handles context switches much slower than the SPOC runtime; given this, it is surprising to see that the Transterpreter is 10% faster than SPOC on PAR startup and shutdown times. This could perhaps be explained by the difference in structure between the two commstime executables. The Transterpreter is a 1257 line run-time interpreting an

---

[5]Numbers generated using *sloccount*, `http://www.dwheeler.com/sloccount/`

Table 2: Context switch and PAR startup/shutdown times on a Sun v480

Implementation	Context switch (ns)	Startup/shutdown (ns)
KRoC 1.0	83	13
SPOC 1.3	572	382
Transterpreter	1245	344

array of 1249 bytes of Transputer byte-code; SPOC compiles the same version of comm-stime into 2898 lines of C (which includes an embedded run-time). Given such differences, anything from the efficiency of the respective schedulers to cache locality could account for this observed performance difference; future work will explore this in greater detail.

5.2.2 Linux/x86

KRoC 1.3 has a context switch time of 114ns on our Linux/x86 test platform, and a PAR startup/shutdown time of 22ns. With a context switch time of 618ns and a PAR cycle time of 200ns, the Transterpreter is, on average, between six and ten times slower than KRoC 1.3.

It is important to note that many new additions to the occam programming language are supported by KRoC 1.3 that are not supported by KRoC 1.0. These new additions include multiple priority levels, mobile channels, and dynamic memory, all of which increase the complexity of the run-time. Additionally, the run-time kernel is no longer hand-crafted assembly; instead, it has been re-written in C [14]. These factors are the most likely explanation for the Transterpreter's relative "improvement" when compared to KRoC 1.3 as opposed to KRoC 1.0.

6 Future Work

We need to achieve unit test coverage in the interpreter, and set up a test harness for running the interpreter on a suite of test cases automatically. The authors acknowledge that this would have ideally driven the implementation of the Transterpreter from the beginning. In terms of growing the interpreter, we will extend the currently supported instruction set to include KRoC's instructions for allocating and using dynamic memory and all its 32 levels of priority.

In addition to supporting additional extensions to occam, we look forward to exploring the use of our run-time on other platforms. Mobile phones, handheld devices, and other ubiquitous computing devices are natural hosts for our portable occam run-time.

Acknowledgments

We would like to thank Fred Barnes for his excellent work on the Kent Retargetable occam Compiler, his willingness to answer questions on all things occam, as well as "real-time" software development to support our needs in compiling occam for 16-bit architectures using the KRoC tool chain. We would also like to thank Dr. Andy King for his comments on an early draft of this paper, our anonymous reviewers, and David Wood, who first suggested "Transterpreter" as a historically appropriate name for our project. Lastly, thanks to our colleagues and friends who listened (suffered) endlessly as we discussed and debated design and implementation issues surrounding the Transterpreter. We claim all remaining errors as our own.

References

[1] Inmos Limited. *occam2 Reference Manual*. Prentice Hall, 1984. ISBN: 0-13-629312-3.

[2] Denis A. Nicole, Sam Ellis, and Simon Hancock. occam for reliable embedded systems: lightweight runtime and model checking. In Jan F. Broenink and Gerald H. Hilderink, editors, *Communicating Process Architectures 2003*, pages 167–172, 2003.

[3] The LEGO Mindstorms homepage, 2004. http://www.legomindstorms.com/.

[4] Inmos Limited. *The occam Portakit Implementors Guide*. Bristol, November 1984.

[5] Markus L. Noga. The legos operating system, Oct 1999. http://brickos.sourceforge.net/.

[6] Peter H. Welch, Gerald H. Hilderink, and Nan C. Schaller. Using Java for Parallel Computing - JCSP versus CTJ. In Peter H. Welch and Andre W. P. Bakkers, editors, *Communicating Process Architectures 2000*, pages 205–226, 2000.

[7] Matthew C. Jadud. Teamstorms as a theory of instruction. In *Systems, Man, and Cybernetics, 2000 IEEE International Conference*, volume 1, 2000.

[8] Julian C. Highfield. A transputer emulator. http://spirit.lboro.ac.uk/emulator.html.

[9] D.C. Wood and P.H. Welch. The Kent Retargetable occam Compiler. In Brian O'Neill, editor, *Parallel Processing Developments, Proceedings of WoTUG 19*, volume 47 of *Concurrent Systems Engineering*, pages 143–166. World occam and Transputer User Group, IOS Press, Netherlands, March 1996. ISBN: 90-5199-261-0.

[10] Frederick R.M. Barnes. *Dynamics and Pragmatics for High Performance Concurrency*. PhD thesis, University of Kent, June 2003.

[11] F.R.M. Barnes. tranx86 – an Optimising ETC to IA32 Translator. In Alan Chalmers, Majid Mirmehdi, and Henk Muller, editors, *Communicating Process Architectures 2001*, volume 59 of *Concurrent Systems Engineering*, pages 265–282, Amsterdam, The Netherlands, September 2001. WoTUG, IOS Press. ISBN: 1-58603-202-X.

[12] Ruth Ivimey-Cook. Legacy of the Transputer. In Barry M. Cook, editor, *Proceedings of WoTUG-22: Architectures, Languages and Techniques for Concurrent Systems*, pages 197–211, 1999.

[13] M. Debbage, M. Hill, S. Wykes, and D. Nicole. Southampton's portable occam compiler (SPOC). In Roger Miles and Alan Chalmers, editors, *Proceedings of WoTUG-17: Progress in Transputer and occam Research*, volume 38 of *Transputer and occam Engineering*, pages 40–55, Amsterdam, April 1994. IOS Press.

[14] J.Moores. CCSP – a Portable CSP-based Run-time System Supporting C and occam. In B.M.Cook, editor, *Architectures, Languages and Techniques for Concurrent Systems*, volume 57 of *Concurrent Systems Engineering series*, pages 147–168, Amsterdam, the Netherlands, April 1999. WoTUG, IOS Press.

[15] Tom Tromey Gary V. Vaughan, Ben Elliston and Ian Lance Taylor. *GNU autoconf, automake, and libtool*. New Riders Publishing, October 2000.

[16] R. Kelsey, W. Clinger, and J. Rees. The revised5 report on the algorithmic language scheme. *Higher-Order and Symbolic Computation*, 11(1), Sep 1998.

[17] F.R.M. Barnes. User Defined Channels in occam. Technical report, Computing Laboratory, University of Kent at Canterbury, April 2002.

[18] David C. Wood. KRoC – Calling C Functions from occam. Technical report, Computing Laboratory, University of Kent at Canterbury, August 1998.

[19] Peter H. Welch and Fred Barnes. Prioritised Dynamic Communicating Processes - Part I. In James Pascoe, Roger Loader, and Vaidy Sunderam, editors, *Communicating Process Architectures 2002*, pages 321–352, 2002.

Communicating Process Architectures 2004
Ian East, Jeremy Martin, Peter Welch, David Duce, and Mark Green (Eds.)
IOS Press, 2004

Adding Mobility to Networked Channel-Types

Mario SCHWEIGLER

ms44@kent.ac.uk / research@informatico.de

Computing Laboratory, University of Kent
Canterbury, Kent, CT2 7NF, UK

Abstract. This paper reports the specification of a sound concept for the *mobility* of network-channel-types in KRoC.net. The syntax and semantics of KRoC.net have also been modified in order to integrate it more seamlessly into the occam-π language. These new features are currently in the process of being implemented. Recent developments in occam-π and KRoC (such as live/dead channel-type-ends and mobile processes) are described, together with their impact on KRoC.net. This paper gives an overview of the recent developments in KRoC.net, and presents its proposed final semantics, as well as the proposed interface between the KRoC.net infrastructure and the KRoC compiler.

1 Introduction and Motivation

Distributed applications are increasingly important in today's world. Infrastructures such as the Grid [1, 2, 3] are specifically designed for the distribution of large computational tasks onto decentralised resources. Many systems supporting the development of distributed applications are built on the paradigm of remote process or method calls. This applies to systems such as CORBA [4], or the Globus Toolkit [5, 6], which is built on Grid technology to provide a basic infrastructure for metacomputing. Other architectures are built on distributed shared memory or tuple spaces, for instance Linda [7] and Java PastSet [8]. Another common approach for developing distributed applications is the Message Passing Interface [9], implemented for instance in the popular LAM/MPI library [10].

KRoC.net is the networking extension of KRoC, the Kent Retargetable occam Compiler [11]. KRoC has been developed at the University of Kent. The programming language it compiles is occam-π, the new dynamic version of the classical occam[1] [12]. Originally targeted at transputer platforms, it was specifically designed for the efficient execution of fine-grained, highly concurrent programs.

The dynamic features of occam-π [13, 14] offer a new way of distributed application development. A well-designed parallel programming language like occam-π can naturally capture the highly parallel 'real world'. This is particularly so if it enables the programmer to use the same concurrency mechanisms for local and distributed applications. Networked services in KRoC.net are represented by *network-channel-types (NCTs)*. These are networked versions of occam-π's mobile channel-types. Thus, distributed occam-π applications can be designed and programmed in the same way as local ones.

KRoC.net has gone through a number of development cycles [15, 16, 17]. Reported here is the planned support for the mobility of NCTs. Supporting this feature, NCTs will be fully transparent in their use; the programmer can communicate over them and move them around just like their local equivalents. We are also incorporating various recent developments in occam-π (such as live/dead channel-type-ends and mobile processes) into KRoC.net.

---

[1] occam is a trademark of ST Microelectronics.

The syntax and semantics of KRoC.net have been modified in order to integrate it more seamlessly into the occam-π language. We have now specified a final semantics for KRoC.net and the interface between the KRoC.net infrastructure and the compiler. Supporting mobility, network-channel-types will be fully exchangeable with their local equivalents so far as the processes using and moving them are concerned (i.e. the networking will be transparent). The final step in the development of KRoC.net will be the completion of the implementation of the KRoC.net infrastructure and its full integration with the KRoC compiler, so that KRoC.net can be part of a future KRoC release.

Section 2 discusses some new features in occam-π that have influenced the design of KRoC.net. Section 3 explains KRoC.net's basic architecture. Section 4 introduces the new concept of network-handles. Sections 5 and 6 discuss KRoC.net's new features in detail. Section 7 summarises the paper and identifies areas for future work.

2   Related Extensions

We have proposed, and partly already implemented, various new features for occam-π. This section gives a summary of those of the new features that have had an impact on the design of KRoC.net in one way or another.

2.1   GATE, HOLE and Dead Channel-Type-Ends

These have been proposed by Welch [18] (and may be added to KRoC in the near future) to tackle a drawback arising from the new dynamic features in occam-π. The classical static occam fixed the design of its process networks (and the channels between the processes) at compile time. It was always obvious over which 'interface' a process would communicate with its environment. With the recently introduced mobile channel-types [13], we have unfortunately also introduced the possibility of hidden communication routes that are not declared in the interface (i.e. the header) of the process.

Previously, the ways in which a process interacted with its environment (e.g. through channels and barriers) could be statically and explicitly listed in the process header. Introducing mobile channel-types means that the set of possible interactions for any process can grow at runtime, so that interactions can take place that were not declared by its interface. This raises specification and security issues that are similar to those found in common OO languages (where aliasing is endemic and the opportunities for object interaction exceed those declared by their public interfaces [19, 20]).

Within our research group at Kent, the following rules have been proposed, for which we now invite feedback from the community. They ensure that there are no hidden interactions between a process and its environment — a property which we call 'structural integrity' — despite the mobility of channel-types:

Definition:

(a) Channel-type-end parameters *may* be qualified as being GATE or HOLE. GATE and HOLE parameters are *live*.

(b) All other channel-type-ends are *dead* (i.e. locally declared channel-type-end-variables and parameters not qualified as GATE or HOLE).[2]

---

[2]This property of channel-type-ends is *static* — each variable is either *always* GATE or *always* HOLE or *always* dead.

Usage:

(c) A process may not communicate over a dead channel-type-end.

Assignment/Communication:

(d) GATE channel-type-end parameters have VAL semantics — they may not be changed inside the process in whose header they are declared.

(e) GATE, HOLE and dead channel-type-ends may be freely assigned/communicated to each other as long as this does not break Rule (d).[3]

Parameter-Passing:

(f) Arguments for GATE parameters may only be live variables — unless the process is being FORKed. If the process is being FORKed, both live and dead arguments are allowed, as long as this does not break Rule (d).[4]

(g) Inside the scope of a CLAIM, a claimed SHARED channel-type-end may be passed as an argument *only* to a non-shared GATE parameter of a process that is not being FORKed.[5]

(h) HOLE parameters are initially undefined when a process starts. Arguments for HOLE parameters may be outer HOLE parameters of matching type which must be currently undefined, or the keyword HOLE. The latter may only be supplied to FORKed processes. HOLE parameters have no return value (i.e. for the calling process they are still undefined when the callee process terminates).

(i) Arguments for dead parameters may be dead or HOLE variables — unless the process is being FORKed. If the process is being FORKed, GATE variables are also allowed as arguments, as long as this does not break Rule (d).

The aim of these rules is that processes only interact with their environment through formally declared live parameters. In the case of HOLE parameters, what they are bound to may change dynamically, but only by explicit action of the processes themselves (by internally assigning or communicating a newly acquired channel-type-end to one of its HOLE parameters). But the external shape of a process does not change — we have structural integrity. There are no undeclared routes into or out from the process.

Additional issues arise from FORKing. It is proposed to restrict forking so that a process cannot fork off another process without the calling process being aware of it. This could be implemented by introducing a 'FORKS' keyword after which a process would declare all possible processes that it (or any subsequently called processes) might fork off (similarly to exceptions and the 'throws' keyword in Java). Since this might be a rather heavy burden for the programmer, we will probably go for a lighter approach. This could be a marker by which a process could be marked as a 'FORKING PROC'. Only FORKING PROCs would then be allowed to fork off other processes or subsequently call other FORKING PROCs.

---

[3]It would, for instance, be possible to assign a SHARED GATE parameter to a dead variable, but it would not be possible to assign a non-shared GATE parameter to another variable because this would leave the GATE parameter undefined, which is not allowed. Nothing can be assigned/communicated to a GATE.

[4]Note that the semantics of passing arguments to parameters of FORKed processes is anyway that of communication. So, this clause conforms with Rule (e).

[5]This forces conformity to the existing rule that inside a CLAIM, a live parameter may only be used for communication; it technically becomes non-shared and its value frozen.

For KRoC.net, the new live/dead property of channel-type-ends is important when it comes to moving NCT-ends. An NCT-end may be allocated on one node, and then passed on to several different nodes before it is actually used for communication. We will be able to increase the performance of KRoC.net by only setting up the network infrastructure and the Generic Protocol Converters (GPCs) [16] for an NCT if an NCT-end is assigned to a live variable. The network infrastructure and the GPCs will not be set up as long as it is assigned to a dead variable, which may be passed on to several different nodes before it ends up in a live variable that actually *is* used for communication.

2.2   Mobile Processes

occam-π's new mobile processes are planned to be supported by KRoC.net as well. That is, it will be possible to move mobile processes to remote nodes via networked channels. The semantics of mobile processes has changed quite significantly compared to the first proposals. Details about these changes and the first steps of their implementation can be found in [14].

Particularly important for KRoC.net is the following:

> The header of a MOBILE PROCess may only contain 'synchronisation objects' like channels, barriers, etc., as well as GATE or HOLE channel-type-ends. It may *not* contain data items or dead channel-type-ends.

This provides a clean interface when it comes to moving mobile processes to remote nodes. When a mobile process, including its workspace, is moved to a remote node, also channel-type-ends stored in this workspace must be moved to the new destination. This would be done in exactly the same way and using the same mechanics as if they were moved directly over a networked channel carrying channel-type-ends (i.e. channel-types may be stretched between nodes). After moving both the mobile process and the channel-type-ends it contains to the new location,[6] all pointers in the process' workspace to channel-type-ends would be updated — the compiler knows where they are in the new location's mobilespace.

3   Architecture

We introduce here some terms used in the rest of this paper:

- A *node* is an occam-π program which is using KRoC.net, i.e. whose main process has declared a network-handle (see Section 4).

- A *network-channel-type (NCT)* is a channel-type that connects several nodes, i.e. whose ends are on more than one node. A *network-channel* is the networked version of a 'classical' occam channel.

- A group of nodes forms a logical *application*. In the non-networked world, node and application would be congruent. In the networked world, an application is made up of several nodes. Nodes can only communicate over NCTs that belong to the same application as they do, and accordingly, each NCT can only connect nodes of the same application.

---

[6]Note that this only applies to dead and HOLE variables. GATE parameters are re-assigned anyway when the mobile process is invoked the next time, therefore it would be pointless to move them to the new location.

- A *Channel Name Server (CNS)* is an external server that administrates applications, nodes and NCTs. Each application has a name that is unique within the CNS by which it is administrated. Within the application, each node and each NCT has a unique name or automatically assigned ID. Each node has to register with a CNS before it can do any network communication. NCTs are either allocated under an application-unique name *explicitly* via the CNS, or *implicitly* by moving ends of locally allocated channel-types to remote nodes.

- The *network-type* is the type of a network infrastructure used by KRoC.net. Every network-type has its own *KRoC.net Manager* (the process managing KRoC.net's network connections). If a node declares a network-handle of a particular network-type, an instance of the respective KRoC.net Manager will be started. Details can be found in Section 4. Currently, TCP/IP is the only supported network-type. However, adding support for others will be relatively easy, as the front-end of the KRoC.net Manager (which the compiler interfaces) is the same for all network-types; just the back-end (the 'network driver') needs to be exchanged.

In summary, KRoC.net allows many network-types, each of which may be served by many CNSes. Each CNS may administrate many different applications. Every application may consist of many nodes which may be connected by many NCTs.

4 Network-Handles

KRoC.net will be released as a library bundled with KRoC. In order to be able to allocate ends of network-channels and NCTs (see Section 5) inside a process, that process must declare a *network-handle* as a GATE parameter in its header. A network-handle is the client-end of the following channel-type declared in the KRoC.net library:

```
CHAN TYPE NET.HANDLE
  MOBILE RECORD
    CHAN NET.HANDLE.REQ req?
    CHAN NET.HANDLE.REPLY reply!
  :
```

The KRoC.net Manager holds the server-end, the user-level program holds the client-end of the 'NET.HANDLE' channel-type. Each communication with the KRoC.net Manager over a network-handle is a sequence of a 'req'uest and a 'reply'. However, these communications are not meant to be done in the user-level code; they are wrapped by special processes.

For all allocations of NCTs, the network-handle is required. This ensures structural integrity, since the calling process will be aware of the fact that the callee might allocate an NCT-end.

4.1 Typing Network-Handles

If the process that declares the network-handle is the *main* process of an occam-π program, the compiler forks off an instance of the KRoC.net Manager to run in parallel with the main process.

For each network-type, there is a separate KRoC.net Manager. In order to know which one to use, the network-handle in the main process must be typed. The compiler can then use the correct KRoC.net Manager depending on the type of the network-handle. Currently, the only supported network-type is TCP/IP, but as the KRoC.net Manager is modular in its design, other types could easily be supported by exchanging the back-end of the KRoC.net Manager.

So, the following code:

```
PROC main (CHAN BYTE keyb, scr, err, GATE NET.HANDLE$TCPIP! net)
   ...  do stuff using 'net'
:
```

would have the semantics of:

```
FORKING PROC main (CHAN BYTE keyb, scr, err, HOLE NET.HANDLE! net)
  NET.HANDLE? net.handle.svr:
  SEQ
    net.handle.svr, net := MOBILE NET.HANDLE
    FORK kroc.net.mgr.tcpip (net.handle.svr)
    ...  do stuff using 'net'
:
```

The '$TCPIP' refers to the network-type. The compiler would in this case use 'kroc.net.manager.tcpip' as the KRoC.net Manager. A network-handle of another network-type could be declared accordingly:

```
PROC main (CHAN BYTE keyb, scr, err, GATE NET.HANDLE$OTHERTYPE! net)
   ...  do stuff using 'net'
:
```

would have the semantics of:

```
FORKING PROC main (CHAN BYTE keyb, scr, err, HOLE NET.HANDLE! net)
  NET.HANDLE? net.handle.svr:
  SEQ
    net.handle.svr, net := MOBILE NET.HANDLE
    FORK kroc.net.mgr.othertype (net.handle.svr)
    ...  do stuff using 'net'
:
```

When a *non-main* process declares a network-handle, it *may* be typed, but it does not have to be. If it is typed, the calling process may only pass a network-handle of the same type to the callee. If a network-handle is not typed, the calling process may pass any network-handle to this parameter, either typed or untyped. So, if a non-main process wants to allocate NCTs, it would declare something like:

```
PROC my.proc (<...>, GATE NET.HANDLE! net, <...>)
   ...  do stuff using 'net'
:
```

where the 'NET.HANDLE' parameter (untyped in this example) could be at any position in the parameter list. In a non-main process, the declaration of a network-handle would *not* cause the forking of the KRoC.net Manager. It is just a parameter to which the calling process can pass its own 'NET.HANDLE' variable as an argument.

4.2 Shared Network-Handles

Network-handles may be SHARED. The normal rules for sharing channel-type-ends apply. If the main process declares a SHARED network-handle parameter:

```
PROC main (CHAN BYTE keyb, scr, err, SHARED GATE NET.HANDLE$TCPIP! net)
  ... do stuff using 'net'
:
```

this would have the semantics of:

```
FORKING PROC main (CHAN BYTE keyb, scr, err, SHARED HOLE NET.HANDLE! net)
  NET.HANDLE? net.handle.svr:
  SEQ
    net.handle.svr, net := MOBILE NET.HANDLE
    FORK kroc.net.mgr.tcpip (net.handle.svr)
    ... do stuff using 'net'
:
```

A SHARED network-handle may be passed to many parallel processes who may then use it to call KRoC.net's special processes (e.g. the allocation processes described in Section 5.4). To do this, the network-handle must be CLAIMed first (cf. Rule (g) in Section 2.1). So, a non-shared network-handle would be used in this way:

```
PROC my.proc (<...>, GATE NET.HANDLE! net, <...>)
  ... declarations
  SEQ
    ... do stuff
    <alloc-proc> (net, <...>)
    ... do more stuff
:
```

whereas a SHARED network-handle would be used in the following way:

```
PROC my.proc (<...>, SHARED GATE NET.HANDLE! net, <...>)
  ... declarations
  SEQ
    ... do stuff
    CLAIM net
      <alloc-proc> (net, <...>)
    ... do more stuff
:
```

4.3 Restrictions

The programmer should use the 'NET.HANDLE' channel-type only in certain ways; this may be enforced by the compiler later. To comply with the rules, user-level code may *only* declare (possibly SHARED) GATE client-ends of that channel-type (which may be network-typed) in the headers of processes. It is not allowed to declare 'NET.HANDLE' channel-type-end-variables that don't meet these criteria. A user-level process may not declare channels carrying 'NET.HANDLE' channel-type-end-variables (which would not make much sense anyway, since only GATE client-end-variables are allowed — into which communication is prohibited anyway, cf. Rule (d) in Section 2.1).

User-level code may not communicate over network-handles directly. The only thing for which network-handles may be used is passing them as arguments to parameters — either to user-level processes (who on their part can do the same) or to KRoC.net's special processes (who then *will* use the network-handle to communicate with the KRoC.net Manager).

5 Network-Channels and Network-Channel-Types

Network-channels and NCTs are the 'backbone' of KRoC.net. KRoC.net uses occam-π's existing paradigm of channels and channel-types as an abstraction on which networked services are built. Channel communication, embedded in the semantics of the CSP calculus [21, 22], is a powerful paradigm for concurrent applications. Therefore KRoC.net uses the same paradigm for distributed applications — which are concurrent by nature. The occam-π programmer will therefore be able to use network-channels and NCTs in the same way as their local equivalents. This transparency is the key requirement in KRoC.net, outweighing all other requirements.

There are two ways to allocate an NCT: explicitly via the CNS, under a name that is unique within the application to which the nodes belong who allocate the NCT's ends; or implicitly, by allocating a channel-type locally, and then sending one of its ends to a remote node. In the latter case, the NCT will be assigned an application-unique ID as soon as it becomes networked. In both cases, no matter how the NCT-ends were originally allocated, their usage (communication, claiming of shared ends, moving of ends) has the usual syntax and semantics. This will all be transparent to the programmer.

5.1 Joining An Application

The first thing which a node must do in order to use KRoC.net is join an application on a CNS. Each node belongs to exactly one application. To join an application, the following process must be called:

```
PROC net.join.app (GATE NET.HANDLE! net, VAL []BYTE cns, app.name, node.name,
                   RESULT INT result, RESULT MOBILE []BYTE full.node.name)
```

- 'net' is the network-handle.

- 'cns' is the name or location of the CNS that administrates the application that the node wants to join. If the string is empty, the default CNS is used. Otherwise, if the string does not contain a '$', it will be regarded as the name of a non-default CNS. If the string has the form '<net-type>$<location>', it will be used to find the CNS directly (without looking at a configuration file).

- 'app.name' is the name of the application that the node wants to join. This can be any name, containing any characters.

- 'node.name' is the name of the node. This can be any name that does not contain '$'.

- 'result' is the return value of the process. It is either an OK or an error message (e.g. if the CNS is not available).

- 'full.node.name' is a return value that contains a unique identifier of the node. With this mechanism, it is possible for identical nodes (with the same name) to join the same application. This could be several 'client nodes' who want to communicate with the same 'server node', or similar architectures. If several nodes with the same name try to join the same application, the CNS will add a unique number to their name, so that they can be distinguished. So, if three nodes named 'darwin' try to join the same application, they will be named 'darwin', 'darwin$1' and 'darwin$2' by the CNS.

The 'net.join.app()' process is implemented by the following sequence of communications over the network-handle:

```
net[req] ! join.app; <cns>; <app-name>; <node-name>
net[reply] ? join.app; <result>; <full-node-name>
```

- '<cns>', '<app-name>' and '<node-name>' are 'MOBILE []BYTE' arrays. The parameters of the 'net.join.app()' process are used for these.

- '<result>' is an 'INT'; '<full-node-name>' is a 'MOBILE []BYTE' array. They are used as the return values of the 'net.join.app()' process.

5.2   Extended Memory Structure For Channel-Types

The memory block of a channel-type, which is located in the dynamic mobilespace of the node and to which the channel-type-end-variables point, is subsequently called *channel-type-block (CTB)*. A traditional (local) channel-type is made up of exactly one CTB. An NCT is made up of several CTBs, namely one CTB on each node where there are end-variables of that NCT. The CTBs of an NCT are connected by the KRoC.net infrastructure.

In order to accommodate the needs of NCTs, KRoC needs to extend the memory structure of CTBs. Currently, a CTB contains the channel-words, the reference-count, and the client-resp. server-semaphores if SHARED. This needs to be extended by the following:

1. A *state-flag* that has one of the following states: *local*, *networked* or *localised*.

2. A *live-reference-count* which counts the number of channel-type-ends held by a GATE or HOLE variable.

3. A *connected-flag* that has one of the following states: *disconnected* or *connected*.

4. A *state-semaphore* that protects the state- and the connected-flag.

5. A pointer to the *NCT-handle* (an 'NCT.HANDLE!' client-end-variable).

6. A pointer to the *client-handle* (a 'CLI.HANDLE!' client-end-variable).

7. A pointer to the *server-handle* (a 'SVR.HANDLE!' client-end-variable).

The possible states of a CTB, as well as the newly introduced handles, are described in the following sections.

5.3   States of a Channel-Type-Block

A CTB can be in several states. The simplest state is the *local* state. In this state, the CTB is in no way connected to the KRoC.net Manager. Communication and claiming of shared ends is done in the traditional way. A CTB can only be in local state if it has been allocated traditionally:

```
THING! thing.cli:
THING? thing.svr:
thing.cli, thing.svr := MOBILE THING
```

In order to use the CTB as part of an NCT, it needs to be in *networked* state. A CTB can enter networked state in the following ways:

- The CTB has been allocated by allocating its end-variable(s) as part of an NCT explicitly via the CNS. Details can be found in Section 5.4. In this case, the CTB starts its life in networked state (it will never be in local state at all, but may become localised — see below).

- The CTB has originally been allocated traditionally, i.e. it was in local state at the beginning. Then an end-variable of the CTB is moved to a remote node over a networked channel. As soon as that happens, the state of the CTB changes to networked.

- The CTB starts its life when an end-variable of an NCT is received by our node (provided that no end-variables of that NCT were present on our node before). Like in the first case, the CTB starts its life in networked state and will never be in local state. Details about the movement of channel-type-ends over networked channels can be found in Section 6.

The last state is *localised*. If a CTB is in localised state, this means that it has been in networked state before, but currently *all* end-variables of the NCT are on our node (i.e. the CTB is currently the only one that the NCT is made up of). If this is the case, the claiming and communication will be like in local state. However, previously set-up network infrastructure and and GPCs will remain in place (hence the distinction between 'local' and 'localised'). A CTB can become localised in the following ways:

- The NCT to which the CTB belongs is *one2one* (i.e. it has a non-shared client-end and a non-shared server-end). Our CTB was referred to by one of the ends. Either the other end was not yet allocated and is now allocated on our node as well; or the other end was on a remote node and now moves (maybe back) to our node.

- The NCT is either *any2one* or *one2any* (i.e. it has one SHARED and one non-shared end) and has been allocated implicitly (not via the CNS). Only the non-shared end has ever been on a remote node. Now the non-shared end moves back to our node.

Note that in any other case (*any2any* NCTs, or explicitly allocated any2one or one2any NCTs, or implicitly allocated any2one or one2any NCTs whose SHARED end was on a remote node before), the CTB cannot enter localised state, because our node can never be sure that no end of this NCT is on a remote node. The reason is that new variables of a SHARED channel-type-end can be created on a remote node at any time (by assigning/communicating existing variables into new ones; or, in the case of explicitly allocated NCTs, by allocating new ones via the CNS). Although it would theoretically be possible to devise a protocol to keep track of these things, in practice this may be very complex and far outweigh the advantages of having the localised state in the first place.

The connected-flag can be in two states: *disconnected* or *connected*. It is used to determine whether the network infrastructure and the GPCs have already been set up. If the CTB is in local state, the connected-flag is always 'disconnected'. As soon as the CTB enters networked state, the run-time system will check the live-reference-count. If it is greater than 0, it will set the connected-flag to 'connected' and set up the network infrastructure and the GPCs. If the live-reference-count was 0 when the CTB entered networked state, as soon it increases the connected-flag will be set to 'connected' and the network infrastructure and the GPCs be set up.

Once the connected-flag is 'connected', it will stay 'connected' as long as the CTB exists. Even if the live-reference-count gets back to 0, the connected-flag will never change back to 'disconnected'. This also means that once the network infrastructure and the GPCs have been set up, they will remain in place until the CTB has been shut down.

If the CTB's state is 'localised', the connected-flag will not be changed even when the live-reference-count changes. It will remain 'connected' or 'disconnected', whichever it was before the CTB entered localised state. When the CTB goes back from localised to networked state and the connected-flag is 'disconnected', the behaviour is the same as if the CTB changes from local to networked state (checking the live-reference-count etc.) If the connected-flag is 'connected' already when the CTB goes from localised to networked state, the connection needs to be confirmed with the KRoC.net Manager. The reason for this, as well as details on connecting CTBs and confirming the connection, can be found in Section 5.6.

The state-semaphore protects the state- and the connected-flag. It must be claimed before changing one of the flags, and during actions that depend on the state of the CTB. Details will be given later in the paper when these actions are discussed.

5.4   Explicit Allocation of NCT-Ends

Explicit allocation of an NCT-end is made by invoking a process such as:

```
PROC net.alloc.one2one.client (GATE NET.HANDLE! net, <CT>! the.cli,
                               VAL []BYTE nct.name, RESULT INT result)
```

This allocates the client-end of a one2one NCT (an NCT with a non-shared client-end and a non-shared server-end). Similar processes exist for the allocation of server-ends, and for any2one, one2any and any2any NCTs.

The first parameter is the network-handle. If a process does not have one, it cannot allocate an NCT-end. This further guarantees our notion of structural integrity — a process cannot establish external connections unless explicitly given that capability. The network-handle is that capability. The other parameters are the channel-type-end being networked, the name for the NCT and a result code. Implementation requires external communication with the CNS, which may fail. In this case the allocation process would return an error.

The full set of allocation processes and details of their parameters and implementation is given in Appendix A.

5.5   Implementation of Network-Channels

Network-channels — i.e. networked single (classical occam) channels — will be implemented as 'anonymous' NCTs that contain exactly one channel. This approach is similar to the implementation of the anonymous SHARED channels discussed in [13].

The following declaration:

```
NET CHAN INT iw!:              -- These network-channel-ends
NET CHAN BOOL br?:             -- must be allocated before
SHARED NET CHAN BOOL sbw!:     -- we can communicate over them!
SHARED NET CHAN INT sir?:
...   allocate iw!, br?, sbw!, sir?
...   use iw!, br?, sbw!, sir?
```

would have the semantics of:

```
CHAN TYPE $anon.INT            -- compiler-generated type
  MOBILE RECORD
    CHAN INT x?:               -- server-end holds reading-end
  :
```

```
CHAN TYPE $anon.BOOL              -- compiler-generated type
  MOBILE RECORD
    CHAN BOOL x?:                 -- server-end holds reading-end
  :

$anon.INT! iw$cli:
$anon.BOOL? br$svr:
SHARED $anon.BOOL! sbw$cli:
SHARED $anon.INT? sir$svr:
...  allocate iw$cli, br$svr, sbw$cli, sir$svr
...  use iw$cli, br$svr, sbw$cli, sir$svr
...  resp. iw$cli[x], br$svr[x], sbw$cli[x], sir$svr[x]
```

where the server-end of the compiler-generated channel-type by definition holds the reading-end of the channel. Before a process can communicate over a network-channel-end, that end needs to be allocated. This is done by allocation processes similar to those for NCT-ends. Details can be found in Appendix A.

Occurrences of network-channel-ends in user-level code are replaced by the compiler by the appropriate generated variables. In parameters, network-channel-ends are replaced by the generated channel-type-end (e.g. 'br?' is replaced by 'br$svr'). When used for communication, they are replaced by the actual channel-field (e.g. 'iw ! 5' is replaced by 'iw$cli[x] ! 5').

5.6 Connecting a Channel-Type-Block

As pointed out in Section 5.3, the connected-flag stores whether the network infrastructure and the GPCs for the CTB have already been set up. As soon as the live-reference-count becomes greater than 0 (which may be instantly after the allocation if the CTB is allocated into a live variable), the CTB must be connected. This is done (automatically by the run-time system) by first claiming the state-semaphore and updating the connected-flag, and then carrying out the following sequence of communications over the NCT-handle stored in the CTB:

```
nct.handle[req] ! connect; <chan-descs>; <cli-claimed>; <svr-claimed>
nct.handle[reply] ? connect; <cli-handle>; <svr-handle>;
                            <write-handles>; <read-handles>
```

- '<chan-descs>' is a 'MOBILE []CHAN.DESC' array whose size equals the number of channels in the CTB. 'CHAN.DESC' is the following record structure[7]:

  ```
  DATA TYPE CHAN.DESC
    RECORD
      BOOL write.read:
    :
  ```

  – 'write.read' specifies whether the channel is a writing-end or a reading-end from the point of view of the server-end of the CTB. It is either 'NET.WRITER' or 'NET.READER'.

---

[7]We implement the channel descriptor as a record, even though it contains only one element at present, in order to be able to easily extend it if necessary (e.g. to support the buffered channels planned for occam-π in the future).

- '<cli-claimed>' and '<svr-claimed>' are 'BOOL's. They specify whether the client-resp. server-end of the CTB is claimed at the moment when it is connected — which can only be the case if the CTB was in local or localised state and has just entered networked state (cf. Section 5.3).

- '<cli-handle>' and '<svr-handle>' are channel-type-ends of type 'CLI.HANDLE!' resp. 'SVR.HANDLE!', which will be stored in the CTB. The server-ends of the client- and the server-handle are held by the KRoC.net Manager.

- '<write-handles>' and '<read-handles>' are dynamic MOBILE arrays whose size equals the number of channels in the CTB. They contain channel-type-ends of type 'WRITE.HANDLE!' resp. 'READ.HANDLE!', who on their part contain the necessary channels to be plugged into the GPCs. (For details on how the GPCs work, refer to [17].) The server-ends of the write- and read-handles are held by the KRoC.net Manager.

The runtime system will then FORK off a DECODE.CHANNEL and an ENCODE.CHANNEL process for each channel in the CTB, and connect them to the reading- resp. writing-ends of the channel-ends in the CTB on the one hand, and to the writing- resp. reading-handles, that are connected to the KRoC.net Manager, on the other hand. When all this is done, the state-semaphore can be released.

5.7   Confirming the Connection of a CTB

If the CTB is in localised state and is already connected, changing back to networked state requires to 'confirm the connection' of the CTB (again, this is done automatically by the runtime system). The reason is that when the CTB is in networked state and connected, the KRoC.net Manager needs to know whether the client- resp. server-end of the CTB is claimed. Confirming the connection is done immediately after changing the state to networked (while the state-semaphore is still claimed), and implemented by the following communication sequence:

```
nct.handle[req]   ! confirm.connect; <cli-claimed>; <svr-claimed>
nct.handle[reply] ? confirm.connect
```

5.8   Shutting Down a Channel-Type-Block

If the reference-count of a CTB becomes 0 (which means that all its end-variables have gone out of scope or been overwritten), the runtime system will send a shut-down request to the NCT-handle:

```
nct.handle[req]   ! shut.down
nct.handle[reply] ? shut.down
```

The KRoC.net Manager will shut down the GPCs connected to the CTB and then send the reply. When the reply is received, the CTB can be deallocated.

Similarly, the entire KRoC.net Manager as such will be shut down by sending a shut-down signal to the network-handle at the very end of the main process.

6   Mobility of NCT-Ends

6.1   Claiming and Releasing NCT-Ends

In order to communicate over NCT-ends, they must be claimed from the KRoC.net Manager. This is done (automatically) by sending a request to the KRoC.net Manager over the client- resp. server-handle. For SHARED ends, this request will be generated at the beginning of a CLAIM block, right after the CTB's client- resp. server-semaphore has been successfully claimed. At the end of the CLAIM block, just before releasing the client- resp. server-semaphore, a release request is sent to the KRoC.net Manager in order to release the end.

Non-shared ends are claimed when the CTB gets connected. They remain claimed as long as they stay on the same node. When a non-shared end is sent to another node (see below), the DECODE.CHANNEL process is responsible for releasing the end before it leaves the old node. When the end is received by the destination node, the ENCODE.CHANNEL process immediately claims it again as soon as it arrives, provided that a connected CTB for that NCT already exists on this node; otherwise the end will be claimed, as pointed out above, when its new CTB gets connected.

The claim and release requests are (automatically) implemented as follows:

```
cli.or.svr.handle[req]   ! claim
cli.or.svr.handle[reply] ? claim

cli.or.svr.handle[req]   ! release
cli.or.svr.handle[reply] ? release
```

When the KRoC.net Manager receives a claim or a release request, it forwards it to the *administration node* of the NCT. Initially, this is the first node that allocates an end of that NCT. The CNS stores the administration node of each NCT. Should that node be shut down, the administration of the NCT will dynamically be moved to another node that holds a CTB that is part of the NCT.

The administration node holds FIFO queues of client-ends and server-ends that have made a claim request. When a previously claimed end is released, the next end in the queue is selected. When this happens, an acknowledgement is sent to the KRoC.net Manager of the node on which the end is located. This acknowledgement contains the current location of the opposite end of the NCT. The KRoC.net Manager then returns a reply over the client- resp. server-handle.

The network link between the nodes of the claimed client-end and the claimed server-end is established dynamically on demand.

6.2   Moving NCT-Ends

The movement of NCT-ends was inspired by the mobile channels in Muller and May's Icarus language [23]. However, implementing mobility for KRoC.net's NCT-ends is more complex because it needs to take into account the special properties of channel-types (e.g. that they are bundles of channels, that the ends may be shared, etc.), as well as KRoC.net's general architecture with the CNS etc.

Moving a channel-type-end is a three phase approach, automated within the KRoC.net infrastructure. Firstly, the DECODE.CHANNEL process reads the channel-type-end from the user-level application. If the CTB is local or localised, it claims the state-semaphore and changes the state to networked. If the state of the CTB was local, an implicit allocation is done via the network-handle, similar to the mechanism for explicit allocation described in Appendix A:

```
net[req]   ! alloc.implicit.sending; <x2x>; <c/s>; <ctb-pointer>
net[reply] ? alloc.implicit.sending; <nct-handle>
```

where '<c/s>' specifies whether a client-end or a server-end is sent away. The other fields have the same meaning as discussed in Appendix A. The KRoC.net Manager will contact the CNS, where the new NCT will be registered under an application-unique ID. This ID is a '$' followed by a number. As with explicitly allocated NCT-ends, the live-reference-count is checked and the CTB is connected/the connection confirmed if necessary when networked state is entered.

In the second stage, DECODE.CHANNEL sends a release request to the KRoC.net Manager if the end is non-shared and the CTB was already networked and connected. Then DECODE.CHANNEL passes the '<ctb-pointer>' to the KRoC.net Manager, together with a flag which indicates that this pointer refers to a channel-type-end rather than a data item. The KRoC.net Manager matches the '<ctb-pointer>' with the name or ID of the NCT to which the CTB belongs. Then it sends a special 'data packet' to the remote node, containing the name of the NCT. On the receiving node, the KRoC.net Manager finds out whether an NCT-end of that name is already located on the receiving node. If yes, it sets '<ctb-pointer>' to the pointer of the matching CTB — otherwise it sets '<ctb-pointer>' to 0. It sets '<is-localised>' to the correct value (i.e. TRUE in the cases mentioned in Section 5.3).

In the last stage, the KRoC.net Manager passes '<nct-name>', '<ctb-pointer>' and '<is-localised>' to ENCODE.CHANNEL. ENCODE.CHANNEL checks whether '<ctb-pointer>' is 0, in which case it allocates a new CTB and sets its initial state to 'networked'. Then it sends an 'implicit allocation' request via the network-handle:

```
net[req]   ! alloc.implicit.receiving; <x2x>; <c/s>; <nct-name>; <ctb-pointer>
net[reply] ? alloc.implicit.receiving; <nct-handle>
```

where '<c/s>' specifies whether a client-end or a server-end has been received. As with explicitly allocated NCT-ends, the live-reference-count is checked and the CTB is connected if necessary.

If the '<ctb-pointer>' received from the KRoC.net Manager was not 0, '<is-localised>' is checked. If it is TRUE, the state-semaphore of the (already existing) CTB would be claimed, the state be set to 'localised', and then the state-semaphore be released. If the (already existing) CTB does not become localised, and if it was already connected and the received NCT-end is non-shared, ENCODE.CHANNEL sends a claim request for the received end to the KRoC.net Manager.

Once this is all done, ENCODE.CHANNEL communicates a channel-type-end pointing to '<ctb-pointer>' to the user-level application.

7   Conclusions and Future Work

This paper has presented the specification of those of KRoC.net's features that were still missing in order for it to be fully transparent. The most important development was the specification of KRoC.net's mobility semantics. Other improvements have been made in order to make the use of KRoC.net as simple and intuitive as possible for the programmer. Wherever possible, we have used existing occam-π syntax and avoided inventing new syntax that would make occam-π more complicated. An example for this is the use of allocation processes rather than the previously proposed new special keywords.

We welcome feedback on all these plans. So far, the basic infrastructure for KRoC.net's network communication has been implemented. The next task will be the implementation of the new features discussed in this paper. This includes both the KRoC.net library, implemented in occam-π, and the compiler-related parts, such as the extension of the CTBs and the special compiler-generated processes.

Finally, when the implementation of KRoC.net will be fully completed, its performance needs to be examined by a new series of benchmarks.

Acknowledgements

The author is very grateful to Fred Barnes for his work on the KRoC compiler and his helpfulness in discussing the various issues arising from the development of KRoC.net and its integration into the KRoC environment. It has always been a great help to be able to rely on him implementing the compiler-related parts of KRoC.net.

The author would also like to thank the other members of the University of Kent's concurrency research group (Peter Welch, David Wood and Christian Jacobsen), as well as Matt Jadud and the anonymous reviewers. Their advice in reviewing this paper and their contributions to our many discussions on the project were very valuable.

References

[1] I. Foster, C. Kesselman, and S. Tuecke. What is the Grid? A Three Point Checklist. *GRIDToday*, July 2002. Available at: http://www-fp.mcs.anl.gov/~foster/Articles/WhatIsTheGrid.pdf.

[2] I. Foster, C. Kesselman, and S. Tuecke. The Anatomy of the Grid: Enabling Scalable Virtual Organizations. *International Journal of Supercomputer Applications*, 2001. Available at: http://www.globus.org/research/papers/anatomy.pdf.

[3] I. Foster, C. Kesselman, J.M. Nick, and S. Tuecke. The Psychology of the Grid: An Open Grid Services Architechture for Distributed Systems Integration. *Global Grid Forum*, June 2002. Available at: http://www.globus.org/research/papers/ogsa.pdf.

[4] Object Management Group. The Common Object Request Broker: Architecture and Specification (CORBA). Technical report, Object Management Group, December 1993. Available at: ftp://ftp.omg.org/.

[5] I. Foster and C. Kesselman. Globus: A Metacomputing Infrastructure Toolkit. *International Journal of Supercomputer Applications*, 1997. Available at: ftp://ftp.globus.org/pub/globus/papers/globus.pdf.

[6] IBM Corporation. Globus Toolkit 3.0 Quickstart, Redpaper. Technical report, IBM Corporation, 2003. Available at: http://www.redbooks.ibm.com/redpapers/pdfs/redp3697.pdf.

[7] Nicholas Carriero and David Gelernter. Linda in Context. *Communications of the ACM*, 32(4):444–459, April 1989.

[8] K.S. Pedersen and B. Vinter. Java PastSet: A Structured Distributed Shared Memory System. In James Pascoe, Peter Welch, Roger Loader, and Vaidy Sunderam, editors, *Communicating Process Architectures 2002*, WoTUG-25, Concurrent Systems Engineering, pages 97–108, IOS Press, Amsterdam, The Netherlands, September 2002. ISBN: 1-58603-268-2.

[9] MPI Forum. MPI-2: Extensions to the Message-Passing Interface. Technical report, MPI Forum, July 1997. Available at: http://www.mpi-forum.org/docs/mpi-20.ps.

[10] Indiana University LAM Team. LAM/MPI User's Guide. Technical report, Indiana University, May 2004. Available at: http://www.lam-mpi.org/download/files/7.0.6-user.pdf.

[11] P.H. Welch and D.C. Wood. The Kent Retargetable occam Compiler. In Brian O'Neill, editor, *Parallel Processing Developments, Proceedings of WoTUG 19*, volume 47 of *Concurrent Systems Engineering*, pages 143–166. World occam and Transputer User Group, IOS Press, Netherlands, March 1996. ISBN: 90-5199-261-0.

[12] Inmos Limited. occam 2.1 Reference Manual. Technical report, Inmos Limited, May 1995. Available at: http://www.wotug.org/occam/.

[13] Frederick R.M. Barnes. *Dynamics and Pragmatics for High Performance Concurrency*. PhD thesis, University of Kent, UK, Canterbury, Kent, CT2 7NF, June 2003.

[14] F.R.M. Barnes and P.H. Welch. Communicating Mobile Processes. In I. East, J. Martin, P. Welch, D. Duce, and M. Green, editors, *Communicating Process Architectures 2004*, WoTUG-27, Concurrent Systems Engineering Series, ISSN 1383-7575, IOS Press, Amsterdam, The Netherlands, September 2004.

[15] I.N. Goodacre. occam NetChans. Technical report, Computing Laboratory, University of Kent at Canterbury, UK, March 2001. Project report.

[16] M. Schweigler. The Distributed occam Protocol — A New Layer on Top of TCP/IP to Serve occam Channels Over the Internet. Master's thesis, Computing Laboratory, University of Kent, Canterbury, UK, September 2001.

[17] M. Schweigler, F.R.M. Barnes, and P.H. Welch. Flexible, Transparent and Dynamic occam Networking With KRoC.net. In J.F. Broenink and G.H. Hilderink, editors, *Communicating Process Architectures 2003*, WoTUG-26, Concurrent Systems Engineering Series, pages 199–224, IOS Press, Amsterdam, The Netherlands, September 2003. ISBN: 1-58603-381-6.

[18] P.H. Welch. Maintaining Structural Integrity in Dynamic Systems. Technical Report UKC-CRG-11-03-2004, Computing Laboratory, University of Kent, Canterbury, UK, March 2004.

[19] T.S. Locke. Towards a Viable Alternative to OO – extending the occam/CSP programming model. In Alan Chalmers, Majid Mirmehdi, and Henk Muller, editors, *Communicating Process Architectures 2001*, volume 59 of *Concurrent Systems Engineering*, pages 329–349, Amsterdam, The Netherlands, September 2001. WoTUG, IOS Press. ISBN: 1-58603-202-X.

[20] P.H. Welch. Process Oriented Design for Java – Concurrency for All. In *PDPTA 2000*, volume 1, pages 51–57. CSREA Press, June 2000. ISBN: 1-892512-52-1.

[21] C.A.R. Hoare. Communicating Sequential Processes. *Communications of the ACM*, 21(8):666–677, August 1978.

[22] C.A.R. Hoare. *Communicating Sequential Processes*. Prentice-Hall, 1985. ISBN: 0-13-153271-5.

[23] Henk L. Muller and David May. A simple protocol to communicate channels over channels. In *EURO-PAR '98 Parallel Processing, LNCS 1470*, pages 591–600, Southampton, UK, September 1998. Springer Verlag.

Appendix A: Allocation Processes

Allocation Processes for NCTs

To explicitly allocate an NCT-end, one of the following allocation processes must be called:

```
PROC net.alloc.one2one.client (GATE NET.HANDLE! net, <CT>! the.cli,
                               VAL []BYTE nct.name, RESULT INT result)
PROC net.alloc.any2one.client (GATE NET.HANDLE! net, SHARED <CT>! the.cli,
                               VAL []BYTE nct.name, RESULT INT result)
PROC net.alloc.one2any.client (GATE NET.HANDLE! net, <CT>! the.cli,
                               VAL []BYTE nct.name, RESULT INT result)
PROC net.alloc.any2any.client (GATE NET.HANDLE! net, SHARED <CT>! the.cli,
                               VAL []BYTE nct.name, RESULT INT result)

PROC net.alloc.one2one.server (GATE NET.HANDLE! net, <CT>? the.svr,
                               VAL []BYTE nct.name, RESULT INT result)
PROC net.alloc.any2one.server (GATE NET.HANDLE! net, <CT>? the.svr,
                               VAL []BYTE nct.name, RESULT INT result)
PROC net.alloc.one2any.server (GATE NET.HANDLE! net, SHARED <CT>? the.svr,
                               VAL []BYTE nct.name, RESULT INT result)
PROC net.alloc.any2any.server (GATE NET.HANDLE! net, SHARED <CT>? the.svr,
                               VAL []BYTE nct.name, RESULT INT result)
```

The process names are fairly self-explanatory. 'one2one' means that the NCT has a non-shared client-end and a non-shared server-end; 'any2one' means that the NCT has a SHARED client-end and a non-shared server-end; etc.

- The first argument is the network-handle; the second argument is a (SHARED or non-shared, depending on the '<...>2<...>' part of the process name) client- or server-end of *any* possible channel-type that is in scope.

- 'nct.name' is the name of the NCT. This can be any name that does not start with '$'.

- 'result' is the return value of the process. It is either an OK or an error message (e.g. if the 'x2x' type is different from a previously allocated NCT-end of the same name, or if one is trying to allocate more than one non-shared end).

Each allocation process is implemented by the following communication sequence:

```
  net[req]   ! alloc; <x2x>; <c/s>; <phash>; <nct-name>
  net[reply] ? alloc; <result>; <ctb-pointer>; <is-localised>
[ net[req]   ! confirm.alloc; <ctb-pointer>
  net[reply] ? confirm.alloc; <nct-handle> ]
```

- '<x2x>' is the 'x2x' type of the channel-type, and carries one of the following constants: 'NET.ALLOC.ONE2ONE', 'NET.ALLOC.ANY2ONE', 'NET.ALLOC.ONE2ANY' or 'NET.ALLOC.ANY2ANY'.

- '<c/s>' specifies whether we want to allocate a client-end or a server-end. It is either 'NET.CLI' or 'NET.SVR'.

- '<phash>' is an 'INT' carrying the protocol-hash of the channel-type. It is determined using the 'PROTOCOL.HASH()' function described in [17].

- '<nct-name>' is a 'MOBILE []BYTE' array carrying the name of the NCT.

- '<result>' is an 'INT' and will be returned as the result of the allocation process. In order for the result to be an OK, the 'x2x' type and the protocol-hash must be the same as for any previously allocated NCT-ends of the same name. This is checked in the CNS, where these values are stored. Also, the client/server property must make sense; e.g. only one client-end can be allocated for a one2x channel-type etc.

- '<ctb-pointer>' is an 'INT' carrying the pointer to the CTB of the channel-type. If on our node there is already a CTB connected to a channel-type of the same name, the KRoC.net Manager will return the pointer to it. If not, it will return 0.

- '<is-localised>' is a 'BOOL' returned by the KRoC.net Manager. If '<ctb-pointer>' is 0, '<is-localised>' is ignored. Otherwise, if '<is-localised>' is TRUE, the state-semaphore of the (already existing) CTB would be claimed, the state be set to 'localised', and then the state-semaphore be released. The only case when this can happen is if the NCT is one2one, and one end has already been on the same node.

- If the '<result>' was an OK and the returned '<ctb-pointer>' was 0, the compiler-generated code would allocate a new CTB, set its initial state to 'networked', and send its pointer back to the KRoC.net Manager.

- The KRoC.net Manager would then return the NCT-handle, which would be stored in the CTB. This handle will then be used to communicate with the KRoC.net Manager with regards to this particular CTB.

The allocation process returns a channel-type-end pointing to '<ctb-pointer>'.

Allocation Processes for Network-Channels

These are the allocation processes for network-channels-ends:

```
PROC net.alloc.one2one.writer (GATE NET.HANDLE! net, <NCE> the.writer!,
                               VAL []BYTE nc.name, RESULT INT result)
PROC net.alloc.any2one.writer (GATE NET.HANDLE! net, SHARED <NCE> the.writer!,
                               VAL []BYTE nc.name, RESULT INT result)
PROC net.alloc.one2any.writer (GATE NET.HANDLE! net, <NCE> the.writer!,
                               VAL []BYTE nc.name, RESULT INT result)
PROC net.alloc.any2any.writer (GATE NET.HANDLE! net, SHARED <NCE> the.writer!,
                               VAL []BYTE nc.name, RESULT INT result)

PROC net.alloc.one2one.reader (GATE NET.HANDLE! net, <NCE> the.reader?,
                               VAL []BYTE nc.name, RESULT INT result)
PROC net.alloc.any2one.reader (GATE NET.HANDLE! net, <NCE> the.reader?,
                               VAL []BYTE nc.name, RESULT INT result)
PROC net.alloc.one2any.reader (GATE NET.HANDLE! net, SHARED <NCE> the.reader?,
                               VAL []BYTE nc.name, RESULT INT result)
PROC net.alloc.any2any.reader (GATE NET.HANDLE! net, SHARED <NCE> the.reader?,
                               VAL []BYTE nc.name, RESULT INT result)
```

'<NCE>' is a 'NET CHAN' network-channel-end as described in Section 5.5. The network-handle, network-channel-name and result parameters are the same as in the allocation processes for NCT-ends. The '.writer' processes are the equivalent of the '.client' processes; the '.reader' processes are the equivalent of the '.server' processes.

Communicating Process Architectures 2004
Ian East, Jeremy Martin, Peter Welch, David Duce, and Mark Green (Eds.)
IOS Press, 2004

A Comparison of Three MPI
Implementations

Brian VINTER[1]
University of Southern Denmark, Campusvej 55, DK-5230 Odense M, Denmark
John M BJØRNDALEN[1], Otto J ANSHUS and Tore LARSEN
University of Tromsø, N-903700 Tromsø, Norway

Abstract. Various implementations of MPI are becoming available as MPI is slowly emerging as the standard API for parallel programming on most platforms. The open source implementations LAM-MPI and MPICH are the most widely used, while commercial implementations are usually tied to special hardware platforms. This paper compares these two open-source MPI-implementations to one of the commercially available implementations, MESH-MPI from MESH-Technologies. We find that the commercial implementation is significantly faster than the open-source implementations, though LAM-MPI does come out on top in some benchmarks.

1. Introduction

MPI is becoming synonymous with parallel programming, and while far more powerful and advanced models such as HPF[1], JCSP.net[2] and PastSet[3] exist, the performance of MPI implementations are crucial to the overall application performance on clusters. Since most applications are based on MPI, several commercial applications are available only in MPI versions. A search for "MPI programming" on Amazon.com yielded 593 books on the subject. A custom MPI implementation is always delivered with dedicated supercomputers, but for cluster-computers, home-built and brand-name systems alike, one must choose from a variety of MPI implementations where MPICH[4] and LAM-MPI[5] are the best known since they are open-source distributions.

Several commercial MPI implementations are also surfacing, where the best known products are ScaMPI from SCALI[6] and MPI/Pro from MPI-Softtech Solutions[7]. The commercial products often claim improved performance over MPICH and a high level of support as the primary reasons why one needs a commercial MPI implementation[6][7].

One newcomer on the commercial MPI scene is MESH-MPI from MESH-Technologies[8]. MESH-MPI is promoted purely on improved performance and is thus an obvious candidate for a comparative study against the open-source implementations. This study is a quantitative performance comparison that determines if and where MESH-MPI improves the performance over MPICH and LAM-MPI.

This paper is organized as follows. Section 2 introduces MPI and section 3 describes the experiment environment: the cluster and various MPI implementations. In section 4, the benchmarks are presented and, in section 5, the experiment results are presented and analyzed. Finally, we draw our conclusions in section 6.

---

[1] This author is also associated with MESH-Technologies

2. Message Passing Interface

The Message Passing Interface, MPI[12], is a controlled API standard for programming a wide array of parallel architectures. Though MPI was originally intended for classic distributed memory architectures, it is used on various architectures from networks of PCs via large shared memory systems, such as the SGI Origin 2000, to massive parallel architectures, such as Cray T3D and Intel paragon. The complete MPI API offers 186 operations, which makes this is a rather complex programming API. However, most MPI applications use only six to ten of the available operations.

MPI is intended for the *Single Program Multiple Data* (SPMD) programming paradigm – all nodes run the same application-code. The SPMD paradigm is efficient and easy to use for a large set of scientific applications with a regular execution pattern. Other, less regular, applications are far less suited to this paradigm and implementation in MPI is tedious.

MPI's point-to-point communication comes in four shapes: standard, ready, synchronous and buffered. A *standard-send* operation does not return until the send buffer has been copied, either to another buffer below the MPI layer or to the network interface, (NIC). The *ready-send* operations are not initiated until the addressed process has initiated a corresponding receive-operation. The *synchronous* call sends the message, but does not return until the receiver has initiated a read of the message. The fourth model, the *buffered* send, copies the message to a buffer in the MPI-layer and then allows the application to continue. Each of the four models also comes in *asynchronous* (in MPI called *non-blocking*) modes. The non-blocking calls return immediately, and it is the programmer's responsibility to check that the send has completed before overwriting the buffer. Likewise a non-blocking receive exist, which returns immediately and the programmer needs to ensure that the receive operation has finished before using the data.

MPI supports both group broadcasting and global reductions. Being SPMD, all nodes have to meet at a group operation, i.e. a broadcast operation blocks until all the processes in the context have issued the broadcast operation. This is important because it turns all group-operations into synchronization points in the application. The MPI API also supports scatter-gather for easy exchange of large data-structures and virtual architecture topologies, which allow source-code compatible MPI applications to execute efficiently across different platforms.

3. Experiment Environment

3.1 Cluster

The cluster comprises 51 Dell Precision Workstation 360s, each with a 3.2GHz Intel P4 Prescott processor, 2GB RAM and a 120GB Serial ATA hard-disk[2]. The nodes are connected using Gigabit Ethernet over two HP Procurve 2848 switches. 32 nodes are connected to the first switch, and 19 nodes to the second switch. The two switches are trunked[3] with 4 copper cables, providing 4Gbit/s bandwidth between the switches, see Figure 1. The nodes are running RedHat Linux 9 with a patched Linux 2.4.26 kernel to support Serial ATA. Hyperthreading is switched on, and Linux is configured for Symmetric Multiprocessor support.

---

[2] The computers have a motherboard with Intel's 875P chipset. The chipset supports Gigabit Ethernet over Intel's CSA (Communication Streaming Architecture) bus, but Dell's implementation of the motherboards use an Intel 82540EM Gigabit Ethernet controller connected to the PCI bus instead.
[3] Trunking is a method where traffic between two switches is loadbalanced across a set of links in order to provide a higher available bandwidth between the switches.

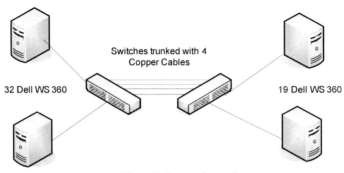

Figure 1: the experiment cluster

3.2 MPICH

MPICH is the official reference implementation of MPI and has a high focus on being portable. MPICH is available for all UNIX flavors and for Windows, a special GRID enabled version, MPICH-G2, is available for Globus[11]. Many of the MPI implementations for specialized hardware, i.e. cluster interconnects, are based on MPICH. MPICH version 1.2.52 is used for the below experiments.

3.3 LAM-MPI

Local Area Multicomputer-MPI, LAM-MPI, started out as an implementation for running MPI applications on LANs. An integrated part of this model was 'on-the-fly' endian-conversion to support different architectures to collaborate on an MPI execution. While endian-conversion still is supported, it is no longer performed per default as it is assumed that most executions will be on homogenous clusters. The experiments in this paper are performed with LAM-MPI 7.0.5.

3.4 MESH-MPI

MESH-MPI is only just released and the presented results are thus brand-new. MESH-MPI is 'yet-another-commercial-MPI', but with a strong focus on performance, rather than simply improved support over the open-source versions. In addition to improved performance, MESH-MPI also promotes true non-blocking operations, thread safety, and scalable collective operations. Future versions have announced support for a special Low Latency Communication library (LLC) and a Runtime Data Dependency Analysis (RDDA) functionality to schedule communication. These functions are not available in the current version which is 1.0a.

4. Benchmarks

This section describes the benchmark suites we have chosen for examining the performance of the three MPI implementations. One suite, Pallas, is a micro-benchmark suite, which gives a lot of information about the performance of the different MPI functions, while the other, NPB, is an application/kernel suite, which describes the application level performance. The NPB suite originates from NASA and is used as the basis for deciding on new systems at NASA. This benchmark tests both the processing power of the system and the communication performance.

4.1 Pallas Benchmark Suite

The Pallas benchmark suite[9] from Pallas GmbH is a suite, which measures the performance of different MPI functions. The performance is measured for individual operations rather than on the application level. The results can thus be used in two ways; either to choose an MPI implementation that performs well for the operations one uses, or to determine which operations performs poorly on the available MPI implementation so that one can avoid them when coding applications. The tests/operations that are run in Pallas are:

- PingPong
  The time it takes to pass a message between two processes and back
- PingPing
  The time it takes to send a message from one process to another
- SendRecv
  The time it takes to send and receive a message in parallel
- Exchange
  The time it takes to exchange contents of two buffers
- Allreduce
  The time it takes to create a common result, i.e. a global sum
- Reduce
  The same as Allreduce *but the result is delivered to only one process*
- Reduce Scatter
  The same as Reduce *but the result is distributed amongst the processes*
- Allgather
  The time it takes to collect partial results from all processes and deliver the data to all processes
- Allgatherv
  Same as Allgather, *except that the partial results need not have the same size*
- Alltoall
  The time it takes for all processes to send data to all other processes and receive from all other processes – the data that is sent is unique to each reciever
- Bcast - the *time it takes to deliver a message to all processes*

4.2 NAS Parallel Benchmark Suite

The NAS Parallel Benchmark, NPB, suite is described as:

> *The NAS Parallel Benchmarks (NPB) are a set of 8 programs designed to help evaluate the performance of parallel supercomputers. The benchmarks, which are derived from computational fluid dynamics (CFD) applications, consist of five kernels and three pseudo-applications. The NPB come in several flavors. NAS solicits performance results for each from all sources.*
> [10]

NPB is available for threaded, OpenMP and MPI systems and we naturally run the MPI version. NPB is available with five different data-sets, A through D, and W which is for workstations only. We use dataset C since D won't fit on the cluster, and also since C is the most widely reported dataset.

The application kernels in NPB are:

- MG – *Multigrid*
- CG – *Conjugate Gradient*
- FT – *Fast Fourier Transform*
- IS – *Integer Sort*
- EP – *Embarrassingly Parallel*
- BT – *Block Tridiagonal*
- SP – *Scalar Pentadiagonal*
- LU – *Lower Upper Gauss-Seidel*

5. Results

In this section we present and analyze the results of running the benchmarks from section 3 on the systems described in section 2. All the Pallas benchmarks are run on 32 CPUs (they run on 2^x sized systems) as are the NPB benchmarks except BT and SP which are run on 36 CPUs (they run on X^2 sized systems).

5.1 Pallas Benchmark Suite

First in the Pallas benchmark is the point to point experiments, the extreme case is the concurrent Send and Recv experiments where MPICH uses more than 12 times longer than MESH-MPI, but otherwise all three are fairly close. MPICH performs worse than the other two and the commercial MESH-MPI loses only on the ping-ping experiment.

The seemingly large differences on ping-pong and ping-ping are not as significant as they may seem since they are the result of the interrupt throttling rate on the Intel Ethernet chipsets which – when set at the recommended 8000, discretises latencies in chunks of 125us, thus the difference between 62.5 us and 125us is not as significant as it may seem and would probably be much smaller on other Ethernet chipsets.

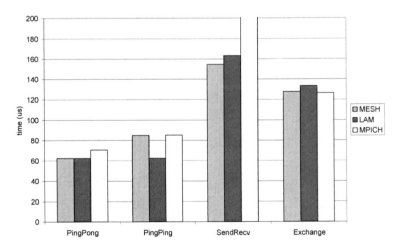

Figure 2: point-to-point latencies from Pallas 0B messages.

Switching to large messages, 4MB, the picture is more uniform and MPICH consistently looses to the other two. LAM-MPI and MESH-MPI are quite close in all these experiments and are running within 2% of each other. The only significant exception is in the ping-ping experiment where LAM-MPI outperforms MESH-MPI with 5%.

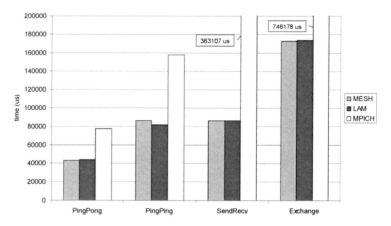

Figure 3: point-to-point latencies from Pallas 4MB messages.

In the collective operations, the small data is tested on 8B (eight bytes) rather than 0B because 0B on group-operations are often not performed at all and resulting times are reported in the 0.05us range, thus to test the performance on small packages we use the size of a double precision number. The results are shown in Figure 4.

In the collective operations, the extreme case is `Allgatherv` using LAM-MPI which reports a whopping 4747us or 11 times longer than when using MESH-MPI. Except for the `Alltoall` benchmark where LAM-MPI is fastest, MESH-MPI is consistently the faster, and for most experiments, the advantage is significant, measured in multiples rather than percentages. The `Bcast` operation, which is a frequently used operation in many applications, shows MESH-MPI to be 7 times faster than MPICH and 12 times faster than LAM-MPI.

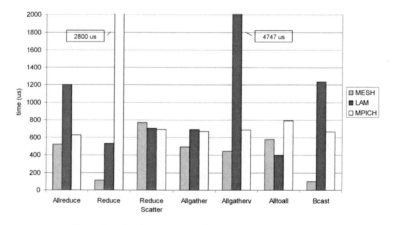

Figure 4: collective Operations latencies from Pallas 8B messages.

For large messages, the results have been placed in two Figures, 5 and 6, in order to fit the time-scale better. With the large messages, MESH-MPI is consistently better than both open-source candidates, ranging from nothing, -1%, to a lot: 11 times. On average MESH-MPI outperforms LAM-MPI with 4.6 times and MPICH with 4.3 times. MESH-MPI is on average 3.5 times faster than the best of the two open-source implementations.

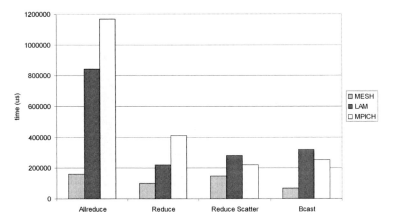

Figure 5: collective Operations latencies from Pallas 4MB messages.

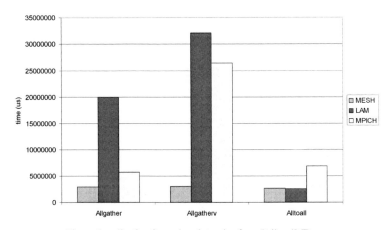

Figure 6: collective Operations latencies from Pallas 4MB messages.

5.2 NPB Benchmark Suite

While micro-benchmarks are interesting from an MPI perspective, users are primarily interested in the performance at application level. Here, according to Amdahl's law, improvements are limited by the fraction of time spent on MPI operations. Thus the runtime of the NPB suite is particularly interesting, since it allows us to predict the value of running a commercial MPI, and it will even allow us to determine if the differences at the operation level performance can be seen at the application level.

The results are in favour of the commercial MPI; MESH-MPI finished the suite 14.5% faster than LAM and 37.1% faster than MPICH. Considering that these are real-world applications doing real work and taking Amdahl's law into consideration, this is significant.

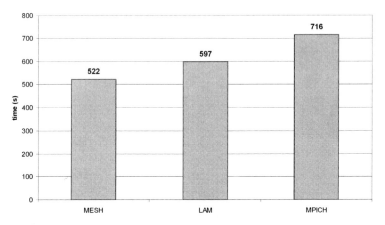

Figure 7: runtime of the NPB benchmark

If we break down the results in the individual applications the picture is a little less obvious and LAM-MPI actually outperforms MESH-MPI on two of the experiments; the FT by 3% and the LU by 6%. Both of these makes extensive use of the Alltoall operation where MESH-MPI has the biggest problems keeping up with LAM-MPI in the Pallas tests.

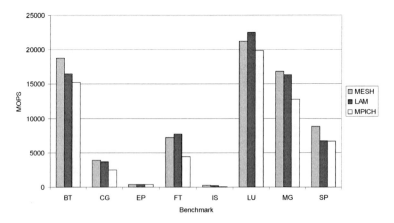

Figure 8: runtime of the individual NPB benchmarks

6. Conclusions

Overall the commercial MPI implementation from MESH-Technologies seems strong and yields results as much as 12 times better than the open source implementations, and at worst 30% worse. The really interesting part is when testing the application level performance, and a 14.5% improvement over the best open-source alternative is significant. Now, MESH-MPI is a commercial product and the obvious question to ask is what is the value of this MPI implementation compared to other computing costs?

If we look at the experiment cluster used in this work the nodes are priced at € 1428 per node. Thus the intrinsic value of a 14.5% improvement in performance is € 206 and € 530 with the improvement of 37.1% in the case of MPICH. Taking the electricity consumption into consideration with each node using 210W and another 25% for cooling the value rises to € 292 and € 749 in Norway and € 386, respectively € 991 in Denmark.

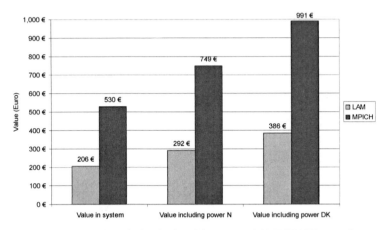

Figure 9: the calculated value of the commercial MESH-MPI per node

Acknowledgements

The authors would like to thank MESH-Technologies for the donation of MESH-MPI for the new cluster installation at the computer science department at Tromsø University. We would also like to thank Morten M. Pedersen for his numerous and detailed comments to this work.

References

[1] An Introduction to High Performance Fortran, John Merlin and Anthony Hey, `ftp://ftp.vcpc.univie.ac.at/vcpc/jhm/jnl/hpf.ps.gz`.

[2] CSP networking for java (JCSP.net). P.H.Welch, J.R.Aldous, and J.Foster. In P.M.A.Sloot, C.J.K.Tan, J.J.Dongarra, and A.G.Hoekstra, editors, Computational Science - ICCS 2002, volume 2330 of Lecture Notes in Computer Science, pages 695-708. Springer-Verlag, April 2002. *See also* `http://www.quickstone.com/xcsp/jcspnetworkedition`.

[3] Brian Vinter, Otto J. Anshus and Tore Larsen. *PastSet A Distributed Structured Shared Memory System*, in the Proceedings of High Performance Computers and Networking Europe, Amsterdam April 1999.

[4] William Gropp and Ewing Lusk and Nathan Doss and Anthony Skjellum, High-performance, portable implementation of the MPI Message Passing Interface Standard, Parallel Computing", Vol 22, no 6, 789- -828, 1996.

[5] Greg Burns and Raja Daoud and James Vaigl, LAM: An Open Cluster Environment for MPI, Proceedings of Supercomputing Symposium, 379--386, 1994.

[6] `hhtp://www.scali.com/`

[7] `http://www.mpi-softtech.com/`

[8] `http://www.meshtechnologies.com`

[9] `http://www.pallas.com/e/products/pmb/index.htm`

[10] `http://www.nas.nasa.gov/Software/NPB/`

[11] `http://www.globus.org/`

[12] David W. Walker. The design of a standard message passing interface for distributed memory concurrent computers. Parallel Computing, 20(4):657–673, March 1994.

Communicating Process Architectures 2004
Ian East, Jeremy Martin, Peter Welch, David Duce, and Mark Green (Eds.)
IOS Press, 2004

137

An Evaluation of Inter-Switch Connections

Brian VINTER and Hans Henrik HAPPE

University of Southern Denmark, Campusvej 55, DK-5230 Odense M, Denmark

Abstract. In very large clusters it is not possible to get Ethernet-switches that are large enough to support the whole cluster, thus a configuration with multiple switches are needed. This work seeks to evaluate the interconnection strategies for a new 300+ CPU cluster at the University of Southern Denmark. The focal point is a very inexpensive switch from D-Link which unfortunately offers only 24 Gb ports. We investigate different inter-switch connections and their impact at application level.

1. Introduction

Cluster computing is today the most widespread architecture for supercomputing for the obvious reason that they offer inexpensive scalable solutions to most computing needs. We have earlier designed and build a 512 CPU cluster[1] based on 100Mb Ethernet. When designing with 100Mb networks a balanced interconnect could be obtained using 24 port 100Mb switches connected through a 1Gb switch, thus getting a 2.4:1 ratio on the internal to external available bandwidth. Today the standard PC is equipped with 1 Gb network interface and thus needs a 10Gb connection for a 24 port switch to keep the same ratio as we achieved on the previous 100Mb system. Unfortunately 10Gb Ethernet is currently targeted for long haul network backbones and thus priced far beyond what is available for cluster computer production.

Ethernet switches are time consuming[8] and the time of passing an Ethernet package through one switch is defined by:

$$T(1) = T(Overhead) + T(Channel) + T(Routing)$$

where T(Overhead) is usually small, less than 2 us, and T(Routing) is less than 0.5 us on most modern switches. That leaves the T(Channel) as the major problem and this is heavily dependent on whether the switch is a 'store-and-forward' type, where the complete package is received at the switch before it is sent on to the receiver, or a 'worm-hole' switch, which forwards the data as they arrive. For a 'store-and-forward' switch we actually get:

$$T(1) = T(Overhead) + 2*T(Channel) + T(Routing)$$

As we expand the number of switches we get:

$$T_{worm-hole}(n) = T(Overhead) + T(Channel) + n*T(Routing)$$
$$T_{store-and-forward}(n) = T(Overhead) + n*(T(Channel) + T(Routing)) + T(Channel)$$

Unfortunately, Ethernet is mainly used for office use where store-and-forward has its advantages; thus worm-hole switches are not available and we have to use store-and-forward switches.

Now another opportunity has presented itself with the introduction of the D-Link 3324 series switch that are 24 port Gb switches with dedicated 10Gb uplink ports. The switch comes in two flavors: 3324sr with two 10Gb uplink ports and 3324sri with six uplinks running at 10Gb. The 3324 series can either be stacked to a height of 12 using only the 3324sr switches to a total of 288 Gb ports. Alternatively a 3324sri can be connected with up to six 3324sr switches to a total of 168 available Gb ports.

We are looking for at solution that scales beyond 300 CPUs – thus none of the solutions intended by D-Link are sufficient for our needs. Fortunately the 3324 is a layer 3 switch that offers link trunking and we thus imagine a system with two times 168 CPUs connected by an 8 Gb trunk. The question then is what is the impact of this?

In section 2, we describe the system used for the experiments. In section 3, the benchmarks are described and, then, the results are analyzed in section 4. Finally, the conclusions are summarized in section 5.

2.   Test System

2.1   Cluster

The experiments are carried out on the SDU Roadrunner cluster, which consists of 48 nodes each with 1.7 GHz Intel Celeron CPU, i845 chipset and 256MB memory. Half the nodes (24) have an Intel Ethernet Express/Pro 1000 gigabit Ethernet adapter in addition to the onboard 100Mb NIC. The experiments will thus be carried out using these machines.

2.2   Switches

The experiments are centered on two D-Link 3324 switches, a 3324sr and a 3324sri. Since the purpose of the experiment is to investigate the effects of using two interconnected switches we choose a scenario where we use 24 nodes which can then be connected to one or two switches. Thus the results of the two-switch experiments can be compared to the performance when running on only one switch.

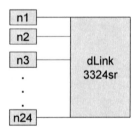

Figure 1: the "flat" model where all nodes are connected to one switch.

An identical experiment will be performed with the regular Gbit switch in Roadrunner, a HP2824, to verify the performance of the switches themselves.

The switches are intended to be interfaced through the dedicated 10Gb link which naturally will be the first alternative to running on one switch. The dedicated 10Gb link maintains the 2.4:1 ratio we have in our existing system which we know to be well balanced for most applications.

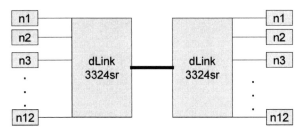

Figure 2: the "10G" model where the nodes are connected to two switches interconnected by a dedicated 10Gb link.

Unfortunately we cannot base the complete system on the 10Gb connections since these are limited to 288 ports in the stacking model and 168 in the star configuration. The 3324 however allows trunking of multiple links between two switches, thus we will also experiment with trunks from eight links, which is the maximum, down to a single link connecting the machines.

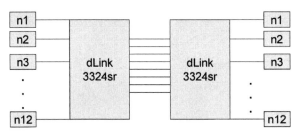

Figure 3: the "8" through "1" model where the nodes are connected to two switches interconnected by a trunk of width 1-8 links.

2.3 Trunking Algorithm

Trunking of ports between Ethernet switches means that the load is distributed across multiple links in order to obtain a higher bandwidth, in essence parallel paths from one switch to another. The 3324 comes with six algorithms for distributing the load over the trunked links. These algorithms really are just hash-keys to map incoming packages to ports. The available keys are IP source, IP destination, IP source and destination, MAC source, MAC destination and finally MAC source and destination. The switch comes with default setting of IP source, which makes good sense since nodes will often have a uniform distribution of IP addresses.

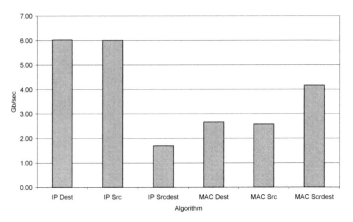

Figure 4: the performance of the different trunking algorithms.

The algorithms were tested with the code shown in Figure 5. The nodes in Roadrunner have contiguous IP addresses and the IP source model seems to fit the performance well, although the absolute result of 6 Gb/sec seems somewhat low. Thus for the remaining experiments we keep the IP source algorithm.

3. Benchmarks

Many benchmarks exists for testing cluster-computer performance, including micro-benchmarks such as Pallas[3], NAS[4] and HPL[5]. We have been designing and building clusters for a while, including the largest cluster within the Nordic countries, Horseshoe[6][7] and have developed a set of benchmarks that represents the type of code that our users run. The user base is 45% chemistry, 25% bio-science, 15% plasma-physics and the remaining 15% is distributed across a quite diverse group of researchers. The benchmark suite is used for testing all aspects of our system including CPU's, compute-nodes, compilers and in this case networking.

3.1 Bandwidth

We test the available bandwidth in two ways, a 'raw' test where a set of NPtcp tests are run in parallel and a structured test where 24 MPI processes exchange 10 messages of each 10MB.

```
partner = (rank+size+size/2)%size;
start=second();
for(i=0;i<10;i++){
  MPI_Irecv(in, dsize, MPI_BYTE, partner, 42, MPI_COMM_WORLD, &flag);
  MPI_Send(out,dsize, MPI_BYTE, partner, 42, MPI_COMM_WORLD);
  MPI_Wait(&flag, (void *)0);
}
stop=second();
if(rank==0)printf("%lf sec\n",stop-start);
```

Figure 5: the simple bandwidth test.

3.2 Monte Carlo Estimate of π

Monte Carlo methods are a widely used group of numerical methods, which involve sampling from random numbers. The Monte Carlo method can be used to solve otherwise intractable problems. Since Monte Carlo applications are based on random events a large number of such events must typically be processed to ensure a realistic result. The Monte Carlo method we use here, Monte Carlo π, is utterly uninteresting in and of itself but exhibits the same behavior as real world Monte Carlo applications as well as the related Las Vegas methods and random walks, all of which are frequently used in physics, biology and finance.

The Monte Carlo estimation of π is embarrassingly parallel, and is included as a sanity-check, if we do not get perfect speedup on this application there is an error somewhere.

3.3 Lower Upper Factorization

To perform the LU decomposition in parallel we basically have two choices, either divide the matrix by rows or by columns. If we divide the system by columns then one processor alone can decide the pivot row and broadcast the pivot to all processors. After this an all-to-all communication phase is needed to create a copy of the active row at all nodes. If the matrix is distributed row-wise then an actual election of the best pivot value is needed. After the election the process that won the election broadcasts its row.

We chose the row-wise solution in order to reduce the large messages to a one-to-all broadcast. Including the partial pivot this means that each iteration use two synchronous group operations, one election of the best divisor and a broadcast of the 'winning' row.

3.4 SOR

Successive Over-Relaxation, SOR, is a frequently used technique for solving very large systems of partial differential equations by successive approximations. The general idea is to approximate each element in a matrix to its neighbors until the sum of all changes within one iteration converges below a given value. The Red-Black checker pointing version of SOR, returns identical results for the same system of equations; independent of the actual computing environment, while at the same time providing sufficient parallelism that real speedup can be achieved. With Red-Black checker pointing, the equation system is divided into alternating red and black points in a chess-board fashion. Updating a red point depends only on black neighboring points and vice versa. Using this, an algorithm is derived where each worker-process updates all its red points and then exchanges red border point values with its neighbors. Each worker then updates its black points and repeats the communication for the black points. At the end of each iteration the global change in the system is calculated and the process continues until the change in the system is below a given threshold.

3.5 WATOR

The WAter TORus world, WATOR, is a classic discrete event simulation[1], and while it provides valuable information in itself we chose to introduce it here for reasons similar to the Monte Carlo π example, namely that it is simple and easy to understand, while still being typical for the class of applications that it represents. Discrete event simulations are widely used to model everything from digital systems to financial forecasts, logistics and traffic simulations.

WATOR is the simulation of a very special world; first of all the planet is not a sphere as most planets we know, rather the planet is shaped as a doughnut, or a torus, which greatly simplifies mapping the world into discrete blocks. As the whole surface of WATOR is covered with water there are only two types of life that we are interested in: fish and sharks.

Fish are simple organisms that move around at random, and at some point when a fish comes of age is will have two children and die itself. A fish can move into any of its neighboring eight squares, given that the square is empty, if all eight neighboring squares are occupied the fish remains in place. At any discrete time step a fish becomes one time-unit older, and once it has come of age it will split into two fish, one of which will go to a neighbor cell while the other stays in the cell where it was born, both new fish is age zero.

Sharks are similar simple creatures, however sharks also need to eat fish in order to survive. At each time-step a shark moves to a random neighboring cell which holds a fish, if there are no fish which neighbors the shark it moves to a random neighboring cell and increases its hunger index, if the hunger index reaches a starvation limit the shark dies, when the shark eats it resets the hunger index to zero. Similar to fish, sharks will at some point get old enough to breed and once this age is reached the shark is replaces by two new sharks, both with age and hunger index zero.

Thus the simulation of one time-step consists of two steps, first all fish are moved, then the sharks, each step issues four asynchronous MPI operations, two send and two receive. The randomness of the application allows us to ignore further synchronization issues.

3.6   Traveling Salesman Problem

The Traveling Salesman Problem, TSP, is a classic representative for the class of global optimization problems. The TSP solution we use in this work is a depth-first branch-and-bound algorithm which makes the parallel version different from the other applications we use by the fact that a static division of the work would result in a highly unbalanced execution. Thus the parallel TSP is implemented as a bag-of-tasks application, a paradigm that does not come natural to the SPMD programming paradigm that MPI is designed around.

The parallel TSP is implemented as a global master process and set of worker-threads on each node, each thread communicates with the master to retrieve jobs and submit results. A job is represented as a set of cities that have already been placed and a set that need to be placed, i.e. a sub-tree. Each job that is sent from the master has the length of the shortest known route piggy-backed and each node maintains one shared instance of the bound value. Since the application is so highly unbalanced in the workload this application use synchronous messages for communication. A scheme for applying asynchronous messages could be developed, but two things talk against it, first of all an asynchronous scheme would place an extra job at each node, which is likely to increase the load-unbalance.

3.7   Matrix Multiplication

Matrix multiplication is frequently used in scientific applications. Although several concurrent and parallel algorithms exist that require extensive communications during the calculation, an alternative approach is to distribute the matrixes coarsely amongst the nodes and broadcast one matrix to all nodes one block at a time.. This approach is similar to the one used in PBLAS [2].

We have chosen a less generic, but more efficient, algorithm where we maintain both A and B in distributed state and thus only need to broadcast one matrix to the other processes. Also, the matrix is not broadcast column by column, but the entire block at once. Each node uses an efficient sub-blocked matrix-multiplication to take advantage of cache-memory.

The MPI solution results in one synchronous broadcast per node in the overall execution. The broadcasts are rather large however and will stress the switch significantly.

4.   Results

4.1   Bandwidth

The first bandwidth test consists of twelve parallel NPtcp runs where nodes 1-12 transmits to nodes 13-24, the test is not synchronized and from the results it is apparent that some of the tests terminate before the last starts. This can be seen from the fact that using one Gb link the test yields 250Mb/sec which cannot be offered to 12 nodes at a time since this would be 3 Gb/sec.[1]

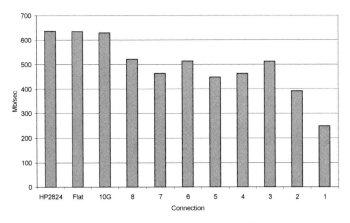

Figure 6: the bandwidth process measured with NPtcp.

The bandwidth test in figure 6 shows a somewhat lower bandwidth but it seems that this is due to the performance of the nodes and the MPI implementation. We are using LAM MPI for these experiments and this can be the reason for the difference in bandwidth between figures 4 and 6. As a sanity check we have run the experiments on the HP2824 switch also and that performs exactly as the D-Link 3324. Thus we can assume that the limited bandwidth is not a result of the switch. This has been verified by running the MPI-bandwidth test on a faster cluster using the lower grade HP2724 switch. In this scenario 8.2 Gb/s was achieved with only 16 nodes.

---

[1] The PCI bus unfortunately has problems breaking the 500Mb barrier on our system.

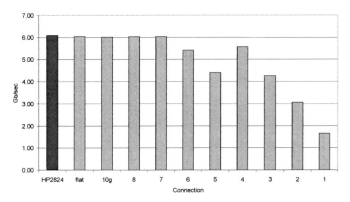

Figure 7: the bandwidth measured with the MPI program from Figure 5.

From the "4-trunk" down to the "1-trunk" we see a linear decrease in throughput which is what one would expect. With one Gb link the throughput is down to 1.7 Gb, less than the maximum of two Gb but still a reasonable performance.

4.2 Applications

The applications all run quite well and only when the bandwidth between the node becomes very low do two of the applications exhibit an actual performance decrease. Figure 8 shows the increased runtime for all the applications when the two switches are connected by a single link. Obviously only the LU and Matrix Multiplication applications are influenced by the limited bandwidth. Interestingly both of these applications depend heavily on broadcasts.

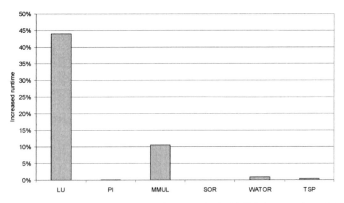

Figure 8: the increased runtime when running on a single Gb link between the switches.

The experiments below were run in two setups; one where MPI was given the nodes in sequence ("linear") and one where they were set up on each side of the switches ("cross").

4.2.1 LU

The LU test fluctuates quite a lot in its execution times, however it is evident that the "linear" boot-sequence performs worse than the "cross" sequence. The poor performance for the "cross" model on the "2-trunk" is hard to explain, but otherwise the "linear" is much worse and when only one link is available runtime increases by almost 45%.

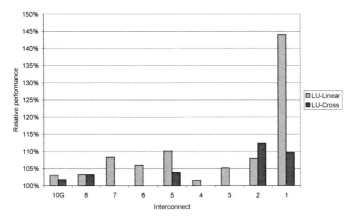

Figure 9: the impact of the interconnect on the LU application.

4.2.2 Matrix Multiplication

The Matrix Multiplication test is not as sensitive to the bandwidth as the LU test but in this experiment it is significant that the "cross" boot-schema performs much worse than the "linear". Once again the "2-trunk" model performs worse than the others but otherwise it is clear that even a 4 Gb connection between the switches is sufficient to satisfy this application.

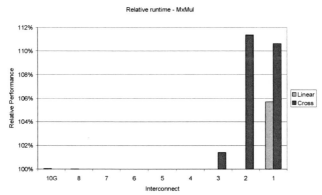

Figure 10: the impact of the interconnect on the Matrix Multiplication.

5. Conclusions

None of the applications exhibit performance degradation above 5% as long as the connection ratio does not drop below 1:6 and most of the applications don't reach any level of degradation at all.

Thus we conclude at we can base our large installation on these cheap switches and propose the layout shown in figure 11. For most jobs we can maintain the 2.4:1 ratio and only when more than 152 CPU's are used will we be forced to attempt the 19:1 ratio. If an application suffers from this ratio it will have to be forced to exist with one of the two "wings" in figure 11 where the 2.4:1 ratio is maintained.

The 10Gb uplinks deliver what was promised and this allows us to maintain the existing 2.4:1 ratio, if we force an application to stay within one 152 CPU segment of the cluster, that we know scales to 652 CPU's today. Thus we dare conclude that since this existing ratio can also be meet here we dare base our new cluster on the D-Link switches.

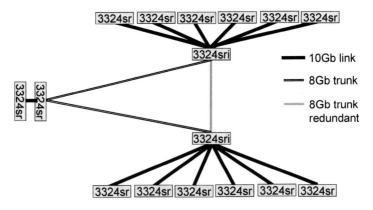

Figure 11: the final 304 port switch design.

Acknowledgements

We would like to thank D-Link for lending us the switches for these experiments.

References

[1] A.K. Dewdney. *Computer recreations*. Scientific American, 250:22–34, 1984.
[2] Almadena Chtchelkanova, John Gunnels, Greg Morrow, James Overfelt, and Robert A. van de Geijn. *Parallel implementation of BLAS: General techniques for level 3 BLAS*. Technical report, The University of Texas at Austin Austin, Texas 78712, 1995.
[3] http://www.pallas.com/e/products/pmb/index.htm
[4] http://www.nas.nasa.gov/Software/NPB/
[5] http://www.netlib.org/benchmark/hpl/
[6] Brian Vinter, *Design and implementation of a 512 CPU cluster as a general purpose SuperComputer*. Proceedings of ParCo 2003, Dresden University of Technology.
[7] http://www.dcsc.sdu.dk/
[8] Cost/Performance evaluation of Gigabit ethernet and Myrinet as Cluster Interconnect, Proceedings of Opnetwork 2000, Washington, DC, August 2000.

Communicating Process Architectures 2004   147
Ian East, Jeremy Martin, Peter Welch, David Duce, and Mark Green (Eds.)
IOS Press, 2004

Observing Processes

A.E. Lawrence

Department of Computer Science, Loughborough University, Leicestershire LE11 3TU, UK.

Abstract. This paper discusses the sorts of observations of processes that are appropriate to capture priority. The standard denotational semantics for CSP are based around observations of traces and refusals. Choosing to record a little more detail allows extensions of CSP which describe some very general processes including those that include priority. A minimal set of observations yields a language and semantics remarkably close to the standard Failures-Divergences model of CSP which is described in a companion paper [1]. A slightly richer set of observations yields a somewhat less abstract language.

1 Introduction

The characterisation of processes by their externally observable behaviour is fundamental in CSP. It is a general principle that processes that cannot be distinguished by observation ought to be identified. An attempt to extend the language should entail a precise elucidation of the nature of observations. The amount of detail in observation determines the level of abstraction.

Once an observational model is established, the way is opened for a process algebra defined by a denotational semantics. The operators of the process algebra are defined compositionally by describing the observations or behaviours in terms of those of their components. This is a mapping from syntax to a representation of behaviour. The accompanying paper [1] is an example for *CSPP*, a CSP like language which includes priority.

The sort of observation envisaged, and the amount of detail included, determines many of the characteristics of the resulting theory. Glabbeek has demonstrated this clearly in a series of papers: [2], [3] and [4]. He produces a taxonomy of various semantics, classified by the sort of observations admitted.

This issue is particularly acute in extending CSP because the semantics for the standard theory uses observations that collect insufficient information to capture priority. Extending the observational model is crucial in adding priority to CSP. In Fidge's approach [5], the standard description of the behaviour of a process was augmented with a *preferences* function. *preferences*(P) is a set of partial orders among events and captures the extra information about priority. However, there is no explicit discussion in [5] about the observational status of preferences. Can processes with different *preferences* always be distinguished? What observations are needed to fully characterize such processes? In Lowe's thesis, [6], a timed and prioritised CSP is presented. The behaviours have the form $(\tau, \sqsubseteq, s)$ where $\sqsubseteq$ is also essentially a partial order on events, at least at any instant. In Lowe's approach, $\sqsubseteq$ carries much of the semantic information: it determines which events can be performed by a process at any instant as well as the extra information needed to capture priority. However, the status of observation is not entirely clear.

CSPP is an attempt to produce an initially untimed simple and intuitive extension of CSP particularly for use in hardware compilation. It is based upon a denotational approach called acceptances which is fundamentally observational, although a thorough examination of its observational status was not conducted initially. Since the semantics is a mapping to observations, the nature of the observations must be clearly established. Then the operators can be defined in terms of the observational behaviours. This paper addresses the first stage: the companion paper [1] shows one version of the second stage.

Following this programme has been very fruitful: examining the observations appropriate for *CSPP* throws light on the approaches by Fidge and Lowe above. More importantly, it became evident that *CSPP* can describe a *far* wider class of processes that those that can be described by priority. It also allowed a simplification and clarification of the axioms.

This paper is intended to be largely self-contained, although many readers will be familiar with *CSPP* from previous papers in this conference series. Some previous exposure to CSP is assumed.

2   Observations

In CSP and most process algebras, the primary notions are those of an event and an environment. Events are observable: that already implies that they are communications with the environment. In CSP there is usually a stronger intuition that an event requires the active participation of the environment. The idea of internal events also arises, but the very term signals that they are not directly observable.

Processes as abstract models of systems are to be characterised by their behaviour: the circumstances in which they perform, or perhaps fail to perform, events needs careful examination. Such behaviour is often formulated in terms of ideal experiments. A process is somehow started, events performed perhaps as the result of some actions by the observer, and the results recorded. Just what is recorded, or what the observer is supposed to be able to distinguish, determines, among other things, the level of abstraction. A thorny issue is that of livelock. How can this be recognised? The halting problem shows that a real observer could never determine in all cases whether a system was in an infinite loop. Nevertheless, we need to represent livelock in decidable cases, so we envisage ideal 'infinite experiments' which can detect this situation.

One of the simplest sort of observation is that of a trace. The only thing that an observer records is the events that a process performs, and the sequence in which they happen. In the context of CSP, the environment must have been willing to perform the recorded events. Indeed, if the trace records are to be useful to describe the process, then all possible offers must be available. If

$$P = (a \rightarrow a \rightarrow Stop) \,\square\, (b \rightarrow b \rightarrow Stop)$$

was not offered the possibility of performing b events, then we would have an incomplete record. Here we have

$$traces\,(P) = \{\langle\rangle, \langle a\rangle, \langle aa\rangle, \langle b\rangle, \langle bb\rangle\}\,.$$

Notice that the empty trace $\langle\rangle$ is included, although one might wonder whether that qualifies as an 'observation' here. Clearly the experimeter has performed at least two experiments: there was one while a copy of the process performed the maximal trace $\langle aa\rangle$ and another for $\langle bb\rangle$. Was this done with the 'same' process? Presumably there were experiments in which other events, c perhaps, were offered. Otherwise, it might be that the process being observed was actually

$$Q = (a \rightarrow a \rightarrow Stop) \,\square\, (b \rightarrow b \rightarrow Stop) \,\square\, (c \rightarrow Stop)\,.$$

So the circumstances of the experiments need clarification. What events are offered? To which copies of the process are offers made? Can a process, especially a quantum process, always be duplicated? When and how may a process silently undergo internal transformations? Is it possible to 'freeze' internal activity? How long are events offered before it is concluded that the process cannot perform an event? In the untimed theories, there is an assumption that if a process can perform an event then it will be accepted eventually. The need to offer an event and maintain that offer until it is either accepted or rejected becomes an important issue in implementing an untimed process. Can an offer be made and then withdrawn and another made?

This paper examines the sorts of observations that are suitable for capturing the behaviour of a class of processes including those which involve the use of priority.

3 Failures

The standard denotational semantics for CSP is based on Failures. These, like traces, are observations of events. The traces are recorded as before, but now the recording is enriched by noting which offers were made and rejected. This is enough to distinguish

$$P = (a \to Stop) \,\Box\, (b \to Stop) \quad \text{from} \quad Q = (a \to Stop) \sqcap (b \to Stop)$$

which share the traces $\{\langle\rangle, \langle a\rangle, \langle b\rangle\}$. A Failure is a pair (s, R) where s is a possible trace of the process in question and R is a refusal set. That is, it is an offer that the process *may* refuse after it has performed s. So Q can refuse the offer $\{a\}$ initially, that is, on the trace $\langle\rangle$: recording the empty trace is now necessary. But P cannot refuse $\{a\}$.

Notice that the information recorded is sparse: only the traces, and *only* the offers that are refused after a particular trace. This is just enough information to distinguish P from Q above, and accounts for the very abstract nature of CSP. This leads to results like

$$(a \to Stop) \,\Box\, (b \to Stop) \sqcap (a \to Stop) \sqcap (b \to Stop) = (a \to Stop) \sqcap (b \to Stop) \quad (1)$$

in standard CSP. The presence of the external choice on the left hand side cannot be unambiguously detected in the presence of the internal choices by such observations.

The standard model for CSP does also record when a process can livelock, or diverge. We admit ideal infinite experiments as a sort of 'observation' to permit that.

4 Priority

Priority is a way of expressing a preference when more than one course of action is available. In the context of process algebra, this involves a selection when more than one event is possible.

Any general theory of shared events which includes priority must address the issue of contention. The decision of whether an event may be performed in general requires arbitration or negotiation: information must be exchanged before an event happens. There must be

1. a declaration;

2. arbitration or negotiation;

3. and a possible action.

A full theory cannot abstract entirely from these matters. In particular, useful systems will normally connect compliant processes to those that employ priority. A compliant process is one which is neutral with respect to available events: it will conform to the preference expressed by a partner. More importantly, compliant processes offer a choice of events to the environment. And since an environment is no more than a way of capturing the behaviour of parallel partners, a theory without compliant processes is deficient. If an enviroment can offer a choice, that must come about because there are processes which can do the same. Clearly the observations must be sufficient to distinguish and characterise compliant processes as well as those which express priority. In this sense, observations of a process have to include some elements of the declaration phase.

The observations of acceptances below seem to be as sparse as possible while fulfilling these requirements. Actually, the declaration phase can be inferred for some classes of processes. The experiments to be performed are similar to those described earlier, but now more details are recorded. The events actually performed are still recorded as traces, but now the offers are also recorded in every case, not just those that are refused. But there is more: in addition, the response is also recorded. That is the records take the form of triples (s, X, Y) where X is an environmental offer made after the process has performed the trace s, and Y is the response. It is most natural to assume that Y is directly observable, and this a very reasonable view of both hardware and software systems that employ priority. However, this is not strictly necessary for one can conduct additional experiments and observe which events can be performed after s and the offer X provided a suitable replication facility is available. This is necessary because nondeterministic processes may have more than one response in the sense that (s, X, Y_1) and (s, X, Y_2) may both be possible, and it must be possible to reliably 'freeze and replicate' if these two responses are to be distinguished properly. The reason why this is not an unreasonable expectation will be clearer in a moment. But it is far simpler and entirely realistic to assume that the responses Y_1 and Y_2 are directly observable which we assume below.

An important point is that the response from a process is reliable. A process that declares to the environment which events it is prepared to perform and then does not honour the commitment is of no use. Processes can be very nondeterministic, and resolve that nondeterminism partially or fully at any time *except* between declaring a response and performing one of the declared events. Processes that do not do that have no place in a system employing priority. In this sense a process must freeze its internal activity between responding to an offer and either performing an event or responding to a further offer. But if an offer is repeated, the process need not give the same response.

Our standard example is $AB = (a \rightarrow Stop) \overset{\leftarrow}{\square} (b \rightarrow Stop)$ which is represented by the triples

$$\{(\langle\rangle, \{a, b\}, \{a\}), (\langle\rangle, \{a\}, \{a\}), (\langle\rangle, \{b\}, \{b\}), (\langle\rangle, \emptyset, \emptyset),$$
$$(\langle a\rangle, \{a, b\}, \emptyset), (\langle a\rangle, \{a\}, \emptyset), (\langle a\rangle, \{b\}, \emptyset), (\langle a\rangle, \emptyset, \emptyset),$$
$$(\langle b\rangle, \{a, b\}, \emptyset), (\langle b\rangle, \{a\}, \emptyset), (\langle b\rangle, \{b\}, \emptyset), (\langle b\rangle, \emptyset, \emptyset)\},$$

when the only events are a and b. An alternative notation for the triple (s, X, Y) is $s : X \rightsquigarrow Y$, so the triples above can be summarised as

$$\langle\rangle : \quad X \quad \rightsquigarrow \quad \{a\} \blacktriangleleft a \in X \blacktriangleright X \cap \{a, b\}$$
$$\langle a\rangle : \quad X \quad \rightsquigarrow \quad \emptyset$$
$$\langle b\rangle : \quad X \quad \rightsquigarrow \quad \emptyset .$$

AB gives priority to $(a \rightarrow Stop)$, so if it is given an offer X which includes both a and b, it will respond with just $\{a\}$. It will only accept b when a is not also offered.

Readers not familiar with *CSPP* may find helpful the contrast between the example of the compliant variant $C = (a \rightarrow Stop) \overset{\leftrightarrow}{\square} (b \rightarrow Stop)$ and

$$\langle\rangle : \quad X \quad \rightsquigarrow \quad X \cap \{a, b\}$$
$$\langle a \rangle : \quad X \quad \rightsquigarrow \quad \emptyset$$
$$\langle b \rangle : \quad X \quad \rightsquigarrow \quad \emptyset$$

When offered both a and b, it replies with the compliant $\{a, b\}$.

To illustrate the exchange of information, which in general may involve arbitration or contention, consider C and AB running in parallel, synchronising on all events: $AB \parallel C$ or explicitly

$$\left((a \rightarrow Stop) \overset{\leftarrow}{\square} (b \rightarrow Stop) \right) \parallel \left((a \rightarrow Stop) \overset{\leftrightarrow}{\square} (b \rightarrow Stop) \right) . \tag{2}$$

If the environment offers $\{a, b\}$ the responses from the two components are $\{a, b\}$ and $\{a\}$, so a occurs. In fact the process in equation (2) is just AB again. In contrast,

$$\left((a \rightarrow Stop) \overset{\leftarrow}{\square} (b \rightarrow Stop) \right) \parallel \left((a \rightarrow Stop) \overset{\rightarrow}{\square} (b \rightarrow Stop) \right) . \tag{3}$$

the two components in equation (3) answer with $\{a\}$ and $\{b\}$ and there is a disagreement. So we have *contention* and may need *arbitration*. Our observational model does not determine the outcome of this priority conflict: that is a matter of the semantics of the operators, primarily of $\parallel$. One answer is given in the second paper [1]: it is deadlock. But there are other versions of *CSPP* in which the result is a nondeterministic choice.

In passing, note that Lowe has very different forms of parallel operators. His parallel operators are always biased, even on shared – synchronised – events: this arises from his desire to remove all except one form of nondeterminism in order to simplify the transition to a probabilistic theory.

In both equations (2) and (3), it is clear that information must be exchanged between the components and the environment to determine which events, if any, can be agreed by the processes. Implementations may involve a scheduler which needs to discover which processes are ready to do what, or arbitration hardware may be involved.

It is in this sense that we contend that there is a need for some abstract form of declaration and arbitration or negotiation in general before events can be selected.

5 Experiments

Ideal experiments are performed on a process: it is made an offer and eventually produces a response which is normally a set of events but may be instead an indication of termination or (perhaps after an infinite wait) of livelock. The environment may now either change the offer, or select an event from the response to jointly perform. If the environment takes the former course and makes another offer, the first offer is termed *hesitant*. Hesitant offers model situations where an environment negotiates with a process to find a mutually agreed event. We noted earlier that the process must be stable when it produces a response in the sense that it is prepared to perform any of the events in that response. But it is allowed to undergo internal transitions when a new offer is made: hiding can produce processes which are naturally understood in this way. Consequently a single copy of a process which has performed a trace s can be nondeterministic about the response to a given offer.

These ideal experiments include observations of infinite duration, and detection of livelock may require such. But some processes with knowledge of their internal construction can immediately declare livelock in appropriate circumstances.

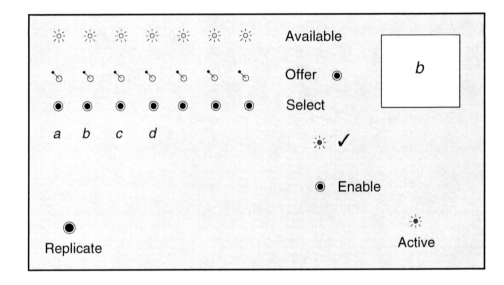

Figure 1: A machine which displays an acceptance matching an offer.

6   A Machine

In [4], [7] and particularly [2] R.J.Glabbeek describes and classifies a series of ideal machines to capture observations of processes. Figure 1 shows a machine in this spirit for observing *CSPP* processes. The machine has three rows: the first labelled *Available*, of lights; the second labelled *Offer*, of switches; and the third labelled *Select*, of buttons. Each column matches an event. The top row of lights displays the events which can be performed in the context of the second row switch settings. Valid processes will only display a light matching a switch which is on. The top row is continuously updated to match the setting of the second row switches while the process is waiting for the environment to initiate an event. That is the function of the third row of buttons. Pressing a single button matching an illuminated *Available* light results in that event happening. The display in this machine is largely redundant, but it shows each event as it occurs as in Glabbeek's machines. The machine has a green light marked ✓. This illuminates when the process inside the machine is prepared to terminate. No other light can be on at the same time as the ✓ light. Pressing the *Enable* button at such a moment will allow termination and end the experiment: ✓ will be shown on the display. Otherwise further offers can be explored. There is also a red light to indicate internal activity: in Glabbeek's machines, this light is green. The *Replicate* button, present in many of Glabbeek's machines, produces a cascade of copies of the machine and its contents in the current state.

It is a misuse of the machine to press a *Select* button when the associated light is off: if the button is so pressed, nothing will happen. The machine might be designed to lock buttons at these times to eliminate this eventuality. If the *Replicate* button is pressed while the active light is off, then the machine and its contents in its current state is copied.

It is clear that the switch setting corresponds to X and the state of the lights to Y in (s, X, Y). The machine is used as follows.

1. When a process starts, the active light is on. Eventually, a response is produced on the event lights including the ✓ light. The active light turns off at this point and enables a

refusal to be recognised. Livelock is recognised in an ideal infinite experiment by the active light staying on.

2. The switches may now be updated in which case the active light turns on at least briefly, and a new response displayed.

3. When a response is displayed and the *Active* light is off, a *Select* button matching an illuminated event light may be pressed: the event then happens. If the $\checkmark$ light is on, then the *Enable* button may be pressed to terminate the experiment. In an ideal infinite experiment, the *Enable* button may be pressed after livelock has been detected: this will also complete the experiment after another infinite time. Some processes with knowledge of their internal construction can predict livelock, and an extra light could be added to the machine to permit this to be passed to the environment as a normal response in a similar way to the $\checkmark$ light.

The recordings made in such experiments are just the (s, X, Y) trace–offer–response triples. The number or order in which the offers are made at a particular s in an experiment is not recorded.

If it is known that a system to be modelled does not involve hesitant offers, then a restricted set of observations can be made. After an event has occurred, the new offer must be set up instantly on the switches. Otherwise an additional *sample* button can be added to introduce each offer. Clearly the set of acceptances collected in such observations will be a subset of those when hesitant offers are included.

7   A Minimal Record: Triples

Recording only the triples as above provides the maximum abstraction with the minimum assumptions about the nature of the processes being observed. Consider the processes

$$
\begin{aligned}
P_1 &= \overleftrightarrow{\{a, u\}} \to \overrightarrow{\{b, v\}} \to Stop \\
P_2 &= \{[\{a\} > \{u\}]\} \to \{[\{b\} > \{v\}]\} \to Stop \\
P_3 &= \overleftrightarrow{\{a, u\}} \to \{[\{b\} > \{v\}]\} \to Stop \,.
\end{aligned}
\tag{4}
$$

The notation $\overleftrightarrow{E} \to P$ is an abbreviation for the compliant prefixing $x : \overleftrightarrow{E} \to P$ which is a process which is prepared to perform any of the events from the set E and thereafter behave like the process P: its initial triples have the form $(\langle\rangle, X, X \cap E)$. If it is offered several events in E, it accepts all of them. So P_1 is a process which is always compliant: initially it is prepared to perform either a or u according to the wishes of its environment. On the next step it will perform either b or v before stopping.

The notation $\{[\{a\} > \{u\}]\} \to P$ is an abbreviation for the biased prefixing $x : \{[\{a\} > \{u\}]\} \to P$ which starts with a preference for a rather than u, so its initial triples have the form $(\langle\rangle, X, \{a\} \blacktriangleleft a \in X \blacktriangleright (X \cap \{u\}))$.

Thus P_2 has the same traces and possible events as P_1, but on the first step it gives priority to a and on the second priority to b. P_3 is like P_1 on the first step, and then behaves like P_2. Now consider $P_1 \sqcap P_2$. If our only observations are of triples, then $P_1 \sqcap P_2$ can behave like P_3. So

$$
P_1 \sqcap P_2 = P_1 \sqcap P_2 \sqcap P_3 \,.
$$

The reason that these processes cannot be distinguished is that the only 'history' in our triples are the traces, and P_1, P_2 and P_3 share these. Should $P_1 \sqcap P_2$ be allowed to behave like

P_3? We may have processes which defer the resolution of internal indeterminism so that the behaviour after each event is only selected at that point, perhaps according to the outcome of a radio-active decay. Then one might argue that a specification $P_1 \sqcap P_2$ should permit a behaviour matching P_3. A less abstract view in which a richer set of records is included is described below. That distinguishes $P_1 \sqcap P_2$ from $P_1 \sqcap P_2 \sqcap P_3$ while still permitting the extreme form of late resolution of nondeterminism to be properly described.

The very abstract approach using just triples is in the spirit of the Failures-Divergences model of standard CSP, has most properties in common, but includes priority. In fact, it goes far beyond processes that can be described with priority or compliance. It describes almost any process that can respond to an offer, produce a reliable response and perform events.

The version of $CSPP$ based on triples constrains processes in the least possible way. The set of triples representing a process P is written as $\mathcal{B}(P)$. The triples have type

$$\mathcal{A} = \{(s, X, Y) \mid s \in \Sigma^* \wedge X \subseteq \Sigma \wedge (Y \subseteq X \vee Y = \{\checkmark\} \vee Y = \{\boldsymbol{X}\})\} . \tag{5}$$

Σ is the set of all possible events, excluding the 'tokens' $\checkmark$ and $\boldsymbol{X}$ which are used to represent termination and livelock. Σ^* is the standard notation for the set of all finite traces, including $\langle\rangle$, drawn from Σ. $\mathcal{B}(P) \subseteq \mathcal{A}$ ensures that the response Y to an offer X is either a subset of the events offered in Y, or is an indication of termination or livelock. The axioms are intended to be minimal:

1. $\langle\rangle \in traces(P)$.

2. There is a triple $(s, X, Y) \in \mathcal{B}(P)$ for each offer X.

3. Traces and responses match properly:
   $s^\frown \langle x \rangle \in traces(P) \Leftrightarrow \exists(s, X, Y) \in \mathcal{B}(P) \bullet x \in Y \cap \Sigma.$

The requirement $\mathcal{B}(P) \subseteq \mathcal{A}$ might be regarded as an additional axiom.

8   Recording History: Behaviours

Recording only the triples (s, X, Y) gives a very abstract form of $CSPP$ which turns out to closely mirror the standard Failure-Divergence semantics of standard CSP. However, there are some slightly disturbing features of the model: in particular, several of the operators including some forms of parallel and sequential composition and hiding fail to distribute over $\sqcap$. This can be understood as a side effect of recording only the traces that lead up to a particular offer and response. Recording a little more information, namely the history of an experiment as the set of responses along a trace turns out to have several advantages. We collect *behaviours* for each experiment. An experiment follows a process along some trace. At each point in the evolution a record of the responses is made. That is, we have a relation, a set of pairs (X, Y) at each point along some trace s. This means that a behaviour b, the record of the evolution along some trace s, is a function $b : \downarrow s \to \left(\mathbb{P}\Sigma \leftrightarrow \overset{\checkmark X}{\mathbb{P}} \Sigma^{\checkmark X} \right)$. The downset $\downarrow s = \{t \mid t \leqslant s\}$ is the set of all prefixes of s: this is a standard notation from the theory of partial orders [8]. $\mathbb{P}S$ is the power set: $\mathbb{P}S = \{U \subseteq S\}$, and $\overset{\checkmark X}{\mathbb{P}} S$ adds the sets $\{\checkmark\}$ and $\{\boldsymbol{X}\}$ so $\overset{\checkmark X}{\mathbb{P}} S = \mathbb{P}S \cup \{\{\checkmark\}, \{\boldsymbol{X}\}\}$. The set of of binary relations between sets S and T is written $S \leftrightarrow T$ so it is an alias for $\mathbb{P}(S \times T)$, [9]. Thus $\mathbb{P}\Sigma \leftrightarrow \overset{\checkmark X}{\mathbb{P}} \Sigma^{\checkmark X}$ is the set of relations consisting of pairs (X, Y) with $X \subseteq \Sigma$ and Y which is either also a subset of Σ, in our case $Y \subseteq X$, or may be one of the singleton sets $\{\checkmark\}$ and $\{\boldsymbol{X}\}$. Hence $b : \downarrow s \to \left(\mathbb{P}\Sigma \leftrightarrow \overset{\checkmark X}{\mathbb{P}} \Sigma^{\checkmark X} \right)$ records the history of the observations of an experiment which ended after the $\{(X, Y)\}$ offer-response relation on s was recorded. A process is characterised as a set of such behaviours.

Once again, the sort of process to be described is not artificially constrained. The axioms are now

1. $t \in \downarrow s \;\Rightarrow\; \downarrow t \lhd b \in \mathcal{B}(P)$.

2. $s \smallfrown \langle x \rangle \in traces(b) \Rightarrow \exists (X, Y) \in bs \bullet x \in Y$
   and
   $s \in traces(b) \wedge \exists (X, Y) \in bs \bullet x \in Y \Rightarrow$
   $\exists b' \in \mathcal{B}(P) \bullet traces(b') = \downarrow(s \smallfrown \langle x \rangle) \wedge b < b'.$

The first axiom requires that we keep records of each prefix of s as a separate experiment. $\lhd$ is domain restriction. The second axiom requires that responses and traces match properly. If the experiment ends when a real event could have been accepted, then there is another behaviour b' which describes the extension of the experiment. As before, the type constraint on $b \in \mathcal{B}(P)$ may be regarded as an extra implicit axiom.

Recording the history of observations in this way now allows us to distinguish $P_1 \sqcap P_2$ from $P_1 \sqcap P_2 \sqcap P_3$ where the processes are given by equation (4). Extreme processes that do not resolve internal nondeterminism until the last moment can still be described, but now we can tell when they are present.

9   Internal and External Nondeterminism

It is evident that the response Y to an offer X is a declaration by a process of which events it is prepared to perform. Whenever the response contains more than one event, this is an invitation to the environment to make a choice. This is an example of *external* nondeterminism. It is an essential feature of useful systems employing priority: it must be possible to arrange synchronisation of events when one partner has a preference.

The tokens $\checkmark$ and $\boldsymbol{X}$ have a special status here. It makes no sense to offer the environment a choice between these pseudo-events and the ordinary 'real' events in Σ. Thus in all our models and experiments, these tokens may only appear as a 'response' as the singletons $\{\checkmark\}$ and $\{\boldsymbol{X}\}$.

Internal nondeterminism is manifested when there is more that one response possible to a given offer X. The standard examples are

$$E = (a \rightarrow Stop) \; \overset{\leftrightarrow}{\Box} \; (b \rightarrow Stop)$$
$$I = (a \rightarrow Stop) \sqcap (b \rightarrow Stop)$$

The compliant E manifests external, and I internal, nondeterminism. Internal nondeterminism is more extreme in that it is outside environmental control.

10   Conclusions

The status of observations which can capture very general processes including those which can express priority have been examined. The minimal axioms that naturally arise for a couple of levels of abstraction have been described. Versions of *CSPP* based on such observations can describe a very wide class of real time systems: some rather irregular processes which cannot be described by any conventional form of priority are included. The companion paper [1], outlines the most abstract of these which bears a remarkable congruence with the standard Failures-Divergence model of CSP.

References

[1] A. E. Lawrence. Triples. In *Communicating Process Architectures – 2004*, volume 62 of *Concurrent Systems Engineering*, pages 157–184, Amsterdam, Sept 2004. IOS Press.

[2] R.J. van Glabbeek. The linear time – branching time spectrum II; the semantics of sequential systems with silent moves (extended abstract). In E. Best, editor, Proceedings *CONCUR'93*, 4th International Conference on *Concurrency Theory*, Hildesheim, Germany, August 1993, volume 715 of LNCS, pages 66–81. Springer-Verlag, 1993.

[3] R.J. van Glabbeek. What is branching time semantics and why to use it? In M. Nielsen, editor, *The Concurrency Column*, pages 190–198. *Bulletin of the EATCS* 53, 1994. Also available as Report STAN-CS-93-1486, Stanford University, 1993, at http://theory.stanford.edu/branching/, and in G. Paun, G. Rozenberg & A. Salomaa, editors: *Current Trends in Theoretical Computer Science; Entering the 21st Century*, World Scientific, 2001.

[4] R.J. van Glabbeek. The linear time – branching time spectrum I; the semantics of concrete, sequential processes. In J.A. Bergstra, A. Ponse, and S.A. Smolka, editors, *Handbook of Process Algebra*, chapter 1, pages 3–99. Elsevier, 2001. Available at http://boole.stanford.edu/pub/spectrum1.ps.gz.

[5] C.J. Fidge. A formal definition of priority in CSP. *ACM Transactions on Programming Languages and Systems*, 15(4):681–705, September 1993.

[6] Gavin Lowe. *Probabilities and Priorities in Timed CSP*. D. Phil thesis, Oxford, 1993.

[7] R.J. van Glabbeek. What is branching time semantics and why to use it? In G. Paun, G. Rozenberg, and A. Salomaa, editors, *Current Trends in Theoretical Computer Science; Entering the 21st Century*. World Scientific, 2001. Also available as Report STAN-CS-93-1486, Stanford University, 1993, at http://theory.stanford.edu/branching/, and in M. Nielsen, editor: *The Concurrency Column, Bulletin of the EATCS* 53, 1994, pp. 190–198.

[8] B.A. Davey and H.A. Priestley. *Introduction to Lattices and Order*. Cambridge University Press, 2nd edition, 2002.

[9] M. J. Spivey. The Z notation: A reference manual. http://spivey.oriel.ox.ac.uk/~mike/zrm/.

[10] C.A.R Hoare. *Communicating Sequential Processes*. Prentice Hall International, 1985.

[11] A.W. Roscoe. *The Theory and Practice of Concurrency*. Prentice Hall, 1998.

Communicating Process Architectures 2004 157
Ian East, Jeremy Martin, Peter Welch, David Duce, and Mark Green (Eds.)
IOS Press, 2004

Triples

A.E. Lawrence

Department of Computer Science, Loughborough University, Leicestershire LE11 3TU, UK.

Abstract. The most abstract form of acceptance semantics for a variant of *CSPP* is outlined. It encompasses processes which may involve priority, but covers a much wider class of systems including real time behaviour. It shares many of the features of the standard Failures-Divergences treatment: thus it is only a Complete Partial Order when the alphabet of events is finite.

1 Introduction

CSPP is a close relative of the process algebra CSP: [1], [2], [3]. It was designed originally to capture priority in the context of hardware compilation using a **occam**-like language. Its development has been informed by the work of the WoTUG community, and explorations of various sorts have been presented regularly in this conference series: [4], [5] [6], [7], [8], [9], [10], [11] and [12]. The intuition and core ideas have not changed and are transparent.

The **occam** community does not need any convincing that CSP is extremely simple and elegant: it well understands that this theoretical underpinning is responsible for the simplicity and power of **occam**. *CSPP* aspires to have the same simplicity and elegance, and to achieve that in the same way: by being properly defined by a mathematical theory. One motivation for its development was to provide the same sort of theoretical underpinning for future **occam**-like languages for co-design.

As with standard CSP, the routine use of the language is quite simple. But setting up a rigorous mathematical theory which covers all the obscure corners is a substantial task. Yet without that theory, we cannot be certain that there is no serious unrecognised trouble waiting to cause disaster.

The mathematical theories underlying process algebras are generally of three sorts: algebraic, operational and denotational. The characteristic flavour of CSP derives from the fact that the first full semantic models were denotational rather than operational: algebraic semantics also played an important role in the development as is evident in [1]. The denotational theories are still regarded as canonical, even though operational semantics have subsequently been developed. [2] gives a comprehensive account of many theories and their interplay.

Denotational semantic theories generally take the form of a mapping from syntax into a mathematical description of behaviour: behaviour which, in principle, is observable. The sorts of observation are not always carefully examined, but in CSP that is usually taken seriously, and can also be regarded as one of the roots of its power and simplicity. The companion paper, [13], is an examination of the observational model underlying *CSPP*.

The scrutiny of the observational basis of *CSPP* has been fruitful: the scope of the language has been extended far beyond systems that exhibit priority or neutrality. The language can now describe almost any system that can be understood to communicate what events it is prepared to perform in any given situation as described in [13]. One might question the relevance of this power in the context of the original design aims for *CSPP*: a foundation for concrete language design. The answer is that the aims have been widened: CSP is probably used mainly to describe and explore the properties of systems which have not themselves been designed with CSP. *CSPP* may eventually be able to play the same role for a wider class of behaviour.

The explicit examination of the observational model also helped elucidate the various denotational approaches that have been explored for *CSPP*. It shows how much detail should be recorded in order to achieve a particular level of abstraction in the resulting dialect. Some readers will see the analogy with, say, the traces and failures models for standard CSP.

This paper presents the most abstract version of *CSPP* based on these developments. The main components of the underlying theoretical model are included.

1.1   The Basic Ideas

Readers familiar with *CSPP* may wish to omit this introductory material. There are three elementary processes in CSP and so also in *CSPP*. *Stop* is the process which does nothing at all, not even terminate. It is usually an error such as deadlock, but as will be abundantly apparent below, it appears very frequently in examples because it so simple.

Skip is the second of the elementary processes and represents termination. In the semantics of CSP, *Skip* is treated as a process which autonomously performs a special event '$\checkmark$'. But in the semantics of *CSPP*, $\checkmark$ is treated as a 'token' rather than as a first class event: it is never 'performed' by a process, instead it is regarded as a signal to the external world. In *CSPP*, it is rather appropriate to say that '*Skip* does nothing, but does it successfully'.

The last process is written as div in CSP and in all except the most recent presentations of *CSPP*. We have recently taken to calling it *Spin* because there are technical connotations of div as the most undefined process which are inappropriate in *CSPP*. But whatever it is called, it represents livelock, a process that is in an uncontrollable sequence of internal actions, usually a loop. In the companion paper, [13], it is explained that in the semantics of *CSPP*, but not in CSP, we introduce a second 'token', which we write as ✗, which we pretend can be 'seen' by an external observer in an ideal infinite experiment.

Stop does nothing at all, not even terminate.

Skip terminates: hands control on to successor.

Spin does nothing at all externally: but it is active internally. Called div in CSP.

Prefixing provides a simple way to build more complex processes from *Stop*, *Skip* and *Spin*. So

- $a \rightarrow Stop$ is a process that performs the event a before stopping;

- $a \rightarrow Skip$ performs the event a before terminating; and

- $a \rightarrow Spin$ does a before typically looping internally for ever.

Another simple way to define a process using prefixing is to write $P = a \rightarrow P$. It is easy to see that this defines a process that will engage in an endless sequence of a events. It is also pretty clear that $Q = a \rightarrow Q$ must define the same process. But can we be sure? We may wonder exactly how we might establish that. What about $P = P$? This does not impose any constraint on P except the implied assumption that P is a process: it is evident that *every* process is a solution. These recursive definitions are at two extremes of a spectrum: one clearly defines a unique process, and the other is satisfied by any process. One may worry about intermediate cases, especially when the recursive equations get complicated. How do we know when there are solutions? Is there some special solution that we should pick when there are several? We can't answer such questions properly without some sort of underlying theory: the more technical later parts of this paper describe one approach.

Note that our examples of recursion above could all be written in the form $P = f(P)$ where f is a function from processes to processes. In the context of $CSPP$, we might write its type as $f : CSPP \to CSPP$. So that $P = a \to P$ matches $f(P) = a \to P$. Solutions to $f(P) = P$ are *fixed points*.

There is a standard mathematical notation for a fixed point of a function f: it is μf or $\mu P \bullet f(P)$. CSP and $CSPP$ use the same notation. Thus the solution of $P = a \to P$ is written $\mu P \bullet a \to P$. Perhaps the most important task in building a theory for any sort of CSP is establishing that fixed points exist with the right properties. Almost all non trivial uses of CSP involve recursion.

Abstraction in the sense of being able to ignore irrelevant or internal detail is a crucial tool for humans. CSP and its derivatives have the powerful notion of *hiding*, examined at length in [12]. The notation is $P \setminus H$ representing a process P where events in the set H are hidden: events from H performed by P become internal, invisible to, and thus uncontrollable by, the outside world. It should be no surprise then that

$$(\mu P \bullet a \to P) \setminus \{a\} = Spin ,$$

which shows how these operations interlock.

There are only 4 basic operations of CSP left. The first is a generalisation of prefixing. $(a \to P_a) \square (b \to P_b)$ is a process which is prepared either to perform the event a and then behave like P_a or to perform b and then behave as P_b. This is where the nature of events as joint actions between partners must be covered. A process P is understood as interacting with its *environment*, primarily by engaging in events which require the cooperation of both parties. Thus $a \to Stop$ cannot perform the event a until such time as the environment cooperates. This single concept covers a typical outermost passive observer who is willing to observe any event as well as parallel partners who may block certain events. The idea of blocking, that is synchronised, communication enters into the semantics of the parallel operators in a crucial way. The real point however is to capture the meaning of a process by external interaction with an agent as in [13].

The choice between a and b in $Q = (a \to P_a)\square(b \to P_b)$ is controlled by the environment in the sense that if it chooses one or the other that fixes the subsequent the behaviour of Q. Of course Q blocks the environment if that only offers another event c initially. For these reasons $\square$ is called external choice. The next operation arises from hiding and external choice and demonstrates more interlocking:

$$((a \to c \to Stop) \square (b \to d \to Stop)) \setminus \{a, b\} = (c \to Stop) \sqcap (d \to Stop) .$$

$\sqcap$ is called internal choice. The environment of the process above has no control over whether the process is prepared to perform c or d: that was determined by whether the event a or b happened internally. In general, $P_1 \sqcap P_2$ may behave like either P_1 or like P_2, but the environment has no influence over the choice.

The remaining ways of composing processes are to place them in parallel, or run them in sequence. $P_1 \| P_2$ is the parallel composition where any events in the set E must be jointly performed by P_1 and by P_2: any other events are interleaved. $P_1 \,\fatsemi\, P_2$ is the process which behaves like P_1 until such time, if ever, that it terminates. If P_1 does terminate, subsequently $P_1 \,\fatsemi\, P_2$ behaves like P_2. Thus $(a \to Skip) \,\fatsemi\, (b \to Stop) = a \to b \to Stop$.

$a \rightarrow P$ performs a when the environment is willing, and then behaves like P.

$\mu P \bullet f(P)$ covers recursion.

$P \setminus H$ has the events in H hidden, internalised.

$P_1 \square P_2$ is external choice: controlled by the environment.

$P_1 \sqcap P_2$ is internal choice.

$P_1 \|_E P_2$ is parallel composition with synchronisation set E.

$P_1 \fatsemi P_2$ is sequential composition.

1.2 *CSPP and Acceptances*

Can $N = (a \rightarrow Stop) \square (b \rightarrow Stop)$ favour a rather than b? Ordinary CSP abstracts away from such issues. The observations on which its semantics are based do not collect sufficient information to answer the question. Both Fidge's approach in [14] and Lowe's in [15] use order relations which can determine that a has greater priority than b.

CSPP is based on a more fundamental observational approach called acceptances. It examines environmental offers and their consequences as described in [13]. But the idea is extremely simple: if we want to know whether N prefers a rather than b, we offer the process both simultaneously, and see which it chooses. The offer is thus $\{a, b\}$ and if the implementation of N is biased in favour of a, it will reply with $\{a\}$. Consequently *CSPP* has a prioritised version of external choice and

$$AB = (a \rightarrow Stop) \overleftarrow{\square} (b \rightarrow Stop)$$

is the process that always gives priority to a. The semantics is captured in the response to offers as $\{a, b\} \rightsquigarrow \{a\}$, $\{a\} \rightsquigarrow \{a\}$, $\{b\} \rightsquigarrow \{b\}$, and $\emptyset \rightsquigarrow \emptyset$ which we can summarise as $X \rightsquigarrow \{a\} \blacktriangleleft a \in X \blacktriangleright X \cap \{b\}$. There is really only this one simple idea in *CSPP* and its defining acceptance semantics. Everything else is just following through the consequences.

Notice that AB is a possible implementation of N in that it is natural to think of N as defined by $\{a\} \rightsquigarrow \{a\}$, $\{b\} \rightsquigarrow \{b\}$ and $\emptyset \rightsquigarrow \emptyset$. The response to $\{a, b\}$ is left partially open: we know that at least one or other of a and b is possible, and AB is one way of satisfying that requirement. Thus AB is better defined than N and its behaviour we suppose is one of those of N. That is AB *refines* N which is written $N \sqsubseteq AB$. N might be regarded as a specification and AB a possible implementation.

We must now come clean and say that there is more than one way of interpreting N in *CSPP*. But to understand that, we need to introduce neutral or *compliant* processes. As first pointed out by Bill Roscoe, most CSP practitioners who do not use **occam** think of N as a neutral process. So far we have only produced a biased version of $\square$. This is where *CSPP* begins to show that it has a far wider scope than just priority. What is the response of a neutral version of N to the offer $\{a, b\}$? The answer is $\{a, b\}$ again: it is happy to do either. So *CSPP* also has $\overleftrightarrow{\square}$ which can be used to write

$$S = (a \rightarrow Stop) \overleftrightarrow{\square} (b \rightarrow Stop)$$

with $\{a, b\} \rightsquigarrow \{a, b\}$, $\{a\} \rightsquigarrow \{a\}$, $\{b\} \rightsquigarrow \{b\}$, and $\emptyset \rightsquigarrow \emptyset$. As noted in [13], it is *incoherent* to have a theory of priority which does not also cover compliance. This is because priority is only of relevance when an environment offers more than one choice of event simultaneously. But what is it that can offer several events? In a theory that only includes biased processes, the answer is nothing. In *CSPP*, the simple answer is, of course, a compliant process. Since the theory extends beyond simple compliance and simple priority, a more correct answer is a process which is at least partially compliant.

The idea of compliance carries with it the notion of *environmental* or *external* nondeterminism. If an environment offers a choice of $\{a, b\}$, it is nondeterministic about which is to be performed. Just as a compliant process is nondeterministic about which event the environment selects from its response. *CSPP* thus distinguishes *internal nondeterminism* which arises mainly from $\sqcap$ and *external nondeterminism* which is necessary in order for priority to be meaningful. Indeed, priority is precisely a means of resolving external nondeterminism.

These ideas percolate through many other operators. Although we have not introduced it above, standard CSP has a more general form of prefixing in which $e : E \to P(e)$ is a process which is prepared to do any of the events in the set E and then behave like the corresponding process $P(e)$ matching the particular event e selected. This is really a form of external choice, so there is a variety of possibilities for preference and lack of preference among the members of E. A simple and useful case is when all the members of E are available compliantly. That is written $e : \overleftrightarrow{E} \to P(e)$.

We take a simple example, $Q = e : \overleftrightarrow{E} \to Stop$, to illustrate how we define the semantics precisely. As in [13], Σ represents a universe of all events that we may wish to consider. We assume here that $E \subseteq \Sigma$, that is, E does not contain the tokens $\checkmark$ or $\textsf{X}$. In *CSPP* it is sometimes convenient to permit those tokens to appear in a prefix set. Before Q has performed any events, the only trace is $\langle\rangle$. Then an offer $X \subseteq \Sigma$ evokes the response $X \cap E$ which is compliant when more than one member of E is in X. We write that as $\langle\rangle : X \rightsquigarrow X \cap E$. The only traces that can be performed thereafter are of the sort $\langle e \rangle$ and then the process refuses everything: $\langle e \rangle : X \rightsquigarrow \emptyset$. We specify all this precisely as the set

$$\mathcal{B}(e : \overleftrightarrow{E} \to Stop) = \quad \{(\langle\rangle, X, X \cap E) | X \subseteq \Sigma\}$$
$$\cup \tag{1}$$
$$\{(\langle e \rangle, X, \emptyset) | e \in E \wedge X \subseteq \Sigma\} \ .$$

$\mathcal{B}$ is the mapping from syntax to a set of behaviours, here triples: this is a denotational semantics. It completely specifies the meaning of $e : \overleftrightarrow{E} \to Stop$. All the definitions later in this paper follow this style.

The other place where priority has a major effect is in the definition of the parallel operations. In $P_1 \|_E P_2$, P_1 and P_2 may themselves express priority, but we are more concerned here with the parallel constructor itself. Synchronised events in E are joint actions of P_1 and P_2 and their selection involves the preferences of the partners. But external nondeterminism arises when both P_1 and P_2 offer unsynchronised events: the situation is exactly the same as for external choice. A parallel operator might always favour P_1: so *CSPP* includes $\overleftarrow{\|}_E$. One can think of $\overleftarrow{\|}_E$ as behaving like $\overleftarrow{\Box}$ on unsynchronised interleaved events, but on every event rather just the initials. The compliant version, $\overleftrightarrow{\|}_E$, is likely to match the intuition of most CSP practitioners. But notice that because CSP abstracts away from preferences, one should really always make the most nondeterministic identification. Thus $\|_E$ in *CSPP* can have any sort of bias or lack thereof and behave quite differently in that respect from event to event. This is in the spirit of CSP as an abstraction, but in practical applications of *CSPP* one nearly always chooses the simpler versions like $\overleftrightarrow{\|}_E$. It should be mentioned that Lowe in [15] uses a very restricted set of parallel operators with a very different semantics from $CSPP$ on the synchronised events.

To summarise, $P_1 \overleftrightarrow{\underset{E}{\|}} P_2$ is simple and the most used parallel operator in $CSPP$. $P_1 \overleftarrow{\underset{E}{\|}} P_2$ is occasionally useful. $P_1 \underset{E}{\|} P_2$ is extremely chaotic in the sense that it permits any sort of resolution or lack of resolution of external nondeterminism. When soft priority, see below in section 3, is in force, $\underset{E}{\|}$ can be identified with the corresponding CSP operator.

1.3 Internal and External Nondeterminism

The major insight in $CSPP$ and acceptances is in distinguishing external from internal nondeterminism. We have seen that external nondeterminism is captured in multiple events present in either an offer or a response (in the pairs $X \rightsquigarrow Y$).

Internal nondeterminism is captured in the usual way: by recording multiple behaviours. Thus $Ex = (a \rightarrow Stop) \overleftrightarrow{\square} (b \rightarrow Stop)$ and $In = (a \rightarrow Stop) \sqcap ((b \rightarrow Stop)$ are represented by the sets

$$\mathcal{B}(Ex) = \quad \{(\langle\rangle, X, X \cap \{a,b\}) \,|\, X \subseteq \Sigma\}$$
$$\cup$$
$$\{(\langle x\rangle, X, \emptyset) \,|\, x \in \{a,b\} \wedge X \subseteq \Sigma\}$$

and

$$\{(\langle\rangle, X, X \cap \{a\}) \,|\, X \subseteq \Sigma\}$$
$$\cup$$
$$\mathcal{B}(In) = \quad \{(\langle\rangle, X, X \cap \{b\}) \,|\, X \subseteq \Sigma\} \quad = \quad \mathcal{B}(a \rightarrow Stop) \cup \mathcal{B}(b \rightarrow Stop) \,.$$
$$\cup$$
$$\{(\langle x\rangle, X, \emptyset) \,|\, x \in \{a,b\} \wedge X \subseteq \Sigma\}$$

In general, internal nondeterminism is represented by the union of behaviours:
$\mathcal{B}(P_1 \sqcap P_2) = \mathcal{B}(P_1) \cup \mathcal{B}(P_2)$.

1.4 Fixed Points: the Heart of a Denotational Semantics.

We have seen that CSP is elegant and sparse with very few operators. $CSPP$ aims for the same qualities, but the inclusion of priority means that some variant decorated versions of the standard operators are needed. In both cases, recursion is the only way to produce non trivial programs: all the other syntax only gives us finite length traces.

Accordingly recursion is at the heart of both theories. It is essential that $\mu P \bullet f(P)$ is well defined, and any restrictions on the function f which may be used are identified. Let $P = a \rightarrow b \rightarrow P$. Successively unwinding this recursion as $P = a \rightarrow b \rightarrow a \rightarrow b \rightarrow P$, $P = a \rightarrow b \rightarrow a \rightarrow b \rightarrow a \rightarrow b \rightarrow P, \ldots$ can be thought of a sequence of more precise specifications for P. $P = a \rightarrow b \rightarrow P$ might potentially be satisfied by any process that at least starts off like $a \rightarrow b \rightarrow \ldots$. Next we admit the subset of those processes that start with $a \rightarrow b \rightarrow a \rightarrow b \rightarrow \ldots$. But these are successive *refinements*. Each unwinding is getting *nearer* to the final fixed point (if there is one). We are 'converging' towards a solution. We can think of this as a succession of successive approximations $A_0 \sqsubseteq A_1 \sqsubseteq A_2 \ldots$. So it is no surprise to discover that we use the refinement partial order as a way to establish that recursions are properly defined. Indeed this is usually the major task in setting up any denotational semantics.

In ordinary convergence, there must be limit points available to which a sequence can converge: that is the space is complete. In partial order theory, the corresponding property of the space is that it be a Complete Partial Order (CPO). Refinement is a partial order, and we prove in section 8.15 that the variant of *CSPP* below is a CPO under a certain condition. It then follows from standard theorems that functions that are monotone in the refinement order have a least fixed point. We show below that all the *CSPP* operators are indeed monotone. If a function is in addition continuous (a partial order analogue of ordinary continuity), then the fixed point of a function can be calculated in a simple way which is essentially the same as we did above with the sequence $A_0, A_1, A_2, \ldots$. Background can be found in [16] and [2] among other places.

1.5 Differences from Earlier Versions of *CSPP*

Earlier versions of the semantics allowed ✓ and ✗ to appear in a response mixed in with ordinary events. So this appeared to offer an environment the possibility of making a choice that might in effect steer a process either towards or away from termination or livelock. Both tokens represent situations that are normally regarded as being outside environmental control, so in the current versions, these tokens may only appear as singletons. In effect, external nondeterminism in these tokens is converted into internal nondeterminism by this change. It only affects some rather obscure situations.

As a result of the examination of the observational status documented in [13], the axioms have been significantly weakened, and the scope of the language very considerably extended. There are now no preconceived notions of how a 'good' process should behave: there is an exception in section 8.16.4. The language is now based simply on observing what a system, however bizarre, does. We only require that responses are reliable. There is some cost in extra complexity of some of the semantic definitions, at least in the most abstract version below.

There is a little freedom left in two areas: how much detail should be recorded in observations which determines the level of abstraction of the resulting dialect; and whether priority conflict results in deadlock or is resolved nondeterministically.

For this paper, both choices have been made on the grounds of simplicity of the underlying semantics. That implies maximum abstraction and hard priority: conflict results in deadlock. The first choice leads to a dialect which is arguably in the spirit of the Failures models for standard CSP, but is a little too abstract for the author's taste. The second is in the spirit of **occam**, but complicates the congruence with standard CSP.

2 An Abstract Variant of *CSPP*

The companion paper, [13], examines the sorts of observations which can be made of processes that can usefully participate in systems that employ priority. Any process that can be regarded as capable of reacting to an environmental offer with a declaration of which events can be accepted, and then reliably and jointly performing one of the accepted events is included. This is a far wider class then just those that employ a straightforward notion of priority.

This version of the language includes

$$P ::= Stop \mid Skip \mid Spin \mid a \to P \mid e : E \to P(e) \mid e : (\alpha) \to P(e) \mid P \,\S\, P$$
$$\mid P \sqcap P \mid P \overset{\leftarrow}{\Box} P \mid P \overset{\leftrightarrow}{\Box} P \mid P \overset{\leftarrow}{\underset{E}{\|}} P \mid P \overset{\leftrightarrow}{\underset{E}{\|}} P \mid P \setminus H \mid \mu P \bullet f(P) \mid P[\![R]\!] .$$

$e : (\alpha) \to P(e)$ is a relational form of prefixing, and provides a syntax for capturing some very irregular processes that are not described by either a priority or absence of a priority: α is a relation. There is no $\top$ process in this version of *CSPP*: it is useful in less abstract versions of the language. *Spin* is usually called div in standard CSP: it is not the bottom of the refinement order here, so the name has been changed to avoid confusion.

The theory below uses *hard* priority for simplicity. The price to be paid is that there is no unique identification of standard external choice $\square$ which accordingly does not appear in the syntax above. There are two maximal, but incompatible, identifications for $\square$:

$$P \square Q = P \overset{\leftrightarrow}{\square} Q \sqcap P \overset{\leftarrow}{\square} Q \quad \text{or} \quad P \square Q = P \overset{\leftrightarrow}{\square} Q \sqcap P \overset{\rightarrow}{\square} Q .$$

Both, of course, are compatible with **occam**. Similarly, there is no unique identification for $\|_E$. However a $\|_E$ is defined below but it should not normally be identified with the corresponding standard operator. In most circumstances, the standard operator would be identified with the compliant version $\overset{\leftrightarrow}{\|}_E$.

The semantics below is all straightforward but because some very irregular processes are admitted few assumptions can be made. It becomes necessary to spell out some conditions in detail. Hiding is by far the most difficult and subtle operator, and the possibility of irregular behaviour needs careful consideration. The existence of least fixed points to define recursion is established for a finite alphabet by showing that *CSPP* is a Complete Partial Order (CPO) under refinement. All operators are monotone, and most distribute over $\sqcap$. There is also a metric so the usual Unique Fixed Point (UFP) theorems hold.

The purpose of this paper is to demonstrate that there is a very abstract version of *CSPP* with a semantics closely analogous to the standard Failures-Divergences model for CSP.

3   Hard and Soft Priority.

Consider

$$\left((a \rightarrow Stop) \overset{\leftarrow}{\square} (b \rightarrow Stop)\right) \| \left((a \rightarrow Stop) \overset{\rightarrow}{\square} (b \rightarrow Stop)\right) .$$

What happens when the environment offers $\{a, b\}$? Soft priority somehow resolves the conflict: some versions of *CSPP* allow the system to 'search' for the largest sub-offers on which the two processes can agree. When there is more than one such sub-offer, there is a non deterministic choice between the options.

However, hard priority is simpler, and arguably more in the spirit of **occam**. In this case, if the two processes cannot agree, the result is deadlock. A difficulty is that $\overset{\leftarrow}{\square}$ and $\overset{\rightarrow}{\square}$ cannot simultaneously refine $\square$ since $((a \rightarrow Stop) \square (b \rightarrow Stop)) \| ((a \rightarrow Stop) \square (b \rightarrow Stop))$ cannot deadlock.

4   Alphabets and Traces

There is a global alphabet Σ of ordinary events: this will be large enough to include all the visible events of any process that we need to describe. Later we will need to restrict it to be finite. We add the pseudo events $\checkmark$ and $\times$ which only occur as singleton responses.

Traces are simply sequences, empty or finite, of events drawn from Σ. $\langle\rangle$ is the empty sequence. The set of all finite traces drawn from Σ is written as $\Sigma^{\cdot}$. Because we need $\langle\rangle$, it is convenient to label the elements of the other traces from 1: such a trace t has type $t : \{1, 2, \ldots, n\} \rightarrow \Sigma$ and we can write $t = \langle t(1), t(2), \ldots, t(n) \rangle$. In this context, it is sometimes useful to implicitly identify $\langle\rangle$ with the empty function $\emptyset$: this is used below, for example in definition 4 on page 166.

$t \frown s$ represents the concatenation of two sequences, so $\langle a,b \rangle \frown \langle c,d \rangle = \langle \rangle \frown \langle a,b,c,d \rangle =$ $\langle a,b,c,d \rangle = \langle abcd \rangle$: we may omit commas when there is no ambiguity.

We also make use of infinite traces which are of the sort $s : \mathbb{N}_1 \to \Sigma$, but only to express certain properties of *finite* traces.

5   Acceptances

As described in the companion paper, we specify the meaning of a process by describing its responses after it has performed some trace of events. Traces are members of Σ^*. Given such a trace s, we record the response Y to an offer X. We sometimes write that as $X \rightsquigarrow Y$ or $s : X \rightsquigarrow Y$ as an equivalent way of expressing the triple (s, X, Y). The offer X is some subset of the alphabet Σ: that is $X \subseteq \Sigma$. And a response Y is a subset of Σ or $\{\checkmark\}$ or $\{\boldsymbol{X}\}$.

Definition 1

- When $X \subseteq \Sigma$, $X^\checkmark$ denotes $X \cup \{\checkmark\}$ and $X^{\checkmark\boldsymbol{X}}$ denotes $X \cup \{\checkmark, \boldsymbol{X}\}$.

- The lone sets of X are $\overset{\checkmark\boldsymbol{X}}{\mathbb{L}}(X) \equiv \{\{\checkmark\} \mid \checkmark \in X\} \cup \{\{\boldsymbol{X}\} \mid \boldsymbol{X} \in X\}$.

- $\overset{\checkmark\boldsymbol{X}}{\mathbb{S}}(X) \equiv \{\emptyset\} \blacktriangleleft X = \emptyset \blacktriangleright \overset{\checkmark\boldsymbol{X}}{\mathbb{L}}(X) \cup \{X \cap \Sigma \mid X \cap \Sigma \neq \emptyset\}$

- $\overset{\checkmark\boldsymbol{X}}{\mathbb{P}} X$ denotes $\mathbb{P}(X \cap \Sigma) \cup \overset{\checkmark\boldsymbol{X}}{\mathbb{L}}(X)$.

- $\overset{\checkmark\boldsymbol{X}}{\mathbb{M}}(X)$ denotes $\{\emptyset\} \blacktriangleleft X = \emptyset \blacktriangleright \left(\overset{\checkmark\boldsymbol{X}}{\mathbb{P}}(X) - \{\emptyset\} \right)$.

Acceptances have type $\Sigma^* \times \mathbb{P}\Sigma \times \overset{\checkmark\boldsymbol{X}}{\mathbb{P}} \Sigma^{\checkmark\boldsymbol{X}}$, which we occasionally identify with

$$\Sigma^* \times \left(\mathbb{P}\Sigma \times \overset{\checkmark\boldsymbol{X}}{\mathbb{P}} \Sigma^{\checkmark\boldsymbol{X}} \right). \tag{2}$$

More specifically, acceptances are members of

$$\mathcal{A} = \{(s, X, Y) \mid s \in \Sigma^* \wedge X \subseteq \Sigma \wedge Y \in \overset{\checkmark\boldsymbol{X}}{\mathbb{P}}(X^{\checkmark\boldsymbol{X}})\} \tag{3}$$

Thus we have a description which is a set $\mathcal{B}P$ of such acceptances $\mathcal{B}(P) \subseteq \mathcal{A}$. $[\![P]\!]$ is the usual notation for the semantic function describing the behaviour of the process P, but $\mathcal{B}P$ is more intuitive here and avoids confusion with the renaming of equation (23) on page 177.

The set of traces of the process is

$$traces(P) = \{s \mid \exists X, Y \bullet (s, X, Y) \in \mathcal{B}P\} \quad \text{or} \quad traces(P) = \text{dom}\, \mathcal{B}P$$

when the type of $\mathcal{B}P$ is taken from (2).

We identify a process directly with its acceptances where the context warrants.

5.1   Acceptances Determine Traces

There are often simple patterns for triples (s, X, Y) representing a process P for a general s. That is, when $s \in traces\,(P)$ then the pattern $(s, X, Y) \in \mathcal{B}\,(P)$. It is sometimes intricate, error prone and laborious to spell out explicitly which s is a trace of P. But that information is already implicit in the acceptances, determined by the events in Y.

Thus, take $B \subseteq \mathcal{A}$ and define

$$
\begin{aligned}
B_0 &= \{(\langle\rangle, X, Y) \in B\} \\
B_{n+1} &= \{(s^\frown\langle e\rangle, X, Y) \in B \mid \exists X', Y' \bullet (s, X', Y') \in B_n \wedge e \in Y'\} \quad \text{for } n \in \mathbb{N}.
\end{aligned}
\tag{4}
$$

The we define the inductive core, $\lfloor B \rfloor$ by

$$
\lfloor B \rfloor \equiv \cup\{B_n \mid n \in \mathbb{N}\} . \tag{5}
$$

Since all traces are finite, when $\mathcal{B}\,(P) \subseteq B$, then $\mathcal{B}\,(P) = \lfloor B \rfloor$. In this context we can say that acceptances determine the traces.

6   Some Definitions

$\#s$ is the length of s: $\#\langle\rangle = 0$ and $\#(t^\frown\langle e\rangle) = \#t + 1$. We extend this notation to acceptances: $\#A = \max\{\#s \mid s \in traces\,(A)\}$ which is well defined when the lengths are bounded. Otherwise $\#A = \infty$.

$s \mid n$ just truncates a trace to a length no more than n whether s is finite or infinite:

Definition 2 $s \mid 0 = \langle\rangle$ *and* $s \mid n = \mathbf{n} \lhd s$ *where* $\mathbf{n} = \{i \mid 1 \leq i \leq n\}$.

Here $\lhd$ is domain restriction: if $f : X \to Y$ is a function then $D \lhd f : X \cap D \to Y$ is the restriction of $f_{|D \cap X}$ with domain $X \cap D$. So $\#(s \mid n) \leq n$.

If S is a set of traces $S \mid n$ contains only the truncated versions:

Definition 3 $S \mid n = \{s \mid n \mid s \in S\}$.

We extend prefixing to allow comparison of a finite with an infinite trace:

Definition 4 *Let* $s \in \Sigma^*$ *and* $t \in \Sigma^\omega$. *Then*

$$
(s \leq t) \iff (s = \langle\rangle \vee \exists n \in \mathbb{N} \bullet s = \mathbf{n} \lhd t)
$$

$\lhd$ above is domain restriction as before: the leading n elements of t match a non-null s above.

Definition 5 $s \setminus H$ *is a trace composed of those elements not in the set H:*

$$
\langle\rangle \setminus H = \langle\rangle \qquad s^\frown\langle x\rangle \setminus H = s \setminus H \blacktriangleleft x \in H \blacktriangleright (s \setminus H)^\frown x
$$

We can extend trace hiding to infinite traces.

Definition 6 *If* $w \in \Sigma^\omega$ *then we write* $w \setminus H = s$ *when*

$$
\forall n \in \mathbb{N} \bullet (w \mid n) \setminus H \leq s \quad \text{and} \quad \forall n \in \mathbb{N} \bullet \exists m \in \mathbb{N} \bullet s \mid n = (w \mid m) \setminus H .
$$

Definition 7 *The down-set* $\downarrow s = \{t \mid t \leq s\}$ *is a standard notion from partial order theory.*

If $A : \mathbb{P}\left(\Sigma^* \times \mathbb{P}\Sigma \times \overset{\checkmark x}{\mathbb{P}}\Sigma^{\checkmark x}\right)$ is a set of acceptances then $A \parallel n$ just represents the acceptances no longer than n:

Definition 8
$$A \parallel n = \{(s, X, Y) \in A \mid \#s \leqslant n\} . \tag{6}$$

The notation $R(|X|)$ means the relational image of a set X. So:

$$R(|X|) = \{y \mid x \in X \wedge x R y\} .$$

Definition 9 *Let $(S, \leqslant)$ be a partial order.* $\mathbf{m}_{\leqslant} : \mathbb{P}S \to \mathbb{P}S$ *is the function that produces the set of maximal elements:*

$$\mathbf{m}_{\leqslant}(\emptyset) = \emptyset$$
$$\mathbf{m}_{\leqslant}(X) = \{x \in X \mid \forall y \in X \bullet x \not< y\} \quad (X \neq \emptyset) .$$

Usually the order is implied and we write $\mathbf{m} : \mathbb{P}S \to \mathbb{P}S$.

Definition 10 *An* atomic *process is one represented by a minimal non empty set of acceptances: any smaller non empty set cannot represent a process. Such processes have a unique response to any offer: they are* internally deterministic.

7 Axioms

The axioms here were briefly described in the companion paper and shown to encompass a very large class of processes. For a set $\mathcal{B}P \subseteq \mathcal{A}$ to describe a process, it must conform to these simple constraints.

Every process performs events only after it has started:

H1: $\langle\rangle \in \textit{traces}(P)$

There is at least one acceptance for every possible offer:

H2: $\forall s \in \textit{traces}\,(P) \bullet \forall X \subseteq \Sigma \bullet \exists Y \in \overset{\checkmark\mathsf{X}}{\mathbb{P}}(X^{\checkmark\mathsf{X}}) \bullet (s, X, Y) \in \mathcal{B}(P)$

The traces of a process are prefix closed, and match the responses:

H3: $\forall s \in \Sigma^{\cdot} \bullet \forall x \in \Sigma \bullet s\,\widehat{}\,\langle x \rangle \in \textit{traces}(P) \Leftrightarrow \exists (s, X, Y) \in \mathcal{B}(P) \bullet x \in Y \cap \Sigma$

One may regard $\mathcal{B}P \subseteq \mathcal{A}$ and properties like $\checkmark \neq \mathsf{X}$ and $\Sigma \cap \{\checkmark, \mathsf{X}\} = \emptyset$ as implicit axioms.

8 Semantics

The main purpose of this paper is to present the details of the semantics of the principal operators of *CSPP*.

8.1 *Stop, Skip and Spin*

Stop, Skip and *Spin* are all similar:

$$
\begin{aligned}
\mathcal{B}\,Stop &= \{(\langle\rangle, X, \emptyset) \mid X \subseteq \Sigma\} \\
\mathcal{B}\,Skip &= \{(\langle\rangle, X, \{\checkmark\}) \mid X \subseteq \Sigma\} \\
\mathcal{B}\,Spin &= \{(\langle\rangle, X, \{\mathsf{X}\}) \mid X \subseteq \Sigma\}
\end{aligned}
\tag{7}
$$

8.2 ⊥

⊥ is the most unpredictable of all processes: it can behave in any fashion at all.

$$\mathcal{B}\bot = \mathcal{A} \tag{8}$$

See equation 3 on page 165 for the definition of $\mathcal{A}$.

8.3 Prefix Choice

Consider $e : E \to P(e)$ with $E \subseteq \Sigma^{\checkmark\chi}$. In general there are many possible initial acceptances

$$\langle\rangle : X \rightsquigarrow \emptyset \blacktriangleleft X^{\checkmark\chi} \cap E = \emptyset \blacktriangleright U$$

where $U \in \overset{\checkmark\chi}{\mathbb{P}}\left(X^{\checkmark\chi} \cap E\right)$ is not empty.

$$\mathcal{B}(e : E \to P(e)) = \left\{(\langle\rangle, X, Y)\middle| X \subseteq \Sigma \wedge Y \in \overset{\checkmark\chi}{\mathsf{M}}\left(X^{\checkmark\chi} \cap E\right)\right\}$$
$$\cup$$
$$\{(\langle e\rangle^\frown s, X, Y)\,|\,e \in E \cap \Sigma \wedge (s, X, Y) \in \mathcal{B}(P(e))\} \tag{9}$$

$\overset{\checkmark\chi}{\mathsf{M}}(X)$ was defined in definition 1 on page 165: the acceptances include all ways of assigning or refraining from assigning priority among the events of E. Subsequent behaviour, if any, depends on the initial event e and matches one of those in $\mathcal{B}P(e)$. Clearly, $P(e)$ is defined on $E \cap \Sigma$, at least.

Example 1 *Usually E in e : E $\to$ P(e) is a set of real events. More general cases include*

1. $x : \{\checkmark\} \to Stop = x : \{\checkmark\} \to P = Skip$ *for any P.*

2. $x : \{\chi\} \to Stop = x : \{\chi\} \to P = Spin$ *for any P.*

3. $x : \{\checkmark, \chi\} \to P = Skip \sqcap Spin$ *for any P.*

4. $x : \{a, \checkmark\} \to Stop = (a \to Stop)\overset{\leftarrow}{\square} Skip \sqcap Skip.$

When subsequent behaviour does not depend on the choice of event as in the examples above, it is natural to omit "$x :$" as in $\{a, b\} \to \{b, c\} \to Stop$.

8.4 Relational Prefix Choice

It does not take much experience using $\mathcal{CSPP}$ syntax to see the utility of notations like $e :$ $(S, [\{a, b\} > \{c\} > \{d\}]) \to P(e)$ to stand for $((a \to P(a))\overset{\leftrightarrow}{\square}(b \to P(b)))\overset{\leftarrow}{\square}(c \to P(c))\overset{\leftarrow}{\square}(d \to P(d))$. More generally $e : (S, \leqslant) \to P(e)$ is a process which initially gives priority to events according to the partial order $\leqslant$ and then behaves like $P(e)$. One might expect that we can always find such a partial order to describe the initial acceptances, but this is not true.

Example 2

$$((a \to Stop)\overset{\leftarrow}{\square}(b \to Stop))\,\overset{\leftrightarrow}{\square}\,((c \to Stop)\overset{\leftarrow}{\square}(b \to Stop)\overset{\leftarrow}{\square}(a \to Stop))$$

has initial acceptances that do not match any partial order:
$\{a, b, c\} \rightsquigarrow \{a, c\}, \{b, c\} \rightsquigarrow \{b, c\}, \{a, c\} \rightsquigarrow \{a, c\}, \{a, b\} \rightsquigarrow \{a, b\}, \dots$ *. In such an order, $\{a, b, c\} \rightsquigarrow$ $\{a, c\}$ would give $b \leqslant a$, but that does not match $\{a, b\} \rightsquigarrow \{a, b\}$ which would require that a and b are incomparable.*

This suggests that a more general form of prefixing may be desirable. The obvious, simple and natural approach is to directly specify an initial acceptance relation, although an acceptance function would be adequate. Relations used in practice are nearly always functions: such prefixes can be called atomic.

$$\mathcal{B}(e : (\alpha) \to P(e)) =$$
$$\{(\langle\rangle, X, Y) \in \mathcal{A} \,|\, X \,\alpha\, Y\} \cup \{(\langle e \rangle^\frown s, X, Y) \,|\, \exists (X', Y') \in \alpha \bullet e \in Y' \cap \Sigma \wedge (s, X, Y) \in \mathcal{B}(P(e))\} \tag{10}$$

where $\alpha : \mathbb{P}\left(\mathbb{P}\Sigma \times \overset{\checkmark\textbf{x}}{\mathbb{P}}(\Sigma^{\checkmark\textbf{x}})\right)$ is an acceptance relation with $\operatorname{dom}\alpha = \mathbb{P}\Sigma$ matching the axioms and respecting $\mathcal{A}$. $P(e)$ is understood to be defined for all the events that can be accepted by α.

The most common use of this notation is atomic. It is when the initial acceptances match a partial order relation $(S, \leqslant)$ on events in which every nonempty subset of S has a maximal element and $\checkmark$ or $\textbf{X}$ may be present only as bottom elements. In such cases

$$\mathcal{B}(e : (S, \leqslant) \to P(e)) =$$
$$\left\{(\langle\rangle, X, \mathbf{m}(S \cap X^{\checkmark\textbf{x}})) \,|\, X \subseteq \Sigma\right\}$$
$$\cup \tag{11}$$
$$\left\{(\langle e \rangle^\frown s, X, Y) \,|\, \exists Z \subseteq \Sigma \bullet e \in \mathbf{m}(S \cap Z^{\checkmark\textbf{x}}) \cap \Sigma \wedge (s, X, Y) \in \mathcal{B}(P(e))\right\}$$

$\mathbf{m} : \mathbb{P}\Sigma^{\checkmark\textbf{x}} \to \mathbb{P}\Sigma^{\checkmark\textbf{x}}$ is the function which selects the maximal elements of a set: see definition 9 on page 167.

Many orders of interest can be expressed in terms of *layers* as in $[\{p\} > \{q, r\} > \{s\}]$: the elements of the component sets are strictly ordered only with respect to members of other sets. This notation is used in some of the examples below:

Example 3 $x : (\{a, b\}, =) \to Stop = a \to Stop \overset{\leftrightarrow}{\square} b \to Stop.$

Example 4 $x : ([\{a\} > \{b\}]) \to Stop = a \to Stop \overset{\leftarrow}{\square} b \to Stop.$

Example 5
$x : ([\{a, b\} > \{c\} > \{d\}]) \to Stop = (a \to Stop \overset{\leftrightarrow}{\square} b \to Stop) \overset{\leftarrow}{\square} (c \to Stop \overset{\leftarrow}{\square} d \to Stop).$

Example 6 $x : ([\{a, b\} > \{\checkmark\}]) \to Stop = (a \to Stop \overset{\leftrightarrow}{\square} b \to Stop) \overset{\leftarrow}{\square} Skip.$

All the examples above are cases when the '$x :$' might have been omitted for brevity: x was not explicitly bound in the bodies, which means that $P(e)$ is a constant function.

8.5 Compliant Prefixing

$e : \overset{\leftrightarrow}{E} \to P(e)$, is defined as $e : (E, =) \to P(e).$

8.6 Internal Choice

$$\mathcal{B}(P_1 \sqcap P_2) = \mathcal{B}P_1 \cup \mathcal{B}P_2 \tag{12}$$

We extend the definition to suitable non empty sets of processes $\mathcal{P}$, writing

$$\mathcal{B}\left(\sqcap \mathcal{P}\right) = \bigcup \{\mathcal{B}P \mid P \in \mathcal{P}\}. \tag{13}$$

To avoid foundational issues, we need to impose a suitable limit on the size of the sets admitted by (13) to ensure the behaviours form a set rather than a proper class. It is then immediately clear that $\sqcap \mathcal{P}$ satisfies the axioms of section 7:

Lemma 1 $\mathcal{B}(\bigcup \mathcal{P})$ *represents a process when $\mathcal{P}$ is a suitable non empty set of processes.*

The following lemmas are not hard to prove:

Lemma 2 *Let $\{P_i : \Sigma \to CSPP\}$ be an indexed nonempty set of process functions. Then $e : E \to \sqcap\{P_i(e) \mid i \in I\} = \sqcap\{e : E \to P_i(e) \mid i \in I\}$.*

Lemma 3 *Let $\{P_i : \Sigma \to CSPP\}$ be an indexed nonempty set of process functions. Then $e : (\alpha) \to \sqcap\{P_i(e) \mid i \in I\} = \sqcap\{e : (\alpha) \to P_i(e) \mid i \in I\}$.*

Lemma 4 *Let $\{P_i : \Sigma \to CSPP\}$ be an indexed nonempty set of process functions. Then $e : (S, \leqslant) \to \sqcap\{P_i(e) \mid i \in I\} = \sqcap\{e : (S, \leqslant) \to P_i(e) \mid i \in I\}$.*

8.7 Compliant External Choice

$$\mathcal{B}(P_1 \overleftrightarrow{\square} P_2) =$$

$$\left\{ (\langle\rangle, X, Y) \,\middle|\, \begin{array}{l} \exists Y_1, Y_2 \in \overset{\checkmark\mathsf{X}}{\mathbb{P}}(\Sigma^{\checkmark\mathsf{X}}) \bullet \\ (\langle\rangle, X, Y_1) \in \mathcal{B}P_1 \wedge (\langle\rangle, X, Y_2) \in \mathcal{B}P_2 \wedge Y \in \overset{\checkmark\mathsf{X}}{\mathsf{S}}(Y_1 \cup Y_2) \end{array} \right\} \tag{14}$$
$$\cup$$
$$\left\{ (\langle x\rangle ^\frown s, X, Y) \,\middle|\, (\langle x\rangle ^\frown s, X, Y) \in \mathcal{B}(P_1) \ \vee \ (\langle x\rangle ^\frown s, X, Y) \in \mathcal{B}(P_2) \right\}$$

$\overset{\checkmark\mathsf{X}}{\mathsf{S}}(X)$ is defined in definition 1 on page 165. It ensures that $\checkmark$ and X can be returned only as singletons if they are present.

Example 7 $(a \to P_1) \overleftrightarrow{\square} (a \to P_2) = (a \to P_1) \sqcap (a \to P_2)$.

Example 8 $Skip \overleftrightarrow{\square} (a \to P) = Skip \sqcap (a \to P) \overleftarrow{\square} Skip$.

Although $Skip \overleftrightarrow{\square} (a \to P)$ looks as if it ought to be compliant on $\langle\rangle$, an environment cannot choose $\checkmark$, so $\checkmark$ cannot be offered as a legitimate *choice*, only as a singleton. ∎[8]

It is clear from the definition that $\overleftrightarrow{\square}$ is associative:

$$P_1 \overleftrightarrow{\square} \left(P_2 \overleftrightarrow{\square} P_3\right) = \left(P_1 \overleftrightarrow{\square} P_2\right) \overleftrightarrow{\square} P_3$$

From standard CSP, we might expect that $P_1 \sqcap \left(P_2 \overset{\leftrightarrow}{\square} P_3\right) = (P_1 \sqcap P_2) \overset{\leftrightarrow}{\square} (P_1 \sqcap P_3)$ but this cannot be true in the presence of priority. The reason becomes clear when we regard the processes as specifications. $(P_1 \sqcap P_2) \overset{\leftrightarrow}{\square} (P_1 \sqcap P_3)$ has a refinement of $P_1 \overset{\leftrightarrow}{\square} P_3$ which is not an implementation of $P_1 \sqcap \left(P_2 \overset{\leftrightarrow}{\square} P_3\right)$. The correct result is

$$P_1 \sqcap \left(P_2 \overset{\leftrightarrow}{\square} P_3\right) \sqsupseteq (P_1 \sqcap P_2) \overset{\leftrightarrow}{\square} (P_1 \sqcap P_3) \tag{15}$$

It is again not hard to establish:

Lemma 5 *Let* $\{P_i : \Sigma \to CSPP\}$ *be an indexed nonempty set of processes. Then* $Q \overset{\leftrightarrow}{\square} \sqcap\{P_i \mid i \in I\} = \sqcap\{Q \overset{\leftrightarrow}{\square} P_i \mid i \in I\}$.

8.8   Prioritised External Choice

$$\mathcal{B}(P_1 \overset{\leftarrow}{\square} P_2) =$$

$$\left\{ (\langle\rangle, X, Y) \,\middle|\, \begin{array}{c} \exists Y_1, Y_2 \subseteq \Sigma^{\checkmark\mathsf{X}} \bullet (\langle\rangle, X, Y_1) \in \mathcal{B}P_1 \wedge (\langle\rangle, X, Y_2) \in \mathcal{B}P_2 \\ \wedge \\ Y = (Y_2 \blacktriangleleft Y_1 = \emptyset \blacktriangleright Y_1) \end{array} \right\}$$

$$\bigcup \tag{16}$$

$$\left\{ (\langle e\rangle^\frown s, X, Y) \,\middle|\, \begin{array}{c} (\langle e\rangle^\frown s, X, Y) \in \mathcal{B}(P_1) \\ \vee \\ \exists X' \subseteq \Sigma \bullet (\langle\rangle, X', \emptyset) \in \mathcal{B}(P_1) \wedge \exists Y_2 \subseteq \Sigma^{\checkmark\mathsf{X}} \bullet \\ (\langle\rangle, X', Y_2) \in \mathcal{B}(P_2) \wedge e \in Y_2 \cap \Sigma \wedge (\langle e\rangle^\frown s, X, Y) \in \mathcal{B}(P_2) \end{array} \right\}$$

Equation (16) simply says that the process always behaves like P_1 unless P_1 refuses in which case it behaves like P_2. It allows P_1 to perform any event, terminate or livelock if it is capable of so doing. When P_1 is active in any sense, it is let loose:

$$\langle\rangle : X \rightsquigarrow U \quad \text{if} \quad P_1 :: \langle\rangle : X \rightsquigarrow U \quad \text{apart from } U = \emptyset$$

P_2 is only allowed to be active when P_1 is not. If P_1 shows any sign of life, even pathological life, it executes. Even if P_2 can perform $\checkmark$ or signal X, it is ignored until all events from P_1 are positively blocked.

Example 9 $(a \to Stop) \overset{\leftarrow}{\square} (a \to b \to Stop) = a \to Stop$

In general, $(a \to P_1) \overset{\leftarrow}{\square} (a \to P_2) = a \to P_1$.   ∎[9]

Example 10 *SKIP guards.*

$Skip \overset{\leftarrow}{\square} (a \to Stop)$ *only has acceptances of the sort:*

$$\langle\rangle : X \rightsquigarrow \{\checkmark\}$$

because $Skip$ *never refuses, so* $Skip \overset{\leftarrow}{\square} (a \to Stop) = Skip$. *And*

```
PRI ALT
  B & SKIP
    P
  a?
    Q
```

is $(Skip \, \overset{\circ}{,} \, P \blacktriangleleft B \blacktriangleright Stop) \overset{\leftarrow}{\Box} (a \rightarrow Q) = P \blacktriangleleft B \blacktriangleright (a \rightarrow Q)$ as we would wish. This gives a denotational semantics for, and so defines, SKIP guards. However,

```
PRI ALT
  a?
    P
  SKIP
    Q
```

is not normally implemented with the semantics of $\overset{\leftarrow}{\Box}$. The reason is that when a? is checked for availability, the process which outputs a is not necessarily involved. This is quite different from the semantics of equation (16) which requires P_1 to positively refuse before P_2 is allowed to execute.

Example 11 Skip and Spin are left multiplicative zeroes of $\overset{\leftarrow}{\Box}$ while Stop is a unit:

$$Skip \overset{\leftarrow}{\Box} P = Skip \qquad Spin \overset{\leftarrow}{\Box} P = Spin \qquad Stop \overset{\leftarrow}{\Box} P = P \qquad P \overset{\leftarrow}{\Box} Stop = P$$

Like its compliant counterpart, $\overset{\leftarrow}{\Box}$ is associative:

$$P_1 \overset{\leftarrow}{\Box} \left(P_2 \overset{\leftarrow}{\Box} P_3 \right) = \left(P_1 \overset{\leftarrow}{\Box} P_2 \right) \overset{\leftarrow}{\Box} P_3$$

Notice however that

$$P_1 \sqcap \left(P_2 \overset{\leftarrow}{\Box} P_3 \right) \sqsupseteq (P_1 \sqcap P_2) \overset{\leftarrow}{\Box} (P_1 \sqcap P_3) \tag{17}$$

because $P_1 \overset{\leftarrow}{\Box} P_3$ and $P_2 \overset{\leftarrow}{\Box} P_1$ are refinements of the right hand side, but not of the left.

Lemma 6 Let $\{P_i : \Sigma \rightarrow CSPP\}$ be an indexed nonempty set of processes. Then $Q \overset{\leftarrow}{\Box} \sqcap\{P_i \mid i \in I\} = \sqcap\{Q \overset{\leftarrow}{\Box} P_i \mid i \in I\}$ and $\sqcap\{P_i \mid i \in I\} \overset{\leftarrow}{\Box} Q = \sqcap\{P_i \overset{\leftarrow}{\Box} Q \mid i \in I\}$.

8.9 Parallels

8.9.1 Interleaving

When $P_1\|P_2$ executes and performs a trace s, then the parallel processes have performed matching traces (s_1, s_2). If $E = \Sigma$, then all events are synchronised and performed jointly by P_1 and P_2. In that case $s_1 = s_2 = s$.

The other extreme is when $E = \emptyset$, so no events are synchronised. That is just standard interleaving: $P_1\|P_2 = P_1 \, \|\| \, P_2$. True concurrency is not part of the present theory.

In general a trace s can arise from more than one pair of traces (s_1, s_2). We call this way of picking events from the s_1 and s_2 to form s generalised interleaving and write $s \in s_1\|s_2$. Clearly $\langle\rangle\|\langle\rangle = \{\langle\rangle\}$.

The following abbreviation captures this:

Definition 11 *Let $s \in \Sigma^{\cdot}$. Then*

Interleaves$(P_1, P_2, s, E) \equiv$

$$
\left\{ f : \downarrow s \to \Sigma^{*2} \left|
\begin{array}{l}
f(\langle\rangle) = (\langle\rangle, \langle\rangle) \\
\wedge \\
\forall\, t \,^\frown\langle x\rangle \in \downarrow s \bullet \exists\, t_1 \in traces\,(P_1) \bullet \exists\, t_2 \in traces\,(P_2) \bullet f(t) = (t_1, t_2) \\
\wedge \\
\left(
\begin{array}{l}
x \in E \Rightarrow \\
\quad\left(
\begin{array}{l}
\exists X, Y_1, Y_2 \bullet \\
(t_1, X, Y_1) \in \mathcal{B}(P_1) \wedge (t_2, X, Y_2) \in \mathcal{B}(P_2) \wedge x \in Y_1 \cap Y_2 \\
\wedge \\
f\left(t \,^\frown\langle x\rangle\right) = (t_1 \,^\frown\langle x\rangle, t_2 \,^\frown\langle x\rangle)
\end{array}
\right) \\
\wedge\; x \notin E \Rightarrow \\
\quad\left(
\begin{array}{l}
f\left(t \,^\frown\langle x\rangle\right) = (t_1 \,^\frown\langle x\rangle, t_2) \wedge t_1 \,^\frown\langle x\rangle \in traces\,(P_1) \\
\vee \\
f\left(t \,^\frown\langle x\rangle\right) = (t_1, t_2 \,^\frown\langle x\rangle) \wedge t_2 \,^\frown\langle x\rangle \in traces\,(P_2)
\end{array}
\right)
\end{array}
\right)
\end{array}
\right. \right\}
$$

The projections of $f \in$ Interleaves(P_1, P_2, s, E) are written as f_1 and f_2 so $f(t) = (f_1(t), f_2(t))$.

Definition 11 has to include a number of details to ensure that irregular processes are handled properly.

8.9.2   General Parallel

$$
\mathcal{B}(P_1 \underset{E}{\|} P_2) = \left\{ (s, X, Y) \left|
\begin{array}{c}
\exists f \in \text{Interleaves}(P_1, P_2, s, E) \bullet \exists Y_1, Y_2 \in \overset{\checkmark \mathsf{X}}{\mathbb{P}}\, X^{\checkmark \mathsf{X}} \bullet \\
(f_1(s), X, Y_1) \in \mathcal{B}(P_1) \wedge (f_2(s), X, Y_2) \in \mathcal{B}(P_2) \\
\wedge \\
Y \in \overset{\checkmark \mathsf{X}}{\mathsf{M}}\Big((Y_1 \cap Y_2 \cap E^{\checkmark}) \cup ((Y_1 \cup Y_2) - E^{\checkmark}) \Big)
\end{array}
\right. \right\}
\tag{18}
$$

$\overset{\checkmark \mathsf{X}}{\mathsf{M}}(X)$ was defined on page 165: see definition 1. In equation (18), Y can be any available nonempty subset or available singleton token.

The difficulty with hard priority here is just the same as that which arises with $\square$: there can be 'unexpected' deadlocks. So $(P_1 \;|||\; P_2) \;|||\; (P_1 \;|||\; P_2)$ can behave like $(P_1 \overset{\leftarrow}{|||} P_2) \overset{\leftrightarrow}{|||} (P_1 \overset{\rightarrow}{|||} P_2)$ at any point and create a deadlock which would not arise in standard CSP. As a consequence, $P_1 \underset{E}{\|} P_2$ should not be identified with the corresponding operator of standard CSP. In most circumstances, $P_1 \overset{\leftrightarrow}{\underset{E}{\|}} P_2$ will be the right identification, although just as for $\square$

$$
P_1 \overset{CSP}{\underset{E}{\|}} P_2 = P_1 \overset{\leftrightarrow}{\underset{E}{\|}} P_2 \;\sqcap\; P_1 \overset{\leftarrow}{\underset{E}{\|}} P_2
$$

and

$$
P_1 \overset{CSP}{\underset{E}{\|}} P_2 = P_1 \overset{\leftrightarrow}{\underset{E}{\|}} P_2 \;\sqcap\; P_1 \overset{\rightarrow}{\underset{E}{\|}} P_2
$$

are more abstract possibilities as well as variants that are not consistent at each step.

Lemma 7 *Equation* (18) *defines a process.*

Proof. Suppose $(f_1(s), X, Y_1) \in \mathcal{B}(P_1) \wedge (f_2(s), X, Y_2) \in \mathcal{B}(P_2)$. Then acceptances of the form $(f_i(s), X', Y'_2)$ exist for all other $X' \subseteq \Sigma$, so all (s, X', Y') triples are present.

The set of acceptances must also satisfy **H3**. Take $s\widehat{}\langle x\rangle \in traces\left(P_1 \| P_2\right)$. That means that

$\exists (s\widehat{}\langle x\rangle, X, Y) \in \mathcal{B}\left(P_1 \| P_2 \atop E\right)$. Suppose $x \in E$. Then there is an $f \in$ Interleaves$(P_1, P_2, s\widehat{}\langle x\rangle, E)$ with $(f_1(s\widehat{}\langle x\rangle), X, Y_1) \in \mathcal{B}(P_1)$ and $(f_2(s\widehat{}\langle x\rangle), X, Y_2) \in \mathcal{B}(P_2)$. From definition 11, there are some sets X', Y'_1 and Y'_2 for which $(f_1(s), X', Y'_1) \in \mathcal{B}(P_1)$ and $(f_2(s), X', Y'_2) \in \mathcal{B}(P_2)$ with $x \in Y'_1 \cap Y'_2$. This shows that there is a Y with $(s, X', Y) \in \mathcal{B}\left(P_1 \| P_2 \atop E\right)$ and $x \in Y$ so the forward implication of **H3** is satisfied when $x \in E$.

When $x \notin E$ the result is even easier to establish because only one parallel partner is involved.

The converse implication of **H3** is obviously satisfied. ⊣

Example 12 *Take P_1, P_2 and Q to be processes with acceptances which include*

$Q :: \langle\rangle :$	$\{a,b\} \rightsquigarrow \{a\}$	$P_1 :: \langle\rangle :$	$\{a,b\} \rightsquigarrow \{a\}$	$P_2 :: \langle\rangle :$	$\{a,b\} \rightsquigarrow \{b\}$
	$\{a,c\} \rightsquigarrow \{c\}$		$\{a,c\} \rightsquigarrow \{a\}$		$\{a,c\} \rightsquigarrow \{a\}$
	$\{b,c\} \rightsquigarrow \{c\}$		$\{b,c\} \rightsquigarrow \emptyset$		$\{b,c\} \rightsquigarrow \{b\}$
	$\{a\} \rightsquigarrow \emptyset$		$\{a\} \rightsquigarrow \{a\}$		$\{a\} \rightsquigarrow \{a\}$
	$\{b\} \rightsquigarrow \{b\}$		$\{b\} \rightsquigarrow \emptyset$		$\{b\} \rightsquigarrow \{b\}$
	$\{c\} \rightsquigarrow \{c\}$		$\{c\} \rightsquigarrow \emptyset$		$\{c\} \rightsquigarrow \emptyset$

$Q :: \langle a\rangle : \quad X \rightsquigarrow X \cap \{a,b,c\}$

$Q :: \langle b\rangle : \quad X \rightsquigarrow X \cap \{a,b,c\}$

$Q :: \langle c\rangle : \quad X \rightsquigarrow X \cap \{a,b,c\}$

$P_1 :: \langle a\rangle : \quad X \rightsquigarrow \emptyset$

$P_2 :: \langle a\rangle : \quad X \rightsquigarrow X \cap \{b\}$

$P_2 :: \langle b\rangle : \quad X \rightsquigarrow \emptyset$

Then $Q \| P_1 :: \langle\rangle : \{a,b\} \rightsquigarrow \{a\}$, so it has a trace $\langle a\rangle$ after which it stops. $Q \| P_2 :: \langle\rangle : \{b\} \rightsquigarrow \{b\}$ provides the only nonempty trace, $\langle b\rangle$, after which it stops. In particular, this process cannot perform the trace $\langle ab\rangle$. However $Q \| (P_1 \sqcap P_2)$ can perform the trace $\langle ab\rangle$. This shows that

$$Q \| (P_1 \sqcap P_2) \neq Q \| P_1 \sqcap Q \| P_2 .$$

The various responses in equation (18) allow, for example, a scheduler to make arbitrary decisions about which events to select in preference to others, perhaps for reasons of efficiency. $P_1 \overset{\longleftrightarrow}{\underset{E}{\|}} P_2$ does not permit that freedom:

$$\mathcal{B}(P_1 \overset{\longleftrightarrow}{\underset{E}{\|}} P_2) = \left\{ (s, X, Y) \left| \begin{array}{c} \exists f \in \text{Interleaves}(P_1, P_2, s, E) \bullet \exists Y_1, Y_2 \in \mathbb{P}\, X^{\checkmark X} \bullet \\ (f_1(s), X, Y_1) \in \mathcal{B}(P_1) \wedge (f_2(s), X, Y_2) \in \mathcal{B}(P_2) \\ \wedge \\ Y \in \mathbb{S}^{\checkmark X}\left((Y_1 \cap Y_2 \cap E^{\checkmark}) \cup ((Y_1 \cup Y_2) - E^{\checkmark}) \right) \end{array} \right. \right\} \quad (19)$$

$\mathbb{S}^{\checkmark X}(X)$ was defined on page 165:

8.9.3 Derived Parallels

As usual there are derived versions.

$$P_X \|_Y Q \;=\; P' \underset{X \cap Y}{\|} Q'$$

where $P' = P \| \text{Run}_X$, $Q' = Q \| \text{Run}_Y$ and $\text{Run}_E = e : E \to \text{Run}_E$. And of course interleaving: $P \,\|\|\, Q \;=\; P \underset{\emptyset}{\|} Q$ and fully synchronised parallel: $\| = \underset{\Sigma}{\|}$.

8.10   Prioritised Parallel

For the form of parallel composition that always favours one partner, we have to refine the notion of interleaving to match because triples like (s, X, Y) only record a very limited history in the trace component s.

Definition 12 *Let $s \in \Sigma^*$. Then*

$$\overleftarrow{\mathsf{Interleaves}}(P_1, P_2, s, E) \equiv$$

$$\left(\left\{ f : \downarrow s \to \Sigma^{*2} \,\middle|\, \begin{array}{c} f(\langle\rangle) = (\langle\rangle, \langle\rangle) \\ \wedge \\ \forall t ^\frown \langle x \rangle \in \downarrow s \bullet \exists t_1 \in traces(P_1) \bullet \exists t_2 \in traces(P_2) \bullet f(t) = (t_1, t_2) \\ \wedge \\ \left(\begin{array}{c} x \in E \Rightarrow \\ \left(\begin{array}{c} \exists X, Y_1, Y_2 \bullet \\ (t_1, X, Y_1) \in \mathcal{B}(P_1) \wedge (t_2, X, Y_2) \in \mathcal{B}(P_2) \wedge x \in Y_1 \cap Y_2 \\ \wedge \\ f(t ^\frown \langle x \rangle) = (t_1 ^\frown \langle x \rangle, t_2 ^\frown \langle x \rangle) \end{array} \right) \\ \wedge \\ \begin{array}{c} x \notin E \Rightarrow \\ \left(\begin{array}{c} f(t ^\frown \langle x \rangle) = (t_1 ^\frown \langle x \rangle, t_2) \wedge t_1 ^\frown \langle x \rangle \in traces(P_1) \\ \vee \\ \left(\begin{array}{c} f(t ^\frown \langle x \rangle) = (t_1, t_2 ^\frown \langle x \rangle) \\ \wedge \\ \exists X, Y_2 \bullet \\ (t_1, X, \emptyset) \in \mathcal{B}(P_1) \wedge (t_2, X, Y_2) \in \mathcal{B}(P_2) \wedge x \in Y_2 \end{array} \right) \end{array} \right) \end{array} \end{array} \right) \end{array} \right\} \right)$$

The projections of $f \in \overleftarrow{\mathsf{Interleaves}}(P_1, P_2, s, E)$ are again written as f_1 and f_2 so $f(t) = (f_1(t), f_2(t))$.

$$\mathcal{B}(P_1 \overleftarrow{\underset{E}{\|}} P_2) = \left\{ (s, X, Y) \,\middle|\, \begin{array}{c} \exists f \in \overleftarrow{\mathsf{Interleaves}}(s, E) \bullet \exists Y_1, Y_2 \in \mathbb{P} X^{\checkmark \mathsf{X}} \bullet \\ (f_1(s), X, Y_1) \in \mathcal{B}(P_1) \wedge (f_2(s), X, Y_2) \in \mathcal{B}(P_2) \\ \wedge \\ Y \in \mathbb{S}\big((Y_1 \cap Y_2 \cap E^\checkmark) \cup \big((Y_2 \blacktriangleleft (Y_1 - E^\checkmark) = \emptyset \blacktriangleright Y_1) - E^\checkmark\big)\big) \end{array} \right\}$$

$$(20)$$

A less explicit way to define $P_1 \overleftarrow{\underset{E}{\|}} P_2$ would just use the ordinary $\mathsf{Interleaves}$ and the $\lfloor B \rfloor$ notation of section 5.1 on page 166 to eliminate the excess traces.

8.11   Sequential Composition

$$\mathcal{B}(P_1 \,\mathring{\,}\, P_2) =$$

$$\{(s, X, Y) \in \mathcal{B}(P_1) \,|\, Y \neq \{\checkmark\}\}$$

$$\cup$$

$$\{(s, X, Y) \,|\, (s, X, \{\checkmark\}) \in \mathcal{B}(P_1) \wedge (\langle\rangle, X, Y) \in \mathcal{B}(P_2)\}$$

$$\cup$$

$$\left\{ (t_1 ^\frown \langle x \rangle ^\frown t_2, X, Y) \,\middle|\, \begin{array}{c} \exists X', Y' \bullet (t_1, X', \{\checkmark\}) \in \mathcal{B}(P_1) \wedge (\langle\rangle, X', Y') \in \mathcal{B}(P_2) \wedge x \in Y' \\ \wedge \\ (\langle x \rangle ^\frown t_2, X, Y) \in \mathcal{B}(P_2) \end{array} \right\}$$

$$(21)$$

The reference to two triples from $\mathcal{B}(P_2)$ in the last set in equation (21) means that distribution over $\sqcap$ is unlikely to hold in all cases, and this proves to be the case.

Example 13 *Take* $\Sigma = \{a, b\}$ *and let* Q *be the rather artificial process that terminates on the offer* $\{a, b\}$ *and refuses all other offers. That is* $Q :: \langle\rangle : \{a, b\} \rightsquigarrow \{\checkmark\}$ *and* $Q :: \langle\rangle : X \rightsquigarrow \emptyset$ *for all other* X. *Write* $P_1 = (a \rightarrow a \rightarrow Stop) \stackrel{\leftarrow}{\square} (b \rightarrow a \rightarrow Stop)$ *and* $P_2 = (b \rightarrow b \rightarrow Stop) \stackrel{\leftarrow}{\square} (a \rightarrow b \rightarrow Stop)$. *Notice that* $Q \, \mathring{,} \, P_1$ *has traces* $\{\langle\rangle, \langle a\rangle, \langle aa\rangle\}$ *and* $Q \, \mathring{,} \, P_2$ *has traces* $\{\langle\rangle, \langle b\rangle, \langle bb\rangle\}$. *However* $Q \, \mathring{,} \, (P_1 \sqcap P_2)$ *has a trace* $\langle ab\rangle$ *so this shows that* $Q \, \mathring{,} \, P_1 \sqcap Q \, \mathring{,} \, P_2 \neq Q \, \mathring{,} \, (P_1 \sqcap P_2)$.

Distribution across $\sqcap$ does work in the other direction:

Lemma 8 *Let* $\{P_i : \Sigma \rightarrow CSPP\}$ *be an indexed nonempty set of processes. Then* $\sqcap\{P_i \mid i \in I\} \, \mathring{,} \, Q = \sqcap\{P_i \, \mathring{,} \, Q \mid i \in I\}$.

The failure to distribute over $\sqcap$ in every case arises from the multiple references to triples from $\mathcal{B}(P_2)$ in equation (21). In effect, the present semantics is too fine grained to guarantee the distribution. The failure is repaired in a more coarse grained semantics in which behaviours representing the histories of experiments are recorded. This yields a slightly less abstract version of $CSPP$, but is not examined further here. The same phenomenon occurs in hiding below.

Notice that we cover processes like $\mu p \bullet (Skip \sqcap a \rightarrow p) \, \mathring{,} \, Q$. And also that it is trivial to check that $Skip \, \mathring{,} \, P = P \, \mathring{,} \, Skip = P$.

8.12   Hiding

Conceptually, $P \setminus H$ is a process with the internal behaviour of P, yet with external 'visible' behaviour which excludes any 'internal' events from the set H. The internal events of H are no longer subject to direct environmental control. Often there are several possibilities for the internal dynamics: the process $P \setminus H$ models them by nondeterminism.

The most natural form of hiding offers the internal hidden events in a compliant way. The version below also allows external hesitant offers.

$$\mathcal{B}(P \setminus H) =$$

$$\left\{ (s \setminus H, X, \{\textbf{X}\}) \,\middle|\, \begin{array}{c} \forall n \in [0, \#s) \bullet \exists X', Y' \bullet (s \mathbin{\downarrow} n, X' \cup H, Y') \in \mathcal{B}(P) \wedge s(n+1) \in Y' \\ \wedge \\ \exists w \in H^\omega \bullet \forall n \in \mathbb{N} \bullet \\ \exists Y' \bullet w(n+1) \in Y' \wedge (s \mathbin{^\frown}(w \mathbin{\downarrow} n), X \cup H, Y') \in \mathcal{B}(P) \end{array} \right\}$$

$$\cup$$

$$\left\{ (s \setminus H, X, Y \setminus H) \,\middle|\, \begin{array}{c} \forall n \in [0, \#s) \bullet \exists X', Y' \bullet \\ (s \mathbin{\downarrow} n, X' \cup H, Y') \in \mathcal{B}(P) \wedge s(n+1) \in Y' \\ \wedge \\ \exists u \bullet u \geqslant s \wedge u \setminus H = s \setminus H \\ \wedge \\ \forall n \in [\#s, \#u) \bullet \exists Y' \bullet (u \mathbin{\downarrow} n, X \cup H, Y') \in \mathcal{B}(P) \wedge u(n+1) \in Y' \\ \wedge \\ \exists Y'' \bullet (u, X \cup H, Y'') \in \mathcal{B}(P) \wedge Y'' \cap H = \emptyset \\ \wedge \\ Y \in \overset{\checkmark X}{\mathbb{P}} \cup \{Y' \mid \exists s' \bullet s \leqslant s' \leqslant u \wedge (s', X \cup H, Y') \in \mathcal{B}(P)\} \end{array} \right\}$$

$$(22)$$

The first set above captures livelock. The second set above references more than one triple in $\mathcal{B}(P)$ and this is why it does not distribute over $\sqcap$. It is however manifestly monotone. $[\#s, \#u) = \emptyset$ when $s = u$ above. u is a 'backstop' ensuring that there is no unbounded sequence of internal actions that might be explored after s. The only way a livelock can appear in the second set is when P can livelock.

Example 14 *Let*

$$P_1 = \overleftrightarrow{\{a, h\}} \to \overleftrightarrow{\{b, h\}} \to \overleftrightarrow{\{c, h\}} \to Stop$$
$$P_2 = \overleftrightarrow{\{e, h\}} \to \overleftrightarrow{\{d, h\}} \to \overleftrightarrow{\{f, h\}} \to Stop$$
and
$$P_3 = \overleftrightarrow{\{a, h\}} \to \overleftrightarrow{\{d, h\}} \to \overleftrightarrow{\{c, h\}} \to Stop$$

Then

$$P_1 \setminus \{h\} : \{a, b, c, d, e, f\} \rightsquigarrow \{a, b, c\}$$
$$P_2 \setminus \{h\} : \{a, b, c, d, e, f\} \rightsquigarrow \{d, e, f\}$$
and
$$P_3 \setminus \{h\} : \{a, b, c, d, e, f\} \rightsquigarrow \{a, c, d\}$$

Since $P_1 \sqcap P_2$ can behave like P_3, it follows that $(P_1 \sqcap P_2) \setminus \{h\} \neq P_1 \setminus \{h\} \sqcap P_2 \setminus \{h\}$.

Lemma 9 *Hiding is monotone: $P \sqsubseteq Q \Rightarrow P \setminus H \sqsubseteq Q \setminus H$.*

Proof. Obvious by inspection of equations (12) and (22). ⊣
    It does not appear that there can be any sensible definition of hiding using the present fine grained semantics which can distribute over $\sqcap$. Sliding requires that we access more than one unit of information to determine responses, and this is incompatible with the distribution. It is interesting to notice how the problem is neatly side-stepped in standard CSP semantics based on Failures by employing 'inverted logic'.

8.13 Renaming

Renaming needs careful definition because one-many renaming introduces additional non determinism. If R is the renaming relation we write $s \; \mathsf{R} \; s'$ to mean that the trace s' is a pointwise renamed version of s. And it is useful to extend it to $\Sigma^{\checkmark \boldsymbol{\times}}$:

Definition 13 $\mathsf{R}^{\checkmark \boldsymbol{\times}} = \mathsf{R} \cup \{\checkmark \mapsto \checkmark, \boldsymbol{\times} \mapsto \boldsymbol{\times}\}$.

If P is a process, $P\llbracket \mathsf{R} \rrbracket$ is the renamed process.

$$\mathcal{B} \, P \llbracket \mathsf{R} \rrbracket = $$

$$\left\{ (s, X, Y) \;\middle|\; \begin{array}{c} \exists t \bullet t \; \mathsf{R} \; s \wedge \exists Y' \bullet (t, \mathsf{R}^\sim \langle\!| X |\!\rangle, Y') \in \mathcal{B}(P) \wedge Y = \mathsf{R}^{\checkmark \boldsymbol{\times}} \langle\!| Y' |\!\rangle \cap X^{\checkmark \boldsymbol{\times}} \\ \wedge \\ \forall n \in [0, \#s) \bullet \exists t \bullet \exists X', Y' \bullet \\ t \; \mathsf{R} \; (s \downharpoonright n) \wedge (t, \mathsf{R}^\sim \langle\!| X' |\!\rangle, Y') \in \mathcal{B}(P) \wedge s(n + 1) \in \mathsf{R}^{\checkmark \boldsymbol{\times}} \langle\!| Y' |\!\rangle \cap X'^{\checkmark \boldsymbol{\times}} \end{array} \right\} \quad (23)$$

    $\mathsf{R}^\sim$ is the reverse relation: the notation is similar to that used in Z. And $\mathsf{R} \langle\!| X |\!\rangle = \{y \mid x \; \mathsf{R} \; y\}$ is the relational image of the set X. The second predicate in equation (23) ensures that **H3** is obeyed: it is needed because the axioms admit some very irregular processes.
    Renaming is clearly monotone.

Lemma 10 *Renaming is monotone: $P \sqsubseteq Q \Rightarrow P\llbracket \mathsf{R} \rrbracket \sqsubseteq Q\llbracket \mathsf{R} \rrbracket$.*

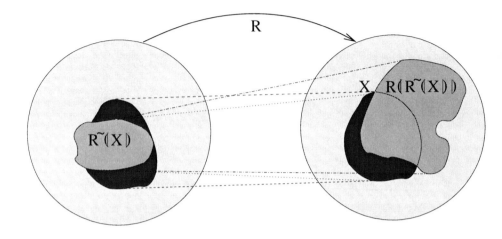

Figure 1: Renaming with R

8.14   Interruption: $P_1 \underset{(i,r)}{\triangle} P_2$

A variant of the usual sort of interrupt operator is defined here with one eye on the evolution of the Honeysuckle language: see [17], [18] and [19].

Let P_1 and P_2 be two processes and i and r two distinguished events. i will represent an interruption, and r can be regarded as a 'return from interrupt'. The intention here is that P_2 is something like a standard interrupt service routine. Denote the alphabets of P_1 and P_2 by αP_1 and αP_2 in the sense that these are the sets of events that the processes can perform. We require that these alphabets be disjoint, and that i is in neither of them. However $r \in \alpha P_2$ since we want P_2 to be able to complete its processing by executing r.

Two standard notations that have not been needed above are $s \downarrow a$ which is the number of occurrences of the event a in the trace s; and $s \upharpoonright E$ which is the subsequence of s consisting of members of the set E. So $s \downarrow i = s \downarrow r$ will determine whether the trace s contains matching pairs of i and r, and so whether we are 'background processing' in P_1 or in the interrupt service routine P_2. And $s \upharpoonright (\alpha P_1)$ will be the portion of s executed by P_1 and similarly for P_2.

Then

$$\mathcal{B}\left(P_1 \underset{(i,r)}{\triangle} P_2\right) = \left\lfloor \left\{ (s,X,Y) \;\middle|\; \begin{array}{c} s \in (\alpha P_1 \cup \alpha P_2 \cup \{i\})^* \\ \wedge \\ (Y = \{i\} \blacktriangleleft i \in X \blacktriangleright (s \upharpoonright (\alpha P_1), X, Y) \in \mathcal{B}(P_1)) \\ \blacktriangleleft s \downarrow i = s \downarrow r \blacktriangleright \\ (s \upharpoonright (\alpha P_2), X, Y) \in \mathcal{B}(P_2) \end{array} \right\} \right\rfloor \tag{24}$$

Recall that $\lfloor B \rfloor$ was defined in section 5.1 on page 166. It avoids the need to be explicit about the set of traces: only the traces that can be 'accepted', starting from $\langle \rangle$, are included.

8.15   Refinement

Refinement is as usual

$$P_1 \sqsupseteq P_2 \;\Leftrightarrow\; P_2 = P_2 \sqcap P_1 \tag{25}$$

which simply maps onto set inclusion on the acceptances:

$$P_1 \sqsupseteq P_2 \;\Leftrightarrow\; \mathcal{B} P_1 \subseteq \mathcal{B} P_2 \tag{26}$$

Proof. Assume $P_1 \sqsupseteq P_2$ or $P_2 = P_2 \sqcap P_1$ from (25) above. Then $\mathcal{B} P_2 = \mathcal{B} P_2 \cup \mathcal{B} P_1$ which gives $\mathcal{B}(P_1) \subseteq \mathcal{B}(P_2)$ immediately. The converse is equally obvious. ⊣

8.15.1 ⊥

The most nondeterministic process which has all possible behaviours is evidently below any other process in this order: it is the least element ⊥ of $\sqsupseteq$.

There is no top process in this version based on triples, although it appears in versions based on behaviours.

8.15.2 Meets and Joins

Let S be a nonempty set of processes. $\sqcap S$ is the obvious candidate to be the meet. *Proof.* First, $\sqcap S$ is an lower bound of S. If $P \in S$, then $\mathcal{B} P \subseteq \mathcal{B}(\sqcap S)$ is an immediate consequence of the definition. But this is $P \sqsupseteq \sqcap S$ so $\sqcap S$ is a lower bound of S.

Second, it is clear that $\sqcap S$ is the supremum of all lower bounds, for any lower bound must contain $\cup \{\mathcal{B} P \mid P \in S\}$. ⊣

If S has a join, then it must match the intersection of the behaviours: $\cap \{\mathcal{B} P \mid P \in S\}$. Unfortunately, this can fail to define a process, as in the pair $(a \rightarrow Stop)$ and $(b \rightarrow Stop)$. With $\Sigma = \{a, b, c\}$, $\mathcal{B}(a \rightarrow Stop) \cap \mathcal{B}(b \rightarrow Stop) = \{\langle \rangle : \{c\} \rightsquigarrow \emptyset, \langle \rangle : \emptyset \rightsquigarrow \emptyset\}$ which is not a process: **H2** is violated.

Theorem 1 *($CSPP, \sqsubseteq$) is a Complete Partial Order when Σ is finite.*

Proof. Let $\mathcal{D}$ be a directed set of processes. It is necessary to show that

$$\mathcal{B}(U) = \cap \{\mathcal{B}(D) \mid D \in \mathcal{D}\}$$

represents a process. When Σ is finite, so also are $\mathbb{P}\Sigma$ and $\overset{\sqrt{x}}{\mathbb{P}} \Sigma^{\sqrt{x}}$. So the number of choices of (s, X, Y) for a fixed s is finite. This observation is used to establish that U satisfies the axioms **H1**, **H2** and **H3** of section 7.

For **H1** suppose that there is no instance of $(\langle \rangle, X, Y) \in \mathcal{B}(U)$. There are only a finite number of such possibilities, so it is possible to construct a finite subset of $\mathcal{D}$ with an upper bound which has no instance of $(\langle \rangle, X, Y)$ for some X and Y. This is a contradiction in that the bound is itself a process satisfying **H1**. Thus U satisfies **H1**.

U must satisfy **H2** by a very similar argument noting that there are only a finite number of choices for Y in (s, X, Y) when s and X are fixed.

Suppose $s^\frown \langle x \rangle \in traces(U)$: we need to show that there is some common $(s, X, Y) \in \mathcal{B}(U)$ with $x \in Y \cap \Sigma$. If we assume the contrary and note the finite number of choices for (X, Y), once again we can construct a finite subset of $\mathcal{D}$ with an upper bound which will fail **H3**. Thus

$$s^\frown \langle x \rangle \in traces(U) \;\Rightarrow\; \exists (s, X, Y) \in \mathcal{B}(U) \bullet x \in Y \cap \Sigma .$$

The converse is obviously satisfied, so U satisfies **H3**.

⊣

8.16   Recursion

8.16.1   Fixed Points from the Refinement Partial Order

$\mu p \bullet f(p)$ denotes a fixed point of the function f. This is often the least fixed point with respect to the refinement order in standard untimed CSP. Theorem 1 establishes $CSPP$ as a CPO. Standard theorems now ensure that every monotone function f has a least fixed point, and so $\mu p \bullet f(p)$ is well defined. All the ordinary operators of $CSPP$ are monotone with respect to the refinement order $\sqsupseteq$: in most cases this follows from the fact that they distribute over $\sqcap$.

If f is *continuous*, that is for every directed set $\mathcal{D}$ of processes, $\bigsqcup f(\mathcal{D})$ exists and is the same as the image of the join of $\mathcal{D}$: $\bigsqcup f(\mathcal{D}) = f(\sqcup \mathcal{D})$, then another theorem gives a more useful formula:

$$\mu p \bullet f(p) = \bigsqcup \{f^n(\bot) \mid n \in \mathbb{N}_0\} . \tag{27}$$

Often there is a unique fixed point, but the results above do not help directly in identifying such cases. A metric exists which is useful in such cases.

8.16.2   Monotone Properties

All of the standard operators are monotone in $\sqsubseteq$: this was shown as each was introduced above. In most cases, the result follows from the the fact that the operators distribute over $\sqcap$, but that is a stronger property. Hiding in particular does not so distribute, but is nevertheless monotone.

Lemma A.1.8 on page 484 of [2] shows that $\mu : (CSPP \xrightarrow{m} CSPP) \to CSPP$ is monotone. $CSPP \xrightarrow{m} CSPP$ denotes the space of monotone functions on $CSPP$ processes. The monotone relation on $CSPP \xrightarrow{m} CSPP$ is defined pointwise:

$$f \sqsupseteq f' \Leftrightarrow \forall P \in CSPP \bullet f(P) \sqsupseteq f'(P) .$$

Hence if $h(Q, P)$ is monotone in both arguments, then $\lambda Q \bullet h(P, Q) \in (CSPP \xrightarrow{m} CSPP)$ so $\lambda P \bullet \mu Q \bullet h(Q, P)$ is also monotone. And similar arguments apply for other forms of which $\lambda P \bullet \mu Q \bullet f_P(Q)$ is perhaps the most general.

In the case of mutual recursion, that is a recursion involving a sequence of functions $\langle f_i \mid i \in I \rangle$ where I is an indexing set, then the standard treatment in [2] applies. So mutual recursion is also monotone and the fixed points are well defined. In applications, I is nearly always a subset of $\mathbb{N}$.

All the elementary functions of $CSPP$ have now been shown to be monotone. Since the composition of monotone functions is itself monotone, this means that all the compound functions in $CSPP$ have least fixed points.

Example 15 $\mu P \bullet Skip \, {}_9^\circ \, P = \bot$ *because* $P = Skip \, {}_9^\circ \, P$ *for every process P.*

8.16.3   Continuity

Once a function is known to be monotone, a least fixed point is guaranteed. If in addition, it is continuous in the partial order, then the constructive equation (27) on page 180 can be used.

When, as in $CSPP$, we have a metric and the function is contracting, then we have the stronger result that iterating from *any* starting point, not just from $\bot$, will converge into a unique fixed point. Given the power of the metric approach, it is not often that *continuity* with respect to refinement is particularly useful.

It is easy to check that $f(|D|)$ is directed when f is monotone and D is itself directed. So $\bigsqcup f(|D|)$ always exists for any $f : CSPP \to CSPP$ and directed set D. And by definition, $f(\bigsqcup D) = \bigsqcup f(|D|)$ for f continuous. If f is monotone, $f(\bigsqcup D) \sqsupseteq \bigsqcup f(|D|)$, because otherwise $f(\bigsqcup D) \sqsubset \bigsqcup f(|D|)$, which would entail some $D \in D$ for which $f(\bigsqcup D) \sqsubset f(D)$ which is a contradiction for monotone f.

So it is only necessary to prove the reverse containment $Bf(\bigsqcup D) \supseteq B \bigsqcup f(|D|)$ to establish continuity.

Lemma 11 $e : E \to \_ = P \mapsto e : E \to P$ *is continuous.*

Proof. We need to show

$$e : E \to \bigsqcup D = \bigsqcup (e : E \to D) \ ,$$

for each directed set D. As we have noted above, it is only necessary to show that $(s, X, Y) \in \bigcap \{B(e : E \to D) \mid D \in D\} \Rightarrow (s, X, Y) \in B(e : E \to \bigsqcup D)$.

From equation (9) on page 168, it is clear that both sets of behaviours coincide when $s = \langle\rangle$, so we need only consider the case $(\langle e \rangle^\frown s, X, Y) \in \bigcap \{B(e : E \to D) \mid D \in D\}$. This means that (s, X, Y) is common to every member $D \in D$. But that gives $(\langle e \rangle^\frown s, X, Y) \in B(e : E \to \bigsqcup D)$ which establishes the continuity. ⊣

Lemma 12 $P \mapsto P \overset{\leftrightarrow}{\Box} Q = Q \overset{\leftrightarrow}{\Box} P$ *is continuous when Σ is finite.*

Proof. Let $(\langle\rangle, X, Y) \in \bigcap \left\{ B\left(D \overset{\leftrightarrow}{\Box} Q\right) \middle| D \in D \right\}$.   From equation (14) on page 170,

$$\exists (\langle\rangle, X, Y_1) \in B(D) \text{ and } \exists (\langle\rangle, X, Y_2) \in B(Q) \text{ with } Y \in \overset{\checkmark\bigstar}{\mathbb{P}}(Y_1 \cup Y_2).$$

Consider first the case when $Y \subseteq \Sigma$ so $Y = Y_1 \cup Y_2$. Since Y is fixed and Σ is finite, there is only a finite number of pairs (Y_1, Y_2) with $Y = Y_1 \cup Y_2$, so this is certainly true when the possibilities for Y_2 are restricted to those available from initials in Q.

Now suppose $(\langle\rangle, X, Y) \notin B\left(\bigsqcup D \overset{\leftrightarrow}{\Box} Q\right)$. Then there must be a finite subset of D with a join which does not contain $(\langle\rangle, X, Y)$, for we can choose a member of D which excludes each possible $(\langle\rangle, X, Y_1)$ in turn. Since D is directed, the join, which contains none of the possible $(\langle\rangle, X, Y_1)$ triples, is a member of D. But that contradicts $(\langle\rangle, X, Y) \in \bigcap \left\{ B\left(D \overset{\leftrightarrow}{\Box} Q\right) \middle| D \in D \right\}$, so there is some common $(\langle\rangle, X, Y_1)$ triple, and $(\langle\rangle, X, Y) \in B\left(\bigsqcup D \overset{\leftrightarrow}{\Box} Q\right)$.

Next suppose $(\langle\rangle, X, \{\checkmark\}) \in \bigcap \left\{ B\left(D \overset{\leftrightarrow}{\Box} Q\right) \middle| D \in D \right\}$. If $(\langle\rangle, X, \{\checkmark\}) \in B(Q)$ then $(\langle\rangle, X, \{\checkmark\}) \in B\left(\bigsqcup D \overset{\leftrightarrow}{\Box} Q\right)$ follows immediately. Otherwise $(\langle\rangle, X, \{\checkmark\}) \in B(D)$ for each $D \in D$ and $(\langle\rangle, X, \{\checkmark\}) \in B\left(\bigsqcup D \overset{\leftrightarrow}{\Box} Q\right)$ again. The same is true for triples of the sort $(\langle\rangle, X, \{\bigstar\})$.

Otherwise, when $(\langle x \rangle^\frown s, X, Y) \in \bigcap \left\{ B\left(D \overset{\leftrightarrow}{\Box} Q\right) \middle| D \in D \right\}$ then either $(\langle x \rangle^\frown s, X, Y) \in B(Q)$ in which case $(\langle x \rangle^\frown s, X, Y) \in B\left(\bigsqcup D \overset{\leftrightarrow}{\Box} Q\right)$ follows immediately, or $(\langle x \rangle^\frown s, X, Y) \in B(D)$ for every D. Again, $(\langle x \rangle^\frown s, X, Y) \in B\left(\bigsqcup D \overset{\leftrightarrow}{\Box} Q\right)$ is an immediate consequence. ⊣   ◆[12]

We omit the proofs of the following lemmas in order to keep this paper within reasonable bounds.

Lemma 13 $P \mapsto P \overset{\leftarrow}{\square} Q$ is continuous when Σ is finite.

Lemma 14 $P \mapsto Q \overset{\leftarrow}{\square} P$ is continuous when Σ is finite.

Lemma 15 $P \mapsto P\|_E Q$ is continuous when Σ is finite.

Lemma 16 $P \mapsto P \overset{\leftrightarrow}{\underset{E}{\|}} Q$ is continuous when Σ is finite.

Lemma 17 $P \mapsto P \overset{\leftarrow}{\underset{E}{\|}} Q$ and $P \mapsto Q \overset{\leftarrow}{\underset{E}{\|}} P$ are both continuous when Σ is finite.

Lemma 18 $P \mapsto P \, {}^\circ_9 \, Q$ and $P \mapsto Q \, {}^\circ_9 \, P$ are both continuous.

Hiding is not in general continuous:

Example 16 *Let $P_m = h^m \to Stop$ be the process that performs m copies of h before stopping. Write $D_n = \sqcap\{P_m \mid m \geqslant n\}$ and note that $D_n \setminus \{h\} = Stop \sqcap Spin$. $\mathcal{D} = \{D_n \mid n \in \mathbb{N}\}$ is a directed set with $\bigsqcup \mathcal{D} = \mu P \bullet h \to P$. Since $\bigsqcup \mathcal{D} \setminus \{h\} = Spin$ and $\bigsqcup\{D_n \setminus \{h\}\} = Stop \sqcap Spin$, hiding is not continuous.*

Lemma 19 $P \mapsto P[\![R]\!]$ is continuous when Σ is finite.

8.16.4 A Stronger Order

The refinement order works well for finite Σ but there is another stronger order:

Definition 14 $P \succcurlyeq Q \equiv \mathcal{B}(P) \subseteq \mathcal{B}(Q) \ \wedge \ clear(Q) \subseteq clear(P)$
where $clear(P) = \{(s, X, Y) \in \mathcal{B}(P) \mid (s, X, \{\pmb{X}\}) \notin \mathcal{B}(P)\}$.

Throughout this paper, we have emphasised that the model is based on pure observation without any notion of what a 'reasonable' process should do. But now we have a reason to restrict our consideration to processes that are not too bizarre: only then does $\succcurlyeq$ become a Complete Partial Order for arbitrary Σ. The additional axiom is light weight: if an event that can be performed is offered on its own, then it may be accepted.

H4: $(s, X, Y) \in \mathcal{B}(P) \ \Rightarrow \ \forall x \in Y \cap \Sigma \bullet (s, \{x\}, \{x\}) \in \mathcal{B}(P)$

$\succcurlyeq$ has the same bottom element as refinement and all the ordinary *CSPP* operators are $\succcurlyeq$-monotone. This order is stronger in that it relates fewer processes: this is exactly the reason why it is a Complete Partial Order when refinement is not. The directed sets that are problematical for refinement need not be considered because the members are not related by $\succcurlyeq$. But for sets that are directed under both orders, the joins are identical: thus $\succcurlyeq$ yields *exactly the same fixed points* as does refinement for recursions. $\succcurlyeq$ is an analogue of Roscoe's alternative order for the Failures-Divergences model described in [20]. It is interesting to discover that $\succcurlyeq$ does not depend upon identifying livelock with the bottom element of the order. More details of $\succcurlyeq$ will be given elsewhere.

8.16.5   A Metric

Another approach to fixed points is via a metric. The big advantage is that it yields *unique* fixed points: these are invaluable in constructing certain proofs. The disadvantage is that it is of little help when there are several fixed points. So the metric and partial order treatments are complementary.

The usual restriction space method is extended here for *CSPP*. A metric is

Definition 15 $d(P_1, P_2) = \inf(\{3^{-n} \mid n \in \mathbb{N} \wedge \mathcal{B}(P_1) \mathbin{\Vert} n = \mathcal{B}(P_2) \mathbin{\Vert} n\} \cup \{3\})$.

Restriction metrics are generally defined using powers of 2. We depart from tradition and use 3 for a technical reason that there is no room to consider here. We merely note that this metric is complete, that prefixing and contracting recursions are contracting, and that the other standard operators apart from hiding are in general non expanding.

9   Conclusions

It has been shown that *CSPP* can be given a simple acceptance semantics which closely mirrors the properties of the standard Failures-Divergences model, while incorporating priority as well as more irregular behaviour. The version of *CSPP* involved is more abstract than those that arise from observation in which records of the histories of experiments are recorded.

I would like to thank Bill Roscoe for a variety of comments which have helped shape *CSPP*, for Jeremy Martin for his initial support, to the referees for spotting a slip and to the CSP and WoTUG communities in general for their interest and input.

References

[1] C.A.R Hoare. *Communicating Sequential Processes*. Prentice Hall International, 1985.

[2] A.W. Roscoe. *The Theory and Practice of Concurrency*. Prentice Hall, 1998.

[3] Steve Schneider. *Concurrent and Real-time Systems*. John Wiley & Sons, Ltd., 2000.

[4] A.E. Lawrence. Extending CSP. In P. H. Welch & A. P. Bakkers, editor, *Proceedings of WoTUG 21: Architectures, Languages and Patterns*, volume 52 of *Concurrent Systems Engineering*, pages 111–131, Amsterdam, April 1998. WoTUG, IOS Press.

[5] A. E. Lawrence. CSPP and event priority. In *Communicating Process Architectures – 2001*, Concurrent Systems Engineering, pages 67–92, Amsterdam, Sept 2001. IOS Press.

[6] A. E. Lawrence. Infinite traces, Acceptances and CSPP. In *Communicating Process Architectures – 2001*, Concurrent Systems Engineering, pages 93–102, Amsterdam, Sept 2001. IOS Press.

[7] A. E. Lawrence. Successes and Failures: Extending CSP. In *Communicating Process Architectures – 2001*, Concurrent Systems Engineering, pages 49–65, Amsterdam, Sept 2001. IOS Press.

[8] A.E. Lawrence. HCSP: Extending CSP for codesign and shared memory. In *Proceedings of WoTUG 21: Architectures, Languages and Patterns*, pages 133–156. WoTUG, 1998.

[9] A.E. Lawrence. Extending CSP - even further. Communicating Process Architectures–2000, 2000. WoTUG.

[10] A. E. Lawrence. Acceptances, Behaviours and infinite activity in CSPP. In *Communicating Process Architectures – 2002*, Concurrent Systems Engineering, pages 17–38, Amsterdam, Sept 2002. IOS Press.

[11] A. E. Lawrence. HCSP, imperative state and true concurrency. In *Communicating Process Architectures – 2002*, Concurrent Systems Engineering, pages 39–55, Amsterdam, Sept 2002. IOS Press.

[12] A. E. Lawrence. Overtures and hesitant offers: hiding in *CSPP*. In *Communicating Process Architectures – 2003*, volume 61 of *Concurrent Systems Engineering*, pages 97–105, Amsterdam, Sept 2003. IOS Press.

[13] A. E. Lawrence. Observing processes. In *Communicating Process Architectures – 2004*, volume 62 of *Concurrent Systems Engineering*, pages 147–156, Amsterdam, Sept 2004. IOS Press.

[14] C.J. Fidge. A formal definition of priority in CSP. *ACM Transactions on Programming Languages and Systems*, 15(4):681–705, September 1993.

[15] Gavin Lowe. *Probabilities and Priorities in Timed CSP*. D. Phil thesis, Oxford, 1993.

[16] B.A. Davey and H.A. Priestley. *Introduction to Lattices and Order*. Cambridge University Press, 2nd edition, 2002.

[17] Ian R. East. Towards a semantics for prioritised alternation. In East and Martin et al., editors, *Communicating Process Architectures 2004*, volume 62 of *Concurrent Systems Engineering*, pages 253–263. IOS Press, 2004.

[18] Ian R. East. Programming prioritized alternation. In H. R. Arabnia, editor, *Parallel and Distributed Processing: Techniques and Applications 2002*, pages 531–537, Las Vegas, Nevada, USA, 2002. CSREA Press.

[19] Ian R. East. The Honeysuckle programming language: An overview. *IEE Software*, 150(2):95–107, 2003.

[20] A.W. Roscoe. An alternative order for the failures model. In *Two Papers on CSP* [27].

[21] Andrew Butterfield and Jim Woodcock. Semantics of prialt in Handel-C. In *Communicating Process Architectures – 2002*, Concurrent Systems Engineering, pages 1–16, Amsterdam, Sept 2002. IOS Press.

[22] Jeremy Malcolm Randolph Martin. *The Design and Construction of Deadlock–Free Concurrent Systems*. PhD thesis, University of Buckingham, 1996.

[23] A.W. Roscoe, editor. *A Classical Mind*. Prentice Hall Series in Computer Science. Prentice Hall, 1994. Essays in Honour of C.A.R. Hoare.

[24] Gavin Lowe. Prioritized and probabilistic models of Timed CSP. Technical Report PRG-TR-24-91, OUCL, 1991.

[25] Gavin Lowe. Prioritized and probabilistic models of timed CSP. *Theoretical Computer Science*, 138(1), 1994. Special Issue on Mathematical Foundations of Programming Semantics conference.

[26] A.W. Roscoe. Unbounded nondeterminism in CSP. In *Two Papers on CSP* [27].

[27] Oxford University Computing Laboratory. *Two Papers on CSP*, number PRG-67 in PRG Technical Monographs, July 1988.

Communicating Process Architectures 2004   185
Ian East, Jeremy Martin, Peter Welch, David Duce, and Mark Green (Eds.)
IOS Press, 2004

C++CSP Networked

Neil BROWN

QinetiQ, Malvern Technology Centre, St Andrews Road,
Malvern, Worcestershire, WR14 3PS, United Kingdom
neil@twistedsquare.com / ncbrown@QinetiQ.com

Abstract. C++CSP is a library for C++ enabling direct implementation of CSP concurrency design. It provides an extended set of CSP primitives that follows the model captured by occam and JCSP, with an API similar to the latter. It runs on most platforms, with efficient realisation for both Windows and Unix/Linux. It was released under the open source Lesser GNU Public Licence in January, 2004. That version supports only concurrency within a single machine. This paper details the development of a network capability for the library and reports some benchmarks, which are encouragingly fast. The design of C++CSP networking follows several of the decisions made for the JCSP Networking Edition (e.g. naming and automatic multiplexing, though not yet a Channel Name Service). Three further extensions to the library (channel poisoning, factories and bundles) are also presented.

1 Background

Communicating Sequential Processes (CSP) [1, 2] is a concurrency model centred around concurrently executing processes that communicate using channels. CSP channels are point-to-point; processes communicate through writing or reading on *channel ends*, rather than the writer having the address of its intended reader. CSP communications are also synchronised. When a channel communication takes place, both parties must engage. When a writer has finished its communication, it knows that its reader has read its message (rather than asynchronous communication, where the writer has no such information). Crucially, a process knows that its internal state cannot be changed behind its back, by being updated through the arrival of messages outside its control.

An advantage of CSP is that the processes do not have to know anything of the delivery mechanism of the channels they are using. Provided that the channels follow CSP channel semantics, their implementation details (e.g. routing) are irrelevant to the processes using them. This means that the channels can be network transparent; two processes will function the same way whether they are communicating using *internal* (on the same machine) channels or over *networked* (between machines) channels.

Due to the limited power of any single machine, distributed computing is an area of huge interest to those involved in high performance computing. Network transparency allows a properly-structured CSP application to run on one computer or on many networked computers in parallel, with little or no change to the program itself. This advantage is particularly useful for problems that have a large variety of scale. For example, machine learning algorithms can operate on data sets that have a huge range of sizes – the smaller data sets can be learnt from using a single machine, but larger problems may require clusters of machines.

Networked computing is not just of interest with relation to high performance computing however. Any client/server application could benefit from the relationship being able to "stretch" over a network with little code change. For example, a GUI client with a server backend could either run in a self contained application on one machine, or it could put the backend on another machine, perhaps shared between many clients.

One year ago, C++CSP was introduced at this conference [3], and at the beginning of this year was released under the Lesser GNU Public Licence [4]. It contained many useful new features such as templated channels and stateful poisoning (see section 2.1), but initially it had no built-in network support. During the intervening year network support has been integrated into C++CSP, and other new features have been added. This paper describes this work, the design decisions that were taken, justification for the decisions and the results that have been achieved with the network component. This paper assumes some familiarity with the basic concepts and API of the core C++CSP library.

2 New C++CSP Features

2.1 Non-poisonable Channel Ends

Stateful poisoning of channels is a feature of C++CSP whereby a process with an end of a channel can poison that channel, causing all successive attempts to use the channel in any form (apart from to poison it) by anyone to throw a PoisonException. However, allowing all processes with a channel end to poison the channel is not always desirable. For example, we may not want *anyone* with a writing end of an any-to-one channel to be able to poison it. To this end, channels also now have noPoisonReader and noPoisonWriter functions that provide channel ends that cannot be used to poison the channel (unlike the ends obtained from the reader and writer functions). Using this mechanism, processes can choose whether the channel ends they pass to their subprocesses can be poisoned or not.

2.2 Channel Factories

When two or more processes function by communicating mostly with each other, it is common to create a parent process that simply creates these two processes and provides an interface to them to the world, hiding the communications that exist solely between the child processes. For example, there might be a process that handles requests to access some data, and an interface process that provides this service to the world in a simple interface. These two processes could then be packaged up into a single server process. A tough decision is what sort of channel to have between the two internal processes. A one-to-one channel would be in keeping with the standard CSP semantics but would make other requests block until the data access process has finished with the request. A buffered channel may be desired instead; but there are multiple types of buffering – various sizes of FIFO, an overwriting buffer, or an infinite size FIFO.

The best solution would be to allow the channel policy to be specified. The channel could not be passed into the constructor as channels themselves cannot be copy-constructed. Pointers to channels could be passed but this constructor-parameter-per-channel approach would not scale well if the policy needed to be specified for a large (or variable) number of channels. Templating the process is possible but would not allow for the decision to be flexibly made at run-time. A buffer type could be passed to the process but this eliminates the possible speed-up from using unbuffered channels, and also does not allow for any future types of channels that may have significantly altered semantics (C++CSP has been designed to allow for such possible future additions). The solution chosen is to use channel "factories".

A class factory (an OOP pattern) is an object that creates other objects. A channel factory is a class that can be used to create channels. Functionality is provided through inheritance, and each channel it creates is guaranteed to have the same lifetime as the factory. This allows channels to last for a long time, but also can make them last beyond the lifetime of their ends. The syntax for the factory is as follows:

```
class SomeProcess : public CSProcess
{
    ChannelFactory<int>* factory;
protected:
    void run()
    {
        Chanin<int> readingEnd;
        Chanout<int> writingEnd_NotPoisonable;
        factory->one2One(&readingEnd,&writingEnd_NotPoisonable,
            true,false);
    }
    ... pass in factory through the constructor
};
```

The one2One method of the channel factory takes the address of the two channel ends to assign to, and also two parameters (with a default value of `true`) to specify whether the reading and writing ends respectively should be poisonable (see the previous section). Channel factories were also implemented in **JCSP.net** [5, 6].

2.3   Channel Bundles

Channel bundles are a concept introduced by **KRoC** [7, 8] (as "channel-types"). A channel bundle is a collection of channel *ends*. Bundling channels allows for easy representation of an interface. For example a process might have two request channels of type string, and a reply channel for each – one of type int and one of type vector<float>. Therefore a channel bundle could be produced to represent this interface containing four items: Chanin<string>, Chanout<int>, Chanin<string>, Chanout< vector<float> >. On its own this would just be a simple struct-like data structure. Channel bundles are reversible though, so the reverse structure of Chanout<string>, Chanin<int>, Chanout<string>, Chanin< vector<float> > could be given to another process wanting to use the original process. In **KRoC**, the bundles are used for mobile channels as follows:

```
CHAN TYPE MYTYPE
  MOBILE RECORD
    CHAN INT in?:
    CHAN INT out!:
    CHAN BOOL extra!:
:

MYTYPE? myin:
MYTYPE! myout:

myin, myout := MOBILE MYTYPE
```

To do the same in C++CSP:

```
typedef
    Bundle< bundle::In<int>,bundle::Out<int>,bundle::Out<bool> >
    MyType;
```

```
One2OneChannel<int> a,b;
One2OneChannel<bool> c;

MyType::Normal myIn(a,b,c);
MyType::Reverse myOut(a,b,c);
```

The constructors of the two bundles can take the actual channels as arguments, and get the channel ends appropriately, to make their use simpler and more elegant.

3   Networked C++CSP – Motivation

Unlike other programming methodologies, such as procedural object-oriented programming, CSP is well-suited to utilising networks because it is naturally network-transparent. Providing that CSP semantics are preserved, CSP processes are able to operate over any transport mechanism, whether it is a CSP kernel on a single machine, or a network between two machines. This is because CSP processes are perfectly encapsulated – there is no shared data between processes. The only way processes can communicate with each other is through recognised CSP primitives such as channels and also barriers and buckets. Barriers and buckets can be built using channels, so for the purposes of this paper only channels will be considered.

C++CSP's University of Kent-based sister technologies, KRoC [7, 8, 9, 10] and JCSP [11, 12] already have networked versions, KRoC.net [13, 14] and JCSP.net [5, 6] respectively. They provide both a proof-of-concept for network-enabling CSP technologies, and also a useful design reference. This allows C++CSP to continue its trend of learning from KRoC and JCSP while also trying to enhance them where possible and appropriate.

4   Networked C++CSP – Aims

Before design work can be undertaken on the networked capability of C++CSP , the aims of the project need to be clarified, to inform our decision-making.

The central goal is to enhance C++CSP by allowing two C++CSP machines[1] to communicate with each other using channels via a network. The primary consideration is utilising TCP/IP sockets for the underlying transport mechanism, as TCP/IP sockets are virtually ubiquitous in modern networking.

The network channels should be easy to use, and should be interchangeable with other channels as much as possible. That is, they should be useable in parallel communications, alternatives, extended rendezvous[15] and so on wherever possible. They should be poisonable, as other channels are. All these aims facilitate network-transparency, the aim being that a process communicating over a network channel should notice no difference from communicating over a standard channel.

It would be easy to state that the network-enabled library should be efficient. There are many measures of efficiency here however. Possible criteria include minimal network latency, maximum data throughput, and minimal loss of speed to the processes the machine is running locally. Which of these is more important than the others depends on the particular application so wherever possible the balance between them should be configurable.

---

[1]In this paper, a machine is defined to be a C++CSP program. Hence two C++CSP machines can run on the same physical machine.

5 Networked C++CSP – Design

The design of the network enhancements to C++CSP consists of many different areas. It is clear that a new component will be needed in the kernel to handle the new consideration of network traffic. This will be referred to as the NET system. Its job is to be the interface between the network and the C++CSP kernel. Its implementation is discussed in section 5.2. The network protocol for channel communications will also need to be decided on – this is described in section 5.3. Finally, consideration needs to be given to the Application Programming Interface (API) for network channels (section 5.1), and the associated issues to do with naming and finding channels (section 5.1.2).

5.1 The Network Class Structure and API

5.1.1 Channel Creation

To create a one-to-one channel and its associated ends the following code can be used:

```
One2OneChannel<int> channel;
Chanout<int> writingEnd = channel.writer();
Chanin<int> readingEnd = channel.reader();
```

This is clearly unsuited to being used for network channels. A network channel is not created entirely on one machine, it is inherently split between the two machines that it communicates between. Therefore allocating the channel as above is not the best solution.

Instead, each machine will allocate its own channel object, where the two channel objects correspond to one actual channel. So one end will have the following code:

```
Net2OneChannel<int> networkChannel;
Chanin<int> readingEnd = networkChannel.reader();
```

The other end will have the corresponding code:

```
One2NetChannel<int> networkChannel;
Chanout<int> writingEnd = networkChannel.writer();
```

These two channels will not be connected as they are above. To correctly connect the two channel objects, we need a shared identifier – a channel name.

5.1.2 Channel Names

Both KRoC.net and JCSP.net opted for using the concept of a "Channel Name Server" (CNS) in their network components. With this system every networked machine took the address of a CNS and queried it for the network address (e.g. IP address and port number) of the machine that corresponded to the name of a channel. This is a similar concept to that of the Domain Name Server (DNS) which is now ubiquitous on the internet.

C++CSP will probably also have this concept included in the near future, but currently there is only a standard explicit connection syntax. A channel name is simply of the form "[NetworkAddress[:PortNumber]/]ChannelName". If the network address is not included, the channel is allocated on the local machine. This means that other machines that connect can request to be connected to this channel, but the channel will not immediately be connected to another machine. At this point use of the channel will block indefinitely until someone connects to it.

If the machine name is included, then the name is effectively a request to connect to a remote channel. The network address (either an IPv4 address or a DNS name) and port number uniquely identify a machine on the network, and the channel name is the channel to connect to on that remote machine. Channel names can contain any ASCII characters above 32, except the / character.

5.1.3 Accepter Channels

The methods described above allow for a single process to connect to a single remote network channel. This will be fine for many scenarios, but will not work for situations where one server process needs to be able to accept connections from a variable number of clients.

To solve this problem, C++CSP supplies *accepter* channels – a concept similar to the socket accept() call. The idea behind accepter channels is that they have a channel name as normal, but for each remote connection, instead of connecting it to the accepter channel, a new channel is created. This mechanism is invisible to the remote process making the connection – it does not know whether it connected to a normal channel or an accepter channel. A suitable syntax for this might have been:

```
Net2OneChannelAccepter<int> accepter;
Net2OneChannel<int> channel = accepter.accept();
```

The accept() call above would of course block until a remote connection was made to this machine. To better fit in with the rest of the library however it is best to make the accepter channel a proper channel (of channels!) as follows:

```
Net2OneAccepterChannel<int> accepter;
Net2OneChannel<int> channel;
accepter.reader() >> channel;
```

There is one remaining issue with this implementation though. In any communication between a client and a server there will inevitably need to be communication in both directions at some point. CSP channels are one-way however, so just by connecting as above, only one way communication would be possible. There are various possible methods for establishing the channel in the other direction.

A second accepter channel for the client to join would not work properly as it cannot be guaranteed that they would join in the same order to match the connections on the two accepter channels, i.e. it would be impossible to tell which connection on accepter channel B was from the same client as one on accepter channel A.

The first channel accepted could be used to send the names of other channels to connect to back to the client. So the client would receive an array of channel names to use, such as "server/input0", "server/output1", but this would be a redundant channel after the connections had all been made. Such an approach is valid, but for some purposes the problem can be solved more efficiently by providing the address of the client to the server when the connection is made, so that the server can connect back to the client. So for example the client connects to the channel "server/ping", the server gets the client address and connects to "client/pong" (see Appendix A for an example of the use of accepter channels).

This mechanism is useful when only one client from a C++CSP machine will be connecting to the server, otherwise name conflicts prevent this mechanism being used. In future, work could be done in the area of connecting entire batches of channels in a single connection attempt.

5.1.4   Channel Transparency

When the original C++CSP library was developed, a decision was taken to have channel ends that provide a consistent API to the channels themselves. While this introduces an extra virtual function call into every channel action, it was considered worthwhile to be able to truly hide the channel type from the process using it. Every channel type uses the same channel end objects, so these ends are all that processes communicating over a channel see. It is up to the parent process to choose the channel type, and pass the channel ends to its child processes appropriately.

At the time of development of the original library this allowed for buffered channels to be used seamlessly in place of normal channels, but with the advent of the networked component of C++CSP, it also allows network channels to be used in place of normal channels.

5.1.5   Data Serialisation and Conversion

Sending data over a network is often not as simple as copying the bytes between two networked machines. A major problem in C++ is that variables are often stored as pointers, references, or complex data structures containing these items. Clearly a pointer is only valid on the machine that it is being used; sending it over the network makes no sense. Another consideration for some systems might be the endianness of the networked machines – if an integer value is to be sent between a little-endian machine and a big-endian machine, it will need to be converted.

The solution to these issues in the networked C++CSP API is to provide a default behaviour for transmitting items across the network (simply copying the bytes), but to allow (and indeed encourage and where possible require) the user to override this. A class, NetConverter is provided:

```
template <typename DATA_TYPE>
class NetConverter
{
public:
    std::pair<const void*,unsigned int> toNet(
        const DATA_TYPE* data);
    unsigned int fromNet(
        DATA_TYPE* data,std::pair<const void*,unsigned int> pr);
};
```

The toNet method converts local data (the data parameter) into raw bytes for sending over the network (the return pair of a pointer to the data, and its size). The fromNet method converts raw bytes (the pr parameter above) back into local data (the data parameter) and returns the amount of bytes it had taken from the buffer. The default converter simply uses memcpy to perform the conversion. This is suitable for "plain old data" types but not for others, so the user is encouraged to provide their own specialisation of the class to handle the conversion.

There are converters supplied for many STL containers (such as string, vector, map) but these are implemented in the safest manner; they convert each data object individually. This is the correct decision for, say, vector< map< int,ComplexDataStructure > > but for vector<float> where there may be millions of floats in the array, it is very inefficient. Therefore if the user is going to be sending such structures, they can (and should) provide a converter for these.

Unfortunately such optimisations cannot be determined by the library itself due to the nature of C++ (and its lack of reflection). The library would explicitly have to supply converters for all situations where a simpler converter would be sensible, and this is not feasible, so it is left to the user of the library. Also, the optimisation may be unwise. For example to convert a `vector<int>` may require converting each `int` individually to change its endianness, so the decision is left to the user.

5.2   The NET System

There are a number of options to consider for how the NET system might interact with the network and the local C++CSP machine. It could use either blocking or non-blocking sockets. Non-blocking sockets would allow the system to avoid making a blocking call, a behaviour that has always been strictly avoided in C++CSP (since blocking would stop the execution of *all* C++CSP processes). However, the behaviour of non-blocking sockets varies a lot between different Unix[2]-clones [16], let alone between them and Windows[3]. This, combined with the messiness of asynchronous notifications that arise from using non-blocking sockets, means that in fact blocking sockets are the better option, due to their simplicity and portability. Blocking on these sockets can actually be avoided by using the `select()` call to check a socket's status before making any send or receive calls.

The NET code can either be in the same thread as the C++CSP machine, or in its own thread. Having it in its own thread seems like the best way to reduce the slow-down effects of checking the network on the main C++CSP processes. It also appeals to the accepted wisdom of having your network code in a separate thread (for example, [17]). This would also allow properly blocking calls to be made without worry of it slowing down the main system.

Initially, the NET system was implemented in a separate thread to the normal C++CSP system. However, it became apparent that communication between the two threads (and all the associated synchronisation) incurred almost as much slow-down as checking the network did. Therefore it seemed that checking the network in the same thread would minimise the network latency without making any difference to the slow-down in the normal system. This claim is explored in a benchmark later on in section 7.2.

5.3   The Protocol

The NET protocol is used between two C++CSP machines. It needs to support the full range of C++CSP (one-to-one, unbuffered) channel semantics. This includes normal communications, parallel communications, extended inputs, alternatives, and poisoning. It must also support making connections to channels (including the previously described accepter channels), and error conditions.

5.4   Semantics

The NET system ensures that it is invisible to processes at the two ends of a networked channel by preserving channel semantics. The NET system does not act like a buffer – it transparently forwards the data across the network, with no change to the synchronisation semantics of the application running on top of it.

5.4.1   Connections

The NET system will multiplex the channels that are connected between two machines over a single socket. No matter how many channels there are between two C++CSP machines,

---

[2]UNIX is a registered trademark of The Open Group
[3]Windows is a registered trademark of Microsoft Corporation

there will only be one actual socket connected between them. This saves the overheads of checking many sockets, but will not affect the data throughput of the channels.

5.4.2 Communication

The simplest protocol for channel communication would be one message per channel communication (from writer to reader). However treating the message being sent as the end of the communication for the writer would allow the writer to continue even if the reader had not read from the channel – a clear violation of CSP synchronised channel communication. The solution is for the reader to send an acknowledgement when the network channel has been read. This simple system allows for all the communication types described above:

- *normal communication*: the writer sends a message with the contents of the communication and then blocks/freezes. The NET system of the reading machine recieves the message and feeds it into the channel. The reader (who may have been waiting, or may arrive at the channel afterwards) then reads the message; the NET system then sends an acknowledgement, which unblocks the writer.

- *extended rendezvous*: the extended rendezvous is a communication where the writer sends a channel communication, and the reader receives it but does not complete the communication (i.e. free the blocked writer) until it has processed the information in some way. This is simple to achieve in the NET system, which simply does not send back its acknowledgement until the reader indicates that the rendezvous is complete.

- *alternatives*: ALTing over a network channel involves placing a "hook" for notification for when a message arrives for the network channel, which can then be used by a guard in an ALT.

- *parallel communication*: performing communications in parallel in C++CSP consists of two phases. The first involves setting up all the communications that are to be performed and the second is suspending the process until all have been completed. So for a parallel output, the writer simply sends the message with the contents of the communication (as in the normal communication) during the setting up phase, and the communication is deemed complete when the acknowledgement is recieved from each reader. A parallel input works similarly, completing when all inputs have arrived.

5.4.3 Channel Identification

It has already been specified that channels will have a name that can be used to make the channel identifiable and unique (within a single machine). So one possibility for identifying the destination channel when a message is sent down the socket would be to provide the channel name. However, C++CSP does not currently impose a limit on the length of channel names, so descriptive names (which should be encouraged to prevent conflicts) would impose a performance penalty for communication. Instead, each end of a networked channel is given a 32-bit *channel ID*, unique within each machine.

5.4.4 Messages

Every message passed between NET systems will take the form of a triple; the channel ID, a size field, and then a stream of data (of that size, except for special messages). The channel ID will always be the ID on the machine to which the message is headed, regardless of the stage of the communication. So a simple communication will put the channel ID on the *destination* machine in the ID field, the size of the data in the size field, and then the data. The receiving machine will then reply (when the communication has been completed) with a message containing the ID of the channel on the source machine, with a special value NetAckType in the size field, and no data.

Each machine maintains a lookup table containing the ID of each channel on the remote machine it is connected to. This way each machine knows which ID to send messages back to on the channel, removing the need to send both a destination and source channel ID with each message. This helps conserve bandwidth.

When a channel is poisoned, a notification is sent to the other end. A poison notification is similar to a reply message – it contains the channel ID (as always, for the message destination end), a special value NetPoisonType in the size field, and no data.

The other message types are the negotiations involved in connecting two ends of a network channel together. To connect to a remote channel, the connecting machine must send a message with the special value RequestChannelConnect_NetChannelId in the ID field, the size field will contain the ID of the channel on the connecting machine, and the data stream will be a null-terminated string containing the name of the channel being connected to. In reply there will be a message with the special value ReplyChannelConnect_NetChannelId in the ID field, the ID of the channel on the replying machine in the size field, and the same string in the data stream.

6   Threading

C++CSP originally used a many-to-many threading model. Each C++CSP program contained one or more threads, which each contained one or more processes. This allowed for considerable flexibility in the library, and the possibility of taking advantage of multi-processor machines. Threads of the same program have a shared address space. This has the advantage of being able to send pointers between threads (rather than sending an entire data structure), although this in turn has the disadvantage of potentially letting the programmer break the CREW (Concurrent-Read, Exclusive-Write) principle. Having multiple programs (communicating via the NET system) would also allow advantage to be taken of multi-processor machines; the only difference would be not having the problematic shared address space, and the speed difference.

There is another issue aside from the speed difference however. Inter-thread communications are done in C++CSP using semaphores. This has the advantage of being portable and generally quick, but there is no portable equivalent of the socket select() call for semaphores that allows multiple semaphores to be checked (and potentially blocked on). This means that communicating via the NET system will scale *much* better than communicating between threads via semaphores. Of course, communicating between threads via the NET system has the same speed as communicating between programs using the NET system.

Therefore to keep the API as simple and clean as possible, C++CSP has been changed back to a single thread for processes to run in, and the advice for those wanting OS-level concurrency on a single physical machine is to run multiple C++CSP machines (programs) on the same physical machine.

6.1   Threading for the NET System

One option for adding the networking would be to run it in a separate thread to our single main thread. However the communication and scheduling overheads for communicating with this thread cause problems. The network process would not (on most operating systems) be able to block while (doing the equivalent of) ALTing between socket events and semaphore events. The only viable thing to do would be to use sockets to communicate between the individual threads and the network thread, which would then communicate using sockets to the remote machines. Clearly this middle-man will only slow the process down for no gain.

Including the network code in the main thread decreases network latency but will also increase the latency of local processes, because of the time taken to check the network. There is a direct trade-off between network latency and local latency, and as such it will be configurable. The benchmarks measuring network latency and local overheads can be found in sections 7.1 and 7.2 respectively.

7 Benchmarks

Previous sections have discussed the API of the networked part of the C++CSP library. The other important factor in distributed computing is the speed of the communications over the network. The following benchmarks were all carried out with a Gentoo GNU/Linux desktop machine with an Athlon 1600+ XP processor and 256MB of SDR RAM as the client (or single machine in single machine benchmarks), and where a second machine was needed as a server, a Windows XP machine with an Athlon 2400+ XP and 512MB of DDR RAM. The machines are connected via a 100Mbps LAN, which had no other load during the tests.

7.1 Latency

7.1.1 Explanation

This benchmark tests the delay involved in communicating between two machines. The easiest way to measure latency is of course a ping test. The time taken to send a (minimal) communication from A to B, and a reply from B to A, is timed by A to form a *ping* time. Usually machines are pinged using ICMP/IP, a protocol designed for such things. ICMP is usually responded to by the system kernel, whereas pinging between two processes over TCP/IP involves extra latency because the message has to pass from the kernel to the user process (which has to be scheduled by the operating system).

7.1.2 Results

A ping test was done between the two test machines, and over 50 runs the average ping time was 718 microseconds. As a comparison, a standard ICMP ping between the machines yielded an average time of 321 microseconds over 50 pings. This is mostly accounted by the extra acknowledgements over the network generated by the C++CSP NET infrastructure (to maintain CSP channel synchronisation), which in this case doubles the network traffic.

A slightly cleaned-up version of the code is provided in Appendix A, as it is a good small example of how to use the networked part of C++CSP.

7.2 Network System Overheads

7.2.1 Explanation

Network system overheads are the amount of time that the network system of C++CSP spends checking the network, i.e. the amount of time "lost" by the local processes because of having the network component running at the same time. The benchmark that will test this runs the

CommsTime benchmark [18] locally, while running a ping client (see the previous benchmark). That client is pinging another machine but, more significantly, is checking the network periodically. These times can then be compared with those from running *CommsTime* without starting up the network component of C++CSP – see Table 1.

7.2.2   Network Overheads Results

Table 1: Results from the Overheads Test

Network-check Frequency	Time Per CommsTime Loop (microseconds)
1 millisecond	2.754
500 milliseconds	2.814
No network	2.753

These timings are of absolute time, not CPU time. The results show that the networked component of C++CSP does not slow down the local processes, even checking a thousand times a second. This is a useful result, because it shows that supporting the network does not "cost" the local processes any significant time.

7.3   Communication Overheads

7.3.1   Explanation

This class of benchmarks measures the time taken up by the communications involved in distributing the computing across multiple machines on the network. This was measured by performing this benchmark with both the server and client on the same machine using normal C++CSP channels, and then running the server and client on separate machines using network channels. So communication overheads encompasses latency and network system overheads, in a realistic example of distributing a computation problem using C++CSP.

The benchmark chosen for this is calculating fourier coefficients. This is done by using the trapezium method of integration. It is an easily parallelisable task, as each calculation of a coefficient is independent of the others. It can therefore show how much difference the network communications are making to the speed of the benchmark.

Benchmarks were run to calculate 10,000 coefficients, splitting them up into work packages (WPs) of 1, 10, 100, 1,000, or 10,000 coefficients. Each coefficient was calculated using either 10, 100 or 1,000 trapeziums – giving a total of fifteen different benchmarks. Each work package requires two communications – one to send the details of the work (40 bytes) to the client, and one from the client to the server with the results ($4*c$ bytes, where c is the number of coefficients calculated in that work package).

These benchmarks were run on the same machine (using normal non-network channels), and then with the server on a different machine across the (100 Mbps) network, so that the client (doing the calculations) is on the same machine for all the tests. The results for all tests were averaged over 50 runs, to eliminate any anomalies from any other background tasks on the machine "stealing" some processor time during the timed tests.

7.3.2   Results – Server and Client on the Same Machine

Table 2 shows the results from running the benchmark on the same machine. The results show that no matter how the work is split, the work scales linearly with the amount of calculation needed.

Table 2: Times from the Same Machine Test (seconds)

Trapeziums	10^0 WPs	10^1 WPs	10^2 WPs	10^3 WPs	10^4 WPs
10	0.085583	0.084918	0.084831	0.086672	0.101007
100	0.818286	0.816175	0.815787	0.817667	0.831389
1000	8.101215	8.098428	8.094989	8.145628	8.105675

This means that the amount of communications that take place make no significant difference to the performance of the system for local channels – an encouraging result for non-networked C++CSP. The one result that deviates slightly from the strictly linear pattern is the test with the greatest number of work packages (only one calculation per work package) and the least calculation per work package (only 10 trapeziums). It makes sense that the communication overheads are mostly likely to show on the test with the smallest computation to communication ratio. Even for this extreme fine granularity, however, the effect is not marked – about 18%.

7.3.3 Results – Server and Client on Different Networked Machines

Table 3 shows the results from this test. It is clear that over the network the results scale both with the number of work packages and the trapeziums. The test with one work package has virtually no network overheads because only two communications are involved. This can be checked by comparing the network result for 1000 trapeziums (i.e. as the problem scales up) with the non-network result – there is only a 0.5% difference. So the one work package result can be used as a base case against which to compare the other networked results (in order to see what difference the greater amount of network communications is making).

Table 3: Times from the Networked Test (seconds)

Trapeziums	10^0 WPs	10^1 WPs	10^2 WPs	10^3 WPs	10^4 WPs
10	0.102680	0.104186	*0.158208*	*0.413571*	*4.108936*
100	0.836837	0.840752	0.877223	*1.231270*	*4.110065*
1000	8.139110	8.148298	8.195977	8.602985	*12.305083*

For higher numbers of trapeziums (i.e. for higher computation to communication ratios), the results are constant for 1, 10 and 100 work packages – so the overheads make no difference for these numbers of work packages (which have a linear relationship with the amount of communication). As the number of work packages climbs towards 10,000, the time taken starts to increase. 10,000 work packages means two network communications for each computation of a coefficient – a very low computation to communication ratio. By comparing the results for 10,000 work packages with those for one work package, it is fairly clear that the communication overheads for 10,000 work packages are around 3 to 4 seconds. Each work package involves four network communications (one each for the request and reply, plus one for each acknowledgement generated by the NET infrastructure), so this overhead is just under 100 microseconds per communication.

It should be noted that these benchmarks are not designed to show application *speed-up* – only network overheads. Farming out the client work (i.e. *all* the computational work) to more than one machine would demonstrate that. Table 3 indicates that near linear speed-up should be obtained for all combinations of numbers of trapeziums and work packages *except* for those whose timings are italicised.

8   Availability

The latest version of the C++CSP library, including all the development covered in this pa-per, is available from the website at http://cppcsp.net/, under the *Lesser GNU Public Licence*.

The latency tests (section 7.1) can be found in the C++CSP distribution in the directory moretest/; the files are ping_server.cpp and ping_client.cpp. They can be run using the ./More_Test -y and ./More_Test -z commands for server and client respectively.

The network system overheads tests (section 7.2) are included in the ping_client.cpp file in the moretest/ directory and the commstime_test.cpp file in the simpletest/ di-rectory, both in the C++CSP distribution. The tests can be run using the ./More_Test -x (using ./More_Test -y for the ping server) and ./Test -j commands.

The communication overhead tests (section 7.3) are located in the fourier_server.cpp and fourier_client.cpp files in the moretest/ directory in the C++CSP distribution. They can be run using ./More_Test -f and ./More_Test -g for the server and client re-spectively.

9   Conclusion

Networked channels have been successfully integrated into C++CSP. The API is similar to the existing C++CSP API and the new network channels are interchangeable with existing channels. Thus, processes do not need to know whether the channel ends they are using belong to normal channels or network channels. This makes it very easy to switch between networked and non-networked versions of C++CSP applications. As home networking and the Internet grow ever more popular, this greatly enhances the usefulness of the C++CSP li-brary.

The *ping* test gave a ping time between two networked processes as double that of an ICMP ping, which itself could be viewed as the maximum possible performance for a ping. This result is still under a millisecond, which can be considered to be an acceptable result. The network overhead test demonstrated that checking the network does not slow down the local processes, which helps remove doubts concerning the possible performance penalty from having the code checking the network in the same thread as the local processes. The last benchmark showed that if the work is divided up into suitably-sized work packages, the performance of distributed computing using networked C++CSP can scale almost linearly.

The (TCP/IP) sockets API provides untyped asynchronous reliable communication be-tween networked machines. The C++CSP network system provides a typed synchronised (reliable and multiplexed) layer on top of the sockets API that abides by CSP semantic rules for channel communication and choice (represented by ALTing). It is hoped that this net-worked C++CSP may provide a useful API and support infrastructure for applications that just want simple networking, as well as for those wanting networked CSP.

One planned addition to the library is the ability to communicate over "raw" TCP/IP sockets. C++CSP network channels are the preferred method of network communication as they observe CSP channel semantics and are typed, but C++CSP programs may need to communicate using an existing protocol on a raw TCP/IP socket (for example, HTTP). Allowing C++CSP programs to use sockets in the same way as channels would enhance the library's usefulness in creating networked applications.

For the future, the provision of *Channel Name Services* (as in KRoC.net and JCSP.net) for a more flexible means of establishing network connections dynamically will be consid-ered. There is also the question of sending channel ends or processes over the network, as discussed in [19, 14].

References

[1] C.A.R.Hoare. Communicating Sequential Processes. In *CACM*, volume 21, pages 666–677, August 1978.

[2] C.A.R.Hoare. *Communicating Sequential Processes*. Prentice-Hall, 1985.

[3] N.C.C. Brown and P.H. Welch. An Introduction to the Kent C++CSP Library. In J.F. Broenink and G.H. Hilderink, editors, *Communicating Process Architectures 2003*, pages 139–156, 2003.

[4] GNU. Lesser GNU Public Licence. http://www.gnu.org/licenses/lgpl.html.

[5] Quickstone Technologies Ltd. JCSP Network Edition Home Page. Available at: http://www.quickstone.com/xcsp/jcspnetworkedition/ Retrieved July, 2004.

[6] P.H.Welch, J.R.Aldous, and J.Foster. CSP networking for java (JCSP.net). In P.M.A.Sloot, C.J.K.Tan, J.J.Dongarra, and A.G.Hoekstra, editors, *Computational Science - ICCS 2002*, volume 2330 of *Lecture Notes in Computer Science*, pages 695–708. Springer-Verlag, April 2002.

[7] P.H. Welch and F.R.M.Barnes. Kent Retargetable occam Compiler Home Page. Available at: http://www.cs.ukc.ac.uk/projects/ofa/kroc/ Retrieved July, 2004.

[8] P.H.Welch and D.C.Wood. The Kent Retargetable occam Compiler. In *Proceedings of WoTUG 19*, volume 47, pages 143–166, March 1996.

[9] F.R.M. Barnes and P.H. Welch. Prioritised Dynamic Communicating Processes: Parts I and II. In James Pascoe, Peter Welch, Roger Loader, and Vaidy Sunderam, editors, *Communicating Process Architectures 2002*, WoTUG-25, Concurrent Systems Engineering, pages 331–380, IOS Press, Amsterdam, The Netherlands, September 2002. ISBN: 1-58603-268-2.

[10] F.R.M. Barnes and P.H. Welch. Prioritised dynamic communicating and mobile processes. *IEE Proceedings – Software*, 150(2):121–136, April 2003.

[11] P.H. Welch. Java Communicating Sequential Processes Home Page. Available at: http://www.cs.ukc.ac.uk/projects/ofa/jcsp/ Retrieved July, 2004.

[12] P.H.Welch. Process Oriented Design for Java: Concurrency for All. In H.R.Arabnia, editor, *Proceedings of the International Conference on Parallel and Distributed Processing Techniques and Applications (PDPTA'2000)*, volume 1, pages 51–57. CSREA, CSREA Press, June 2000.

[13] Mario Schweigler, Fred M.R. Barnes, and Peter H. Welch. Flexible, Transparent and Dynamic occam Networking With KRoC.net. In J.F.Broenink, editor, *Communicating Process Architectures – 2003*, volume 61 of *Concurrent Systems Engineering*, pages 107–126, Amsterdam, The Netherlands, September 2003. (WoTUG), IOS Press.

[14] M. Schweigler. Adding Mobility to Networked Channel-Types. In I. East, J. Martin, P. Welch, D. Duce, and M. Green, editors, *Communicating Process Architectures 2004*, WoTUG-27, Concurrent Systems Engineering, ISSN 1383-7575, pages 201–218, IOS Press, Amsterdam, The Netherlands, September 2004.

[15] F.R.M.Barnes and P.H.Welch. Prioritised Dynamic Communicating and Mobile Processes. *IEE Proceedings-Software*, 150(2):121–136, April 2003.

[16] Geoffrey Lee. Non-blocking sockets. http://www.wychk.org/~glee/non-blocking.html.

[17] Sun Microsystems. How To Use Threads. http://java.sun.com/products/jfc/tsc/articles/threads/threads1.html.

[18] Roger M.A. Peel. A Reconfigurable Host Interconnection Scheme for Occam-Based Field Programmable Gate Arrays. In Alan G. Chalmers, Henk Muller, and Majid Mirmehdi, editors, *Communicating Process Architectures 2001*, volume 59 of *Concurrent Systems Engineering*, pages 179–192, IOS Press, Amsterdam, The Netherlands, September 2001. IOS Press.

[19] F.R.M. Barnes and P.H. Welch. Communicating Mobile Processes. In I. East, J. Martin, P. Welch, D. Duce, and M. Green, editors, *Communicating Process Architectures 2004*, WoTUG-27, Concurrent Systems Engineering, ISSN 1383-7575, pages 201–218, IOS Press, Amsterdam, The Netherlands, September 2004.

Appendix A: Ping Example Code

```
class PingClientTester : public CSProcess {      // client
protected:
    void run() {
        ... read in server address into the string connectTo
        Net2OneChannel<std::string> chanIn("pong");
        One2NetChannel<std::string> chanOut(connectTo + "/ping");

        while (true) {
            chanOut.writer() << ourName;
            chanIn.reader() >> theirName;
            sleepFor(Seconds(1));                 // 1 second delay between pings
        }
    }
};

class PingHandler : public CSProcess {           // server
public:
    Net2OneChannel<std::string> n2o;
    One2NetChannel<std::string> o2n;
protected:
    void run() {
        Chanout<std::string> out(o2n.writer());
        Chanin<std::string> in(n2o.reader());

        try {
            while (true) {
                in >> theirName;
                out << ourName;
            }
        }
        catch (PoisonException e) {}
        in.poison();  out.poison();
    }
};

class PingServerTester : public CSProcess {
protected:
    void run() {
        Barrier barrier(1);
        Net2OneAccepterChannel<std::string> accept("ping");

        while (true) {
            PingHandler* ph = new PingHandler(mn);
            std::pair<Net2OneChannel<std::string>*,std::string> pr(&ph->n2o,"");

            accept.reader() >> pr;

            try {
                ph->o2n.connect(pr.second + "/pong");
                spawnProcess(ph,&barrier);         // only spawn if there is no poison
            }
            catch (PoisonException) {
                ph->n2o.reader().poison();
            }
        }
    }
};
```

Communicating Process Architectures 2004
Ian East, Jeremy Martin, Peter Welch, David Duce, and Mark Green (Eds.)
IOS Press, 2004

Communicating Mobile Processes

Fred R.M. BARNES and Peter H. WELCH

Computing Laboratory, University of Kent,
Canterbury, Kent, CT2 7NF, England.

{frmb, phw}@kent.ac.uk

Abstract. This paper presents a new model for mobile processes in occam-π. A process, embedded anywhere in a dynamically evolving network, may suspend itself mid-execution, be safely disconnected from its local environment, *moved* (by communication along a channel), reconnected to a new environment and reactivated. Upon reactivation, the process resumes execution from the same state (i.e. data values and code positions) it held when it suspended. Its *view* of its environment is unchanged, since that is abstracted by its synchronisation (e.g. channels and barriers) interface and that remains constant. The environment behind that interface will (usually) be completely different. The mobile process itself may contain any number of levels of dynamic sub-network. This model is simpler and, in some ways, more powerful than our earlier proposal, which required a process to terminate before it could be moved. Its formal semantics and implementation, however, throw up extra challenges. We present details and performance of an initial implementation.

1 Introduction

occam-π is a sufficiently small language to allow experimental modification and extension, whilst being built on a language (classical occam) of proven industrial strength. It integrates the best features of CSP [1, 2] and the π-calculus [3], focussing them into a form whose semantics is intuitive and amenable to everyday engineering by people who are not specialised mathematicians — the mathematics being built into the language design, its compiler, run-time system and tools, so that users benefit automatically from that foundation. The new dynamics broadens its area of direct application to a wide field of industrial, commercial and scientific practice.

Our earlier model [4] for mobile processes requires them to terminate before they could be moved. This gives a simple and intuitive semantics for activation:

```
SEQ
  c ? x              -- mobile process arrives
  x (...)            -- process x (...) runs from start to finish
  d ! x              -- mobile process departs
```

and a relatively simple implementation. However, for there to be a purpose behind these mobiles, they have to be able to maintain some (passive) state that survives their termination, movement and reactivation. To achieve this necessitates a *class-like* syntax for those mobile processes, involving private fields (for persistent state), constructors (for initialising that state) and methods (for activation). Such mobiles do not suffer the problems associated with object-orientation — such as leaky encapsulation, aliasing and concurrency blindness — and may be interesting in their own right. A denotational semantics for them, based on Hoare and He's *Unified Theories of Programming* [5], has been constructed that naturally supports system development and verification by refinement from formal specifications [6]. Accordingly, we are likely to combine this earlier model with the new one and we show in sections 2 and 3.1 below how this combination may be done cleanly. Readers unfamiliar with this earlier model may safely ignore these comparisons.

Our new proposal has a slightly less crisp semantics for mobile process activation:

```
SEQ
    c ? x               -- mobile process arrives
    x (...)             -- process x (...) runs from somewhere to somewhere
    d ! x               -- mobile process departs
```

where the *somewheres* are either the *start* of the process, a *suspension-point* or *termination*. The value of the process variable 'x', after it has been input, is (the CSP expression) P/t, where P is the original process and t is the trace it has executed so far (and elsewhere!).

Process types are as in [4] — just PROC header templates. A MOBILE process implementing such a type has an extra primitive it can invoke — 'SUSPEND'. When that happens, the activation '*early terminates*', retaining its state and program counters. This corresponds to a strong occam intuition: that it is very powerful to express process state as a combination of its data values *and* where it is in its code.

The process may now be moved by normal communication down a channel carrying its process type. It may then be reactivated by the receiving process, after plugging it into a local environment. The process resumes execution from where it suspended with its own state unchanged, but with its external synchronisations bound to the new environment[1].

1.1   Implementation Issues

When thinking how to support mobile processes a long time ago, we were concerned about the danger of race hazard between asking a process to suspend and its subsequent movement — how could we be sure it had really suspended (and was not in the middle of some crucial transaction with its current environment)? Note, however, the tenses in the abstract of this paper. Mobile processes have to SUSPEND themselves — they are not suspended by their environment, which would simply not be safe. External processes may ask a mobile to suspend, but the mobile must do it itself and may take its time. When it suspends, control automatically passes to the process that activated it, which may now safely move it.

We are particularly grateful to the insight Tony Hoare gave us for handling a mobile process that has gone parallel internally. Our earlier model handled this by waiting for full termination — i.e. a multi-way synchronisation on the termination event of all internal processes. So, treat SUSPEND also as a multi-way synchronisation bound to all the internal processes — they *all* have to suspend for the whole mobile to suspend. For implementation, we just need a CSP event (an occam-π 'BARRIER') reserved in the workspace of any mobile process. To reactivate the mobile, all its suspended processes will be on the queue held by that event — easy!

Well, not quite that easy. Processes — even mobile processes — are very lightweight mechanisms in occam-π and, currently, are not location independent. A complete occam-π system is, of course, location independent but individual processes have many things addressed relative to the base of the whole system, not the individual process. Moving a process to a new memory space (or 'CLONE'-ing it) means that its workspace is allocated elsewhere and pointers will have to be adjusted. Moving processes across soft channels to a process in the same memory space is no problem.

---

[1]The allowed parameters are restricted to synchronisation types only — e.g. channels and barriers (see section 2.2).

Of course, we have to arrange a '*graceful*' suspension by all the processes within a mobile. If one sub-process gets stuck on an internal communication while all its sibling processes have suspended, we have deadlock. Fortunately, there is a standard protocol for safely arranging this parallel suspend — it's the same as arranging for parallel termination [7]. This is left for the mobile application to implement; it's not our concern as mobile process language designers. We will think about providing language support for such distributed decisions. But that is orthogonal to the issue of mobile processes.

1.2 Structure of this Paper

Section 2 describes how mobile processes are declared, initialised and activated. The 'mobile' aspect of these mobile processes — i.e. moving them around a process network — is described in section 3.

Section 4 discusses some of the potential applications of this technology, with respect to existing "mobile agent" ideas and practice.

An overview of the implementation of these mobile processes is given in section 5. Section 6 draws some preliminary conclusions and lays out intended future directions for this work.

2 Defining Mobile Processes

Mobile processes may be defined in one of two ways. The first, described in [4], allow a single mobile process to support multiple *implementations* of *process-types*. That method of defining a mobile process allows the various implementations to share the state that persists between activations. That state must be declared outside of the individual implementations, however. Process-types provide the type system for mobile processes, and describe the interface to that process. For example:

```
PROC TYPE IO IS (CHAN INT in?, out!):
```

This declares a process-type called 'IO', whose implementations must match the 'PROC'-style signature given, i.e. one INT input channel and one INT output channel — the formal parameter names need not match. Like other types in occam, two similarly structured but differently named process-types are not considered compatible.

The second method of defining a mobile process, described here, only allows a single implementation. This can be viewed as a 'shorthand' syntax for single-implementation mobile processes declared using the first method — and where there is no shared state. Instead of writing, for example:

```
MOBILE PROC integrate                                -- earlier model
    ... persistent/shared state (in this case, empty)
  IMPLEMENTS IO (CHAN INT in?, out!)
    ... process body
  :
```

we would instead write:

```
MOBILE PROC integrate (CHAN INT in?, out!) IMPLEMENTS IO    -- new model
    ... process body
  :
```

Note that 'CONSTRUCT' blocks (section 2.1 and [4]) are not needed for these mobiles, since there is no shared or persistent state to initialise.

Furthermore, the "IMPLEMENTS IO", is not strictly required. The compiler can check this when a mobile process is allocated. It also permits a single mobile process to support multiple implementations, provided that the formal-parameters are compatible. For example:

```
MOBILE IO p:
SEQ
  p := MOBILE integrate
  ...  process using p
```

The type of 'p' is always well-known — occam-π does not support type polymorphism — thus the compiler can easily (and statically) check that 'IO' matches the formal parameters of 'integrate' at the point of its allocation (the 'MOBILE' assignment). The declaration of the mobile 'integrate' process might be simplified even further to an ordinary 'PROC' declaration. For example:

```
PROC integrate (CHAN INT in?, out!)
  ...  process body
:
```

This allows any PROC to be *mobilised*, providing its interface matches the corresponding process-type. However, there are arguments that it may be good programming practice always to include an 'IMPLEMENTS' when declaring a mobile process — as well as identifying explicitly that the process is 'MOBILE'. We may specifically require the latter to enable some optimisations planned for later stages of our implementation.

2.1   Allocating Mobile Processes

As shown above, mobile processes are dynamically allocated using a special form of assignment. This follows in a similar way to other 'MOBILE' allocations, e.g. for dynamic mobile arrays [8] and mobile channel-types [9, 10]. The 'fuller' version of mobile processes (described in [4]) requires the separately declared and persistent state to be initialised using a 'CONSTRUCT' block. This is called at the point of allocation, passing any parameters given. For example, consider the following mobile process definition:

```
MOBILE PROC integrate
  INT total:              -- persistent state

  CONSTRUCT (VAL INT i)
    total := i

  IMPLEMENTS IO (CHAN INT in?, out!)
    ...  process body
:
```

A variable of the 'IO' type could be allocated with:

```
MOBILE IO p:
SEQ
  p := MOBILE integrate (0)
  ...
```

The simplified version of mobile processes presented here does not need this type of alloca-tion. Allocation is simply "p := MOBILE integrate", without any parameters. Initialisa-tion of any internal state follows the normal (and natural) pattern of being the first thing the process does the first time it is activated

Following the allocation of a mobile process, the process variable ('p' in the above code fragment) is used purely in terms of its process-type (e.g. 'IO'), not the process that created it (e.g. 'integrate'). The only data relating to 'integrate' stored inside 'p' are the process entry-point, run-time memory requirements and a pointer to a 'workspace-map' for the pro-cess. These are, of course, not the concern of the programmer using these mobiles. Details are covered in section 5.

Figure 1 shows this process ('p') from its own point of view. The channels are not real channels as such, rather they are placeholders for channels that will be "plugged in" when the process is activated — discussed in the following section.

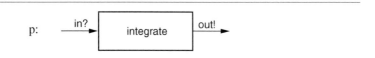

Figure 1: Value of mobile process variable 'p' after allocation of 'integrate'

2.2   Activating Mobile Processes

Mobile processes are *activated* by applying the process variable to a set of local arguments. This binds the mobile process to a *local* environment for the duration of the activation. For example:

```
CHAN INT to.p, from.p:
PAR
  local.environment (to.p!, from.p?, ...)

  MOBILE IO p:
  SEQ
    ...  p acquires some value
    p (to.p?, from.p!)
    ...
```

Figure 2 shows this mobile process active and connected to a local environment.

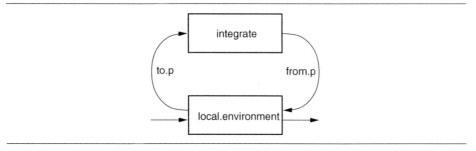

Figure 2: Active mobile 'integrate' process

3   Communicating Mobile Processes

Mobile processes in occam-π follow the semantics of existing mobiles — they are *moved* rather than *copied*, when assigned or communicated. They also share parts of the existing implementation for mobiles (section 5).

Figure 3 shows an example process network containing two processes connected by a channel. In this example, the channel carries mobile processes:

```
CHAN MOBILE IO c:
PAR
  A (c!)
  B (c?, ...)
```

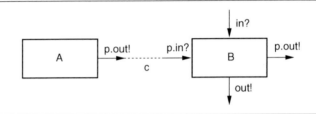

Figure 3: Process network for communicating mobile processes

The 'A' and 'B' processes are implemented such that 'A' creates a new mobile process and communicates it to 'B', that then activates it. For example:

```
PROC A (CHAN MOBILE IO p.out!)      PROC B (CHAN MOBILE IO p.in?, p.out!,
  MOBILE IO p:                                 CHAN INT in?, out!)
  SEQ                                 MOBILE IO v:
    p := MOBILE integrate             SEQ
    p.out ! p                           p.in ? v
    -- p is no longer defined           v (in?, out!)
  :                                     p.out ! v
                                        -- v is no longer defined
                                    :
```

Note that the 'B' process is unaware of the actual implementation — it only knows how to connect with the process (given by the 'IO' process-type). This is one reason why it may turn out to be good programming practice to indicate explicitly what process-type a mobile process implements (e.g. "IMPLEMENTS IO"). That way, 'B' can at least be sure that the process it has in its 'v' variable is one that was intended to implement 'IO' — as opposed to a process whose interface is structurally the same, but whose behaviour is entirely different (as that could lead to deadlock when interfacing with the process). Section 3.2 examines this in more detail.

3.1   Suspending Mobile Processes

A serial implementation of 'integrate' involves a "WHILE TRUE" loop. For a mobile process, this would normally mean that once activated the process would never terminate. For most applications of such a mobile, this would be undesirable.

The mobile processes described in [4] support suspend/resume through explicitly persistent state that survives termination and re-activation. For example:

```
PROC TYPE IO.SUSPEND IS (CHAN INT in?, out!, CHAN BOOL suspend?):

MOBILE PROC integrate.suspend.0
  INT total:                        -- persistent state

  CONSTRUCT ()                      -- simple constructor
    total := 0

  IMPLEMENTS IO.SUSPEND (CHAN INT in?, out!, CHAN BOOL suspend?)
    INITIAL BOOL running IS TRUE:
    WHILE running
      PRI ALT
        BOOL any:
        suspend ? any
          running := FALSE
        INT v:
        in ? v
          SEQ
            total := total + v
            out ! total
  :
```

This is adequate for many purposes, even though the syntax is slightly cumbersome. One of the reasons for defining mobile processes this way is so that state may be shared between several implementations — this 'integrate.suspend.0' has only one. There is a further, more subtle, problem however — if the mobile process goes parallel internally, those parallel processes must be shut-down before the mobile process can terminate.

The mobile processes described here, which need no special support for persistent state, cannot suspend through termination — all its state would go out of scope and be lost! Instead, a mechanism for explicitly suspending a process mid-execution is provided. The above process, for example, now becomes:

```
MOBILE PROC integrate.suspend.1 (CHAN INT in?, out!, CHAN BOOL suspend?)
IMPLEMENTS IO.SUSPEND
  INT total:
  SEQ
    total := 0
    WHILE TRUE
      PRI ALT
        BOOL any:
        suspend ? any
          SUSPEND                   -- suspend process
          -- re-activates here
        INT v:
        in ? v
          SEQ
            total := total + v
            out ! total
  :
```

If control reaches the SUSPEND line, the process suspends execution, retaining all local state and its resumption address (in much the same was as it does when de-scheduled) but returns control to its invoking process. The invoking process may communicate the mobile to a new location, where the receiving process may re-activate it by invocation on its own set of arguments. The mobile then resumes execution from where it suspended with its local state unchanged. The channels bound to its parameters will (usually) be different — but that is of no concern to the mobile, whose semantics are defined with respect to its parameters and not the actual arguments supplied.

We believe that the mechanism for 'integrate.suspend.1' is a little clearer and more natural than that for 'integrate.suspend.0'.

3.2 Mobile Contracts

PROC TYPE interfaces define only the *connections* that are required and offered by the mobile. They do not define *how* those connections are used nor, indeed, how the values generated by the mobile relate to values received. We have just described three levels of specification that refine each other: the most general being the *Connection* (defined by the PROC TYPE), then the *Contract* (definable by a CSP specification of the behaviour of the mobile in terms of the events parameterised by its PROC TYPE), and finally the *Function* (definable by a Z specification of the mobile as a state machine). These all integrate nicely into the Circus algebra of Woodcock et al. [11].

For the safety of both the mobile process itself and its hosting environment, a *Connection* specification is insufficient. For flexibility, a *Function* specification is too constraining — we want to allow differently functioning mobiles (e.g. with successive bug-fixes) to be delivered to and activated in any host environment. Otherwise, mobile processes offer nothing new; we could have a static (conventional) process and just move around passive data.

A *Connection* interface is insufficient because the hosting environment needs to be sure that a mobile process will behave properly when invoked (connected) to its local environment — i.e. that it will not cause deadlock or livelock, will not starve any local processes of its attention and will suspend when asked. Of course, reciprocal promises by the hosting environment are equally important to the mobile. We call those promises a *Contract*.

CSP is sufficiently rich to enable the specification of such good behaviours. Model checkers (such as FDR [12]) are sufficiently powerful to check that *Contract* conforming hosts and mobiles will indeed be safe.

We are looking to boost the PROC TYPE of a mobile to include such a contract. For example, a contract on 'IO.SUSPEND' might be that it is a *server* on its 'in?' and 'suspend?' channels, responding to an 'in?' with an 'out!' and to a 'suspend?' with *suspension*. This could be strengthened to indicate its priorities for service. Or weakened to specify just its traces. Or weakened further to require only that the number of 'in?' events in a trace can never be less than the number of 'out!' events and that a 'suspend?' may only occur when the number of 'in?' events equals the number of 'out!' events.

A behaviour we may want to prohibit in such a *Contract* is that of a 'suspend?' (and, therefore, suspension) occurring in-between an 'in?' and its corresponding 'out!'. That way the host environment will know that the mobile will not suspend with an answer outstanding[2].

Without such a contract, an 'IO.SUSPEND' mobile could arrive that always refuses its 'kill?' channel (and could never be removed by its host!) or starts with an 'out!' (and deadlocks with its host!).

We are considering extending the definition of PROC TYPEs to include some level of contract that the compiler can verify against implementing mobiles — but this is outside the scope of this paper. We note that these notions of behavioural contract would be valuable for *all* PROCs, mobile or not mobile.

---

[2]Note that this behaviour is honoured by 'integrate.suspend.1' above.

3.3 Suspending Mobile Networks

The 'IO.SUSPEND' implementing processes given above are toy examples, but they illustrate mobiles that offer services and gather information. They have also been chosen because their base function (a running-sum integrator) can be implemented as a simple feedback network of *stateless* processes — and is a common teaching example.

We use it here to illustrate suspending a mobile that has gone parallel. The *graceful termination* [7] algorithm can be modified to provide secure distributed suspension. However, that algorithm was not concerned with saving state information — it was only concerned with termination for which the subsequent state of the processes was irrelevant! Here, we must take care to preserve state (in this case, the running total) *and* to honour a minimum level of the contract described in the previous section (i.e. that suspension must not come between an 'in?' and its matching 'out!').

There are many ways to to do this, figure 4 shows one.

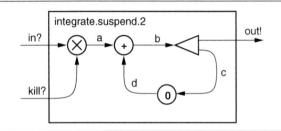

Figure 4: Suspendable parallel mobile integrator

The code for this parallel version of the integrator is:

```
PROTOCOL OK.INT IS BOOL; INT:

MOBILE PROC integrate.suspend.2 (CHAN INT in?, out!, CHAN BOOL suspend?)
IMPLEMENTS IO.SUSPEND

  CHAN OK.INT a, b, c:
  CHAN INT d:
  PAR
    suspend (in?, kill?, a!)
    plus.suspend (a?, d?, b!)
    delta.suspend (b?, c!, out!)
    prefix.suspend (0, c?, d!)
  :
```

The 'OK.INT' protocol tags INTs with a boolean, indicating whether the data carried is a *suspend* signal or *live* data. All sub-processes in the network remain stateless. The feedback loop holds the state of the whole mobile network — even during suspension (the propogating *suspend* signal carrying that state). Channel 'd' could have been 'OK.INT' as well. However, since 'prefix.suspend' only ever outputs *live* data, this has been optimised to just 'INT'.

The 'suspend' process monitors its inputs and reacts in an obvious way:

```
PROC suspend (CHAN INT in?, CHAN BOOL kill?, CHAN OK.INT out!)
  WHILE TRUE
    PRI ALT
      BOOL any:
      kill ? any
        SEQ
          out ! FALSE; 0          -- suspend signal
          SUSPEND
      INT x:
      in ? x
        out ! TRUE; x             -- live data
  :
```

Note that it prioritises its service in the same way as the serial (and stateful) 'integrate.-suspend.1'. The 'plus.suspend' is a simple modification to the standard adder process:

```
PROC plus.suspend (CHAN OK.INT in.0?, CHAN INT in.1?, CHAN OK.INT out!)
  WHILE TRUE
    BOOL b:
    INT x.0, x.1:
    SEQ
      PAR
        in.0 ? b; x.0
        in.1 ? x.1
      IF
        b                              -- live data received
          out ! TRUE; x.0 + x.1        -- send live data
        TRUE                           -- suspend signal received
          SEQ                          -- send suspend signal ...
            out ! FALSE; x.1           -- (carrying the running-sum)
            SUSPEND
  :
```

Note: the graceful termination algorithm requires waiting for the 'kill' signal to return, discarding other data that arrives. For this application, we know that no other data exists, so that only the suspend signal would return. That return has been optimised away here. This also means that this component does not need to remember the running-sum state ('x.1') and remains stateless. The remaining processes now write themselves:

```
PROC delta.suspend (CHAN OK.INT in?, out.0!, CHAN INT out.1!)
  WHILE TRUE
    BOOL b:
    INT x:
    SEQ
      in ? b; x
      IF
        b                          -- live data received
          PAR
            out.0 ! TRUE; x        -- send live data
            out.1 ! x              -- send data
        TRUE                       -- suspend signal received
          SEQ                      -- send suspend signal ...
            out.0 ! FALSE; x       -- (carrying the running-sum)
            SUSPEND
  :
```

```
PROC prefix.suspend (VAL INT n, CHAN OK.INT in?, CHAN INT out!)
  SEQ
    out ! n
    WHILE TRUE
      BOOL b:
      INT x:
      SEQ
        in ? b; x
        IF
          b                       -- live data received
            SKIP
          TRUE                    -- suspend signal received
            SUSPEND
          out ! x                 -- send data
  :
```

So, the running-sum state is actually held in 'prefix.suspend' when the mobile network is moved. From the point of view of 'prefix.suspend' it is *stateless* — i.e. it retains no data between its cycles. Within each cycle, it just reacts to the input received with an output — albeit with a suspension point in-between, depending on the type of input received.

The 'integrate.suspend.2' mobile network gracefully suspends when its environment offers a 'suspend' signal. It does this without deadlocking (which would certainly occur if the sequence of output communication and suspension were reversed in any of its component processes). In fact, the output and suspend operations could safely be run in PAR by all sub-processes *except* for 'prefix.suspend' (where deadlock would result since the output would never be accepted).

This shows the care that needs to be taken in devising and implementing a safe suspension of all processes in a mobile network. However, this is a different responsibility from the actual mobile suspend mechanism. Responsibility for the former rests, for the moment, on the application engineer. We are investigating design (and, hopefully, language) rules to assist.

Finally, we note that initiation of a SUSPEND need not only come from the environment of the mobile. It could be a unilateral decision by the mobile itself (subject, of course, to satisfying any declared behavioural contract with its current environment) or initiated by the mobile and negotiated with its environment.

4 Applications

The most commonly understood meaning of the term "mobile agent" is primarily that of code and data mobility, as described by White in [13]. The main focus of which is on mobility of code and data between nodes in a distributed system, and where the infrastructure for handling mobile agents is provided largely by the application and libraries, not by the language itself. As noted by Jansen and Karygiannis in [14], there are many security issues relating to mobile agents, that should be addressed by any system wishing to support these agents. Generally, these can be divided into two categories — those that relate to the environment (e.g. admittance of an agent for execution) and those that relate to the agent (e.g. its interaction with the environment once 'connected').

The mobile processes of occam-π can provide an equivalent functionality[3]. Furthermore, mobile processes offer a comparatively secure implementation, as a direct consequence of using the occam-π language. For example, there is no way mobiles can access resources

---

[3]At the time of writing, there is no support for migration of mobile processes over networks. We hope to implement this in the near future, however (section 6).

to which their hosts do not explicitly provide connection. Connection and activation of the mobile is wholly under the control of the host.

4.1   Mobile Agents and Agent Platforms

Within the wider "mobile agent" community, an *agent* is the mobile (as expected), and an *agent platform* is the environment in which that mobile agent executes. This maps cleanly onto occam-π — agents are mobile processes and the agent platform is any process that activates a mobile. Mobile processes may also activate other mobiles, becoming "agent platforms" themselves.

The agent platform exists for two main purposes: firstly, to allow agents to interact with the system providing the agent platform; secondly, to allow agents to interact with each other. occam-π can support both types of interaction easily. When activated, mobile processes attach to the local environment (providing 'agent – platform' interaction), and that environment may allow agents to interact with each other (providing 'agent – agent' interaction). Within occam-π, agents may also form links directly between each other — the platform then serves as a mechanism to allow agents to find each other.

Figure 5 shows an example mobile agent system, where the 'platforms' could either be processes in a single system, or distributed over a network. Within the scope of other research (investigation and modelling of nanite assemblies on a grand scale) we are exploring systems containing millions of 'agent' processes and 'platforms'.

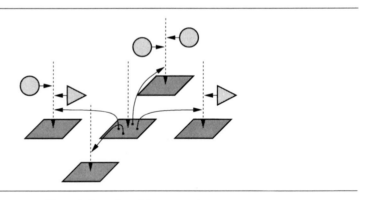

Figure 5: Example mobile agent system

In such systems, each 'platform' is a process constructed into a *matrix* of processes defining the topology of the space over which mobile agent processes roam. The matrix nodes are (mostly passive) servers, in touch with neighbouring nodes and on which arriving agents register. An agent attaches to one matrix node at a time, through which it can sense the presence of other agents and, hence, connect and interact as it chooses (using agent-specific protocols to avoid deadlock).

Matrix-agent protocols will be generic. Agents may enrol and resign from local (or global) barrier synchronisations to maintain a sense of time — as well as move and reproduce according to their own rules. Matrix nodes may also have their own agenda, allowing them to be pro-active in reshaping the space they define (e.g. through the creation of worm-holes) for more exotic environments.

We want to investigate the emergent properties of the system as a whole, rather than the behaviour of individual processes. This will require very large numbers of mobile processes — our current aspirations are for the order of 10^8 processes. The usefulness of networked distribution here is in increasing the overall size of the system. However, we have to take care to minimise the effects of latency as processes migrate between nodes.

Another practical example of the use of mobile agents in distributed systems is in organising meetings, for example. When someone wishes to schedule a meeting, they send out an agent to a 'calendar' platform. This agent then waits for other user's agents to 'check-in' with the calendar, and negotiates suitable times. In practice, agents may need to remain connected to the calendar for some time — to wait for other agents and the finally decided (meeting) time. This leads to other issues, such as how a user's agent finds its way back to the user — the user may have moved. One possible solution would be a 'directory' platform, that can direct agents back to their user — users update a local directory whenever they connect or disconnect, and this information propagates between directories over time. As long as users migrate more slowly than their agents, such a system will work. Such issues are beyond the scope of this paper, however.

We are also exploring the use of mobile processes (as an agent mechanism) in RMoX [15], where having such mechanisms at the operating-system level may be useful — both for application and inter-RMoX use.

4.2 Security

Within the wider mobile-agent community, there is a good deal of concern for the security of mobile agents and agent based systems, as discussed in [14, 16] and [17]. This section covers *some* of these issues. Broadly, these security considerations fall into two categories: those affecting the integrity of the overall system; and those affecting the integrity of individual agents and agent-platforms.

Integrity of the overall system is outside the scope of this paper. Processes that activate mobile agents may safely assume that the agent is valid — because that agent was either created locally or came from another part of the system. Correspondingly, an agent may assume that whoever activates it was meant to do so. In a networked environment, possibly connected using public networks (e.g. the internet), the part of the system that manages network connections is responsible for ensuring the integrity of data communicated over networked channels (where the data may be 'serialised' mobile processes). This may involve proper (public/private key) authentication and encryption.

Of course, we could create a system that freely admits mobile processes from open network connections. Such a system would be open to many of the potential abuses that afflict mobile-agent systems in general. The use of occam-π in the construction of agents allows some of this threat to be minimised. Instead of communicating a serialised agent whole, the (source) code for the process could be sent, along with the saved state of the agent, and used to re-create the agent locally. The occam-π compiler can make certain guarantees about code it compiles, that compilers for many other languages cannot — e.g. that the code is generally safe and interacts with its environment in the intended way.

The use of a synchronisation-only interface to mobile processes limits many of the threats associated with existing agent systems. The widespread use of sequential programming languages (such as C) has led to a generally sequential interfacing for mobile agents. This would typically be realised using a "procedure-call" style activation of agents, that limits basic interactions to input on procedure call and output on procedure return. Concurrent interaction is still a possibility, but requires non-standard (or non-language controlled) code. One possible option would be to use RPC [18], as suggested in [16]. This does not (directly) permit the use of synchronisations between an agent and its environment, however.

The use of a synchronisation interface separates the activation of a mobile process from interaction with it, although the two are closely related — and there is (theoretically) no limit to the amount of interaction that may occur during a single activation. To ensure correctness of those interactions, the 'TRACES' extension described in [19] could be used — although this is unsupported by the current occam-π compiler. This extension would enable to the compiler to check that both the agent and its environment conform to some pre-defined pattern of interaction (by specifying the CSP *traces* of those interactions). This mechanism, once implemented, will be able to define an important part of the *Contract*, described in section 3.2.

5   Implementation

Supporting the mobile processes as described here has required reasonably large modifications to the occam-π compiler used by KRoC [20, 21]. The most complex of these modifications is supporting the 'SUSPEND' functionality — which if not carefully managed could result in disaster (e.g. new activations contaminated with an old environment).

Mobile process variables (e.g. "MOBILE IO p") are implemented in a similar way to mobile channel-end variables — a single word in the process workspace that points to a block of dynamically allocated memory. This dynamically allocated block, ranging from 12 to 16 words in size, contains general information about the process, pointers to the process memories, and a *barrier* [22] that is used to hold suspended processes. Figure 6 shows the structure of this mobile-process descriptor.

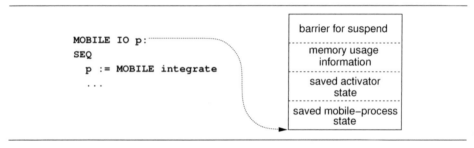

Figure 6: Structure of mobile-process descriptor

Mobile processes that do *not* suspend require very little special treatment — to the point where their activations are treated as ordinary PROC calls. However, once that mobile process has terminated, it may not be re-activated. This is implemented by setting the *reactivation-address* of the terminated process to code that raises a run-time error, or in 'stop' error-mode, deschedules the process attempting the activation.

Processes that *do* suspend require a certain amount of special treatment, largely in the code-generator. Because a mobile process may suspend mid-execution, there is a potential problem with parameters that have been abbreviated internally. Returning to the earlier parallel 'integrate', for example:

```
MOBILE PROC integrate.suspend.2 (CHAN INT in?, out!, CHAN BOOL suspend?)
IMPLEMENTS IO.SUSPEND
  CHAN OK.INT a, b, c:
  CHAN INT d:
  PAR
    suspend (in?, kill?, a!)
    plus.suspend (a?, d?, b!)
    delta.suspend (b?, c!, out!)
    prefix.suspend (0, c?, d!)
  :
```

When this code is activated for the first time, it sets up a network of sub-processes, connecting channels in the interface to those sub-processes. The usual implementation of channel parameter-passing (and abbreviations) is to simply copy the channel-pointer. When the sub-processes 'SUSPEND', the mobile process is shut-down and control returns to the activating process. A subsequent reactivation may be to a different environment, that would render the interface originating channel-pointers inside 'plus.suspend', 'delta.suspend' and 'int.suspend' useless — as they contain channel addresses that came from the environment of the first activation.

This problem is solved by adding an extra layer of indirection in the implementation of channel-parameters. That is, instead of passing a channel-address as a parameter, a *pointer* to the channel-address is passed. This does not apply to the activation, however — that gets channel-pointers for channel parameters. When setting up the sub-processes, the compiler passes addresses that are inside the workspace of the mobile process, for both external and local channels. Local channels require an additional address temporary, since they are the channel themselves.

Inside the sub-processes, the indirect channel-pointers must be dereferenced before communication is attempted. Three new ETC [23] 'specials' have been added for this, that dereference the virtual-transputer A, B and C registers respectively. These instructions are generated immediately prior to communication. The compiler could produce the same result using the traditional "LDNL 0" (load non-local at word offset 0). This, however, would require a more substantial modification to the compiler, that is currently largely unaware of general pointers-to-pointers.

5.1 Suspending Mobile Processes

The idea to collect suspended parallel processes on a barrier — in order to support suspension of entire process networks, rather than just a single process — was suggested by Tony Hoare and documented in [24]. When a mobile process is initially created, the barrier's 'enrolled' count is set to 1. The compiler automatically generates code to enroll and resign parallel processes as they are created and destroyed. When the last parallel process 'SUSPEND's, or resigns, it will complete the barrier and return control to the activating process. When reactivated, the processes blocked in the barrier are put back on the run-queue.

The code that enrolls processes on a barrier is relatively trivial — the barrier count is incremented by $n-1$, where n is the number of parallel processes. The code that synchronises (on 'SUSPEND') and resigns processes from a barrier is not trivial, since both may complete the barrier synchronisation. Rather than being generated in-line, this code is built into the run-time library (written in '*virtual transputer*' assembly language). Compile-time constants required by the code (e.g. offset of the 'count' field within the barrier) are made available as pre-processor variables. Having this code external to the compiler reduces the complexity of the compiler and size of the generated code, at the expense of a slightly longer run-time. However, having the operation identified explicitly (by a procedure call) allows for future optimisation — the native-code translator (tranx86) *could* replace the procedure call with an optimised native-code version of the operation.

5.2 Implementing Mobile Process Communication

For communication and assignment of mobile processes, existing mobile-related code and instructions are used. Within a single system, communication and assignment are simply the moving of a pointer (to the mobile-process descriptor) between processes (or variables in the case of assignment). As with other dynamic mobiles, "old" processes are freed rather than being moved into source of the communication or assignment — as happens for static mobiles.

Mobile processes can be duplicated using the 'CLONE' operator. This returns a copy of the mobile process operand, that is left defined. Supporting 'CLONE' requires knowledge about the workspace (and possibly vectorspace and mobilespace) layout of the process, so that any pointer values are correctly adjusted and other dynamic (mobile) state also 'CLONE'd (a *deep* copy). The one restriction is that any mobile process containing an *unshared* channel-bundle end may not be cloned — because that channel-bundle end cannot be duplicated using 'CLONE' (since that would break its *unshared* semantics!).

'Serialisation' of mobile processes is possible using the built-in 'ENCODE.CHANNEL' and 'DECODE.CHANNEL' processes, that were developed for KRoC.net [25]. 'DECODE.CHANNEL' would input a mobile process, then output a dynamic mobile BYTE array containing the position-independent state of the process, in addition to general information about the process, e.g. memory-requirements and a reference to the code that implements the process. The serialised state although position-independent, will still be architecture and layout dependant — e.g. the byte-ordering in words and the layout of individual variables in the process's workspace. Thus when communicating mobile processes between heterogeneous architectures, some (non-trivial) conversion may be required.

5.3   Performance

The implementation of mobile processes is, on the whole, very lightweight. At the time of writing, the parts of the implementation that are in place are still somewhat experimental, and so have not been optimised.

Measured on an 800 MHz Pentium-III, the time required to create and destroy a basic process (that does not take any visible parameters) is around 450ns — and when the dynamic memory required is immediately available from one of the free-memory lists. Including a complete activation raises the time to around 550ns, giving an approximate activation-deactivation time of 100ns.

Including a SUSPEND and activating the process twice takes approximately 920ns. Thus, the time required to suspend a process and then reactivate it is approximately 370ns.

These times are for a very simple process — that does not have either vectorspace or mobilespace. For more complex mobile processes (e.g. those that take parameters) the time required to activate the process will increase.

6   Conclusions and Future Work

This paper has described a new model for mobile processes in occam-π, that provides code and channel mobility (ideas from the π-calculus) with the discipline and rigour of occam and composable semantics of CSP. Mobile processes complement mobile channels [4, 9, 10] the occam-π programmer with powerful new tools for directly, safely and efficiently capturing the dynamic aspects of complex large-scale systems — e.g. multi-layer modelling of micro-organisms and their environments (the *In Vivo* ⇔ *In Silico* Grand Challenge [26, 27]) and process migration (agents) in distributed systems.

Currently, there is limited support for creating 'CLONE's of a mobile process. This, and 'serialisation' using 'DECODE.CHANNEL' or other means, requires the suspend process to be made independent of its location in memory. In order to do this, the run-time system (or compiler-generated code) needs a *memory-map* for each of the process's memories that contain pointers — i.e. workspace, vectorspace and optionally mobilespace. The compiler-side of KRoC.net [28] will also require this support so that it may transport mobile processes between separate memory-spaces.

At the time of writing, the compiler produces this information for some, but not all, pointer-types in the process workspace — CLONE works for very basic processes. We hope to complete this support, and therefore support for CLONE and serialisation in the near future.

Acknowledgements

We are grateful to Tony Hoare for his insights and advice on suspending parallel process networks [24]. We also wish to thank colleagues and other members of the concurrency research group, in particular David Wood, Christian Jacobsen and Mario Schweigler for their input and advice.

The authors would additionally like to thank the anonymous reviewers for their feedback on an earlier revision of this paper.

References

[1] C.A.R. Hoare. *Communicating Sequential Processes*. Prentice-Hall, 1985. ISBN: 0-13-153271-5.

[2] Steve Schneider. *Concurrent and Real-time Systems — The CSP Approach*. Wiley and Sons Ltd., UK, Baffins Lane, Chichester, UK, 2000. ISBN: 0-471-62373-3.

[3] R. Milner, J. Parrow, and D. Walker. A Calculus of Mobile Processes – parts I and II. *Journal of Information and Computation*, 100:1–77, 1992. Available as technical report: ECS-LFCS-89-85/86, University of Edinburgh, UK.

[4] F.R.M. Barnes and P.H. Welch. Prioritised dynamic communicating and mobile processes. *IEE Proceedings – Software*, 150(2), April 2003.

[5] C.A.R. Hoare. Unified Theories of Programming. Technical report, Oxford University Computing Laboratory, July 1994. Available at: http://users.comlab.ox.ac.uk/tony.hoare/publications.html.

[6] Xinbei Tang and Jim Woodcock. Travelling processes. In Dexter Kozen, editor, *The 7the International Conference on Mathematics of Program Construction*, Lecture Notes in Computer Science, Stirling, Scotland, UK, July 2004. Springer-Verlag. To Appear.

[7] P.H. Welch. Graceful Termination – Graceful Resetting. In *Applying Transputer-Based Parallel Machines, Proceedings of OUG 10*, pages 310–317, Enschede, Netherlands, April 1989. Occam User Group, IOS Press, Netherlands. ISBN 90 5199 007 3.

[8] F.R.M. Barnes and P.H. Welch. Mobile Data, Dynamic Allocation and Zero Aliasing: an occam Experiment. In Alan Chalmers, Majid Mirmehdi, and Henk Muller, editors, *Communicating Process Architectures 2001*, volume 59 of *Concurrent Systems Engineering*, pages 243–264, Amsterdam, The Netherlands, September 2001. WoTUG, IOS Press. ISBN: 1-58603-202-X.

[9] F.R.M. Barnes and P.H. Welch. Prioritised Dynamic Communicating Processes: Part I. In James Pascoe, Peter Welch, Roger Loader, and Vaidy Sunderam, editors, *Communicating Process Architectures 2002*, WoTUG-25, Concurrent Systems Engineering, pages 331–361, IOS Press, Amsterdam, The Netherlands, September 2002. ISBN: 1-58603-268-2.

[10] F.R.M. Barnes and P.H. Welch. Prioritised Dynamic Communicating Processes: Part II. In James Pascoe, Peter Welch, Roger Loader, and Vaidy Sunderam, editors, *Communicating Process Architectures 2002*, WoTUG-25, Concurrent Systems Engineering, pages 363–380, IOS Press, Amsterdam, The Netherlands, September 2002. ISBN: 1-58603-268-2.

[11] J.C.P. Woodcock and A.L.C. Cavalcanti. The Semantics of Circus. In *ZB 2002: Formal Specification and Development in Z and B*, volume 2272 of *Lecture Notes in Computer Science*, pages 184–203. Springer-Verlag, 2002.

[12] Formal Systems (Europe) Ltd., 3, Alfred Street, Oxford. OX1 4EH, UK. *FDR2 User Manual*, May 2000.

[13] Jim White. Mobile agents white paper, 1996. General Magic. `http://citeseer.ist.psu.edu/white96mobile.html`.

[14] Wayne Jansen and Tom Karygiannis. NIST special publication 800-19 – mobile agent security. Technical report, National Institute of Standards and Technology, Computer Security Division, Gaithersburg, MD 20899. U.S., 2000. `http://citeseer.ist.psu.edu/jansen00nist.html`.

[15] F.R.M. Barnes, C.L. Jacobsen, and B. Vinter. RMoX: a Raw Metal occam Experiment. In J.F. Broenink and G.H. Hilderink, editors, *Communicating Process Architectures 2003*, WoTUG-26, Concurrent Systems Engineering, ISSN 1383-7575, pages 269–288, IOS Press, Amsterdam, The Netherlands, September 2003. ISBN: 1-58603-381-6.

[16] Wayne A. Jansen. Countermeasures for Mobile Agent Security. *Computer Communications, Special Issue on Advances in Research and Application of Network Security*, November 2000.

[17] David Chess, Colin Harrison, and Aaron Kershenbaum. Mobile agents: Are they a good idea? In Jan Vitek and Christian Tschudin, editors, *Mobile Object Systems: Towards the Programmable Internet*, volume 1222 of *Lecture Notes in Computer Science*, pages 25–45. Springer-Verlag, April 1997.

[18] A.D. Birrell and B.J. Nelson. Implementing Remote Procedure Calls. *ACM Transactions on Computer Systems*, 2(1):39–59, February 1984.

[19] Frederick R.M. Barnes. *Dynamics and Pragmatics for High Performance Concurrency*. PhD thesis, University of Kent, June 2003.

[20] P.H. Welch and D.C. Wood. The Kent Retargetable occam Compiler. In Brian O'Neill, editor, *Parallel Processing Developments, Proceedings of WoTUG 19*, volume 47 of *Concurrent Systems Engineering*, pages 143–166. World occam and Transputer User Group, IOS Press, Netherlands, March 1996. ISBN: 90-5199-261-0.

[21] P.H. Welch, J. Moores, F.R.M. Barnes, and D.C. Wood. The KRoC Home Page, 2000. Available at: `http://www.cs.ukc.ac.uk/projects/ofa/kroc/`.

[22] Peter H. Welch and David C. Wood. Higher Levels of Process Synchronisation. In A. Bakkers, editor, *Parallel Programming and Java, Proceedings of WoTUG 20*, volume 50 of *Concurrent Systems Engineering*, pages 104–129, Amsterdam, The Netherlands, April 1997. World occam and Transputer User Group (WoTUG), IOS Press. ISBN: 90-5199-336-6.

[23] M.D. Poole. Extended Transputer Code - a Target-Independent Representation of Parallel Programs. In P.H. Welch and A.W.P. Bakkers, editors, *Architectures, Languages and Patterns for Parallel and Distributed Applications, Proceedings of WoTUG 21*, volume 52 of *Concurrent Systems Engineering*, pages 187–198, Amsterdam, The Netherlands, April 1998. WoTUG, IOS Press. ISBN: 90-5199-391-9.

[24] P.H. Welch. UKC-CRG-01-04-2004: Suspending Networks of Parallel Processes. Technical report, Computing Laboratory, University of Kent at Canterbury, UK, March 2004.

[25] M. Schweigler, F.R.M. Barnes, and P.H. Welch. Flexible, Transparent and Dynamic occam Networking with KRoC.net. In J.F. Broenink and G.H. Hilderink, editors, *Communicating Process Architectures 2003*, WoTUG-26, Concurrent Systems Engineering, ISSN 1383-7575, pages 199–224, IOS Press, Amsterdam, The Netherlands, September 2003. ISBN: 1-58603-381-6.

[26] R. Sleep. In Vivo ⇔ In Silico: High fidelity reactive modelling of development and behaviour in plants and animals, May 2003. Available from: `http://www.nesc.ac.uk/esi/events/Grand_Challenges/proposals/ViSoGCWebv2.pdf`.

[27] P.H. Welch. Infrastructure for Multi-Level Simulation of Organisms, March 2004. Available from: `http://www.nesc.ac.uk/esi/events/Grand_Challenges/gcconf04/submissions/42.pdf`.

[28] M. Schweigler. Adding Mobility to Networked Channel-Types. In I. East, J. Martin, P. Welch, D. Duce, and M. Green, editors, *Communicating Process Architectures 2004*, WoTUG-27, Concurrent Systems Engineering, ISSN 1383-7575, IOS Press, Amsterdam, The Netherlands, September 2004.

Communicating Process Architectures 2004
Ian East, Jeremy Martin, Peter Welch, David Duce, and Mark Green (Eds.)
IOS Press, 2004

Dynamic BSP: Towards a Flexible Approach to Parallel Computing over the Grid

Jeremy M. R. MARTIN

Oxagen Limited, 91 Milton Park, Abingdon, Oxon OX14 4RY, UK

Alexander V. TISKIN

Department of Computer Science, University of Warwick, Coventry CV4 7AL, UK

Abstract. The Bulk Synchronous model of parallel programming has proved to be
a successful paradigm for developing portable, scalable, high performance software.
Originally developed for use with traditional supercomputers, it was later applied to
networks of workstations. Following the emergence of grid computing, new programming models are needed to exploit its potential. We consider the main issues relating
to adapting BSP for this purpose, and propose a new model *Dynamic BSP*, which
brings together many elements from previous work in order to deal with quality-of-
service and heterogeneity issues. Our approach uses a task-farmed implementation of
supersteps.

1 Introduction

The BSP parallel computation model [1, 2] is very simple. It assumes that there is a set
of p processors, each capable of performing s operations per second. The processors are
connected by a communication fabric, which can communicate one data item to or from
every processor in the time it takes each processor to perform g floating-point operations. It
can also perform a global handshake synchronisation of all the processors in the time it takes
each processor to perform l floating-point operations.

The BSP programming model is also very simple. Execution of a BSP program is divided
into *supersteps*, each separated by global synchronisations. A superstep consists of each
processor doing some calculation on local data *and/or* communicating some data by direct
memory transfer to other processors. The global synchonisation event guarantees that all
communication of data has completed before the commencement of the next superstep.

Perhaps the most useful feature of BSP is the ability to construct *cost functions* of the parameters (s, p, l, g) in order to predict the performance and scalability of parallel algorithms
across different hardware platforms. This can be done prior to implementation. Tables of approximate values for these parameters are available for a wide range of machines [3, 2]. There
have been a number of successful case-studies of using BSP in practice (see for instance [4]).

BSP was originally intended for use within a reliable, homogeneous, dedicated parallel
computing environment, rather than with the unpredictable and variable resources that are
associated with grid computing [5]. However, it is such an attractive model for programmers,
that it is surely worthy of consideration as to whether it can be adapted for use in the grid
environment.

2 Previous Work

There are three main areas where the grid deviates from the BSP model.

1. *Processor heterogeneity*: variation between grid nodes of available computation power, either due to architectural differences, or due to time-dependent resource sharing issues. If a BSP program were run on a heterogeneous cluster, the progress of the overall computation would be constrained by the rate of the slowest processor. In some cases, we could consider getting around this problem by using sophisticated domain decomposition techniques to achieve better load balancing. However, this would make both programming and cost modelling substantially harder, which is against the spirit of the original BSP philosophy.

2. *Network heterogeneity*: significant variation of communication performance between nodes. Previous work has suggested that progress of a BSP program is usually constrained by the slowest communication link in the network [6].

3. *Reliability and availability*: processors may fail intermittently or be withdrawn unexpectedly by the service provider. This may lead to a variation in processor count during execution.

Let us consider existing published work in this field and assess where it has attempted to deal with the above issues.

Vasilev [7] has developed the BSPGRID model for grid-based parallel algorithms, by extending the BSPRAM model of Tiskin [8]. A BSPGRID computer is a collection of processor-memory units, a shared memory considered to be of unlimited capacity (which is likely to be implemented as a collection of disk units), and a global synchronisation mechanism. Unlike the standard BSP model, there is no persistence of data at processor nodes between supersteps — the contents of all local memories are discarded at the end of each superstep.

The amount of memory at each processor is considered to be limited, so for large problem sizes where the total amount of available memory at the processor nodes is insufficient, the concept of virtual processors is used. This means that each physical processor may be required to perform the work of multiple virtual processors sequentially in a particular superstep. The issue of processor reliability and availability is addressed by allowing the number of available physical processors to vary between supersteps. There is a recovery protocol for the case when processors may fail unexpectedly during a superstep: an additional synchronisation barrier is introduced, and the work of failed processors is rescheduled after the barrier.

A centralised global shared memory would lead to a communication bottleneck at the master processor, therefore any implementation of BSPGRID is likely to implement virtual shared memory distributed over the grid. Such an implementation would need to be made easy to use and fault-tolerant.

BSPGRID has a cost model consisting of the following parameters:

- M — the amount of memory per processor in words;

- g — the cost of shared memory accesses per word;

- l — the cost of synchronisation;

- N — the problem size in words.

The model is used to predict two cost functions for an algorithm: time and work. The time cost of an algorithm is the optimal execution time that could be achieved if enough real processors are applied to the problem, whereas the work cost is the processor-time product of the algorithm. The model does not consider the issues of network and processor heterogeneity, apart from variation in the amount of available memory at each node. A static and uniform allocation of virtual processors to physical processors is performed at each superstep.

Work by Goldschleger et al. [9, 10] describes development of a grid middleware infrastructure InteGrade, and implementation of BSP using that system. It is particularly focussed on provision of a virtual BSP computer to a user by allocation of idle resources within an organisation. There is no treatment of heterogeneity, but it is reported that work is in progress to support fault tolerance via a checkpoint and recovery protocol. The system is based on the Oxford BSP toolkit [11], and is claimed by the authors to be the first grid implementation of BSP.

Mattsson and Kessler [12] describe implementation of a BSP-based virtual shared memory programming language for grid computing. It supports a hierarchical extension to the BSP paradigm with localised supersteps. Other hierarchical extensions of BSP and a discussion of the localised approach can be found in various sources in the literature, including earlier work by the present authors [6, 13].

Nibhanupudi and Szymanski [14] have developed a fault-tolerant version of BSP, which works by running multiple redundant peers for each BSP processor. The peers are able to take over whenever the original process is assumed to have failed. They have developed a complex arbitration protocol to manage this, since it is hard to detect that a process has failed and is not merely slow.

The Satin system by van Nieuwpoort et al. [15] allows dynamic processes in the form of "pure" (side-effect free) function calls, scheduled by work stealing. Our proposed approach is more flexible, allowing more general process types and scheduling strategies. Tiskin [13] proposed a mechanism for dynamic process management in the BSP model, using both SPMD parallelism and dynamic processes. Our approach is conceptually simpler and easier to program, since it involves only one of these parallelism types (dynamic processes).

Rosenberg, Adler and Gong [16, 17] have investigated in depth the matter of optimally scheduling a bag of similar tasks to a heterogeneous network of processors. They have compared mathematically the predicted performance of using a FIFO communication protocol with that of a BSP communication protocol, in order to distribute tasks and gather results. This work is highly relevant to optimisation of the implementation of a superstep within a model such as BSPGRID.

3   Towards a New Approach: Dynamic BSP

Although there has clearly been substantial progress concerning grid implementation of BSP, we have seen that there is no single approach which would address all of our major concerns. Here we present a significant modification to the BSPGRID approach, which will enable us to address the heterogeneity issues, as well as fault-tolerance. It will also offer us a more flexible programming model, with the ability to spawn additional processes within supersteps as and when required.

There has been considerable success in utilising the internet to solve embarrassingly parallel problems using task-farms, for instance by the application of screen savers performing drug-protein docking simulations on vast numbers of personal computers [18]. Task-farming has also been proposed as a general programming paradigm for grid computing, e.g. in [19].

The essence of our new approach is to use the task-farm model to implement BSP supersteps, where the individual tasks correspond to virtual processors (see Figure 1). A task-

Standard BSP computation

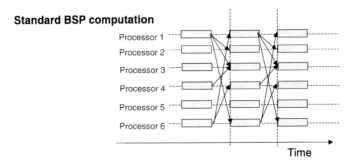

Dynamic BSP computation

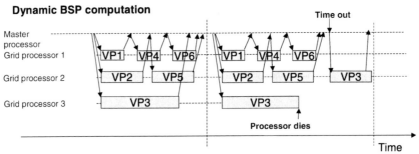

Figure 1: Standard BSP compared with Dynamic BSP

farm implementation of BSP has been suggested previously by Sarmenta [20], whose paper recognises that this approach suffers from the data bottleneck, unless the computation is embarrassingly parallel. We propose a mechanism of avoiding the data bottleneck.

Our model consists of:

- a master processor (task server);

- worker processors; and

- a data server (which can either be implemented as distributed shared memory or remote/external memory).

In each superstep there is a bag of virtual processors to be run on a pool of available physical processors. The computation and communication performance of each processor is considered to be variable, but we do assume a certain minimum level of available memory at each node, as with BSPGRID.

The master processor is responsible for task scheduling, memory management, and resource management. At the beginning of each superstep, a virtual processor number is distributed to each physical processor, which then has the responsibility to retrieve local data from the data server, perform the required computations, write back the modified data, and then inform the master processor that it has finished the task. The master processor maintains a queue of pending virtual processors and dynamically assigns them to waiting physical processors. As soon as the all the virtual processors have been executed on a particular superstep, the global shared memory is restored to a consistent state and the next superstep commences.

Using the task farm approach, the problem of heterogeneity across the grid can be concealed by choosing the number of virtual processors to far exceed the number of physical processors. This approach is sometimes known as *parallel slackness*, and complements explicit heterogeneous extensions to the BSP model, such as the ones by Williams and Parsons [21], and Morin [22].

3.1 Fault Tolerance

If a physical processor fails to complete its task within a reasonable time, then it is considered to have died, and its work is reallocated to another physical processor *within the same superstep*. Also the master process is at liberty to seek additional resources at any point to expand the processor pool. This approach to fault-tolerance is likely to be less computationally expensive than the generic Unix process migration mechanism proposed by Hill et al. [23].

3.2 Creation of Child Processes

Dynamic BSP allows the number of virtual processors to vary not only between supersteps but also *during* supersteps. Hence we may allow them to spawn other virtual processors (which would be useful for example to implement divide-and-conquer algorithms). Since the master processor still has to keep control, a virtual processor has to send a message to the master to spawn one or more children, and is then descheduled. The master will reschedule the requesting processor once all its children have terminated. There can be no data redistribution within supersteps, therefore the new virtual processor can only see a snapshot of the global data as it was at the beginning of the superstep, together with local state inherited from its parent. A traditional superstep would only allow one level of spawning, but within a task farm implementation arbitrarily many levels of descendant processors can be spawned, as long as data redistribution is not required.

The master processor generates tasks (virtual processors) and can either execute them (if they are small enough), or pass them on to workers. Workers can spawn new tasks, which must be registered with the master. Tasks may contain remote data references, and can transmit data to and from the data server. Additionally, sometimes it may be convenient that the data server can perform by request simple data-parallel computations without passing the data to the master or workers.

3.3 Memory Bottleneck

The main barrier to scalability with both BSPGRID and Dynamic BSP is the implementation of the global shared memory. To avoid a bottleneck, the data would need be distributed and treated similarly to BSPRAM model. Virtual processors would be decoupled from their data, but they would also need a mechanism of knowing where their data is (potentially distributed across several physical processors), and be able to access it bypassing the master processor. There would also need to be a separate fault-tolerance mechanism for the data, requiring replication and/or check-pointing such as implemented by Nibhanupudi and Szymanski [14].

3.4 Cost Model

The standard cost model for BSP would appear to be suitable for dynamic BSP, despite the fact that the g and l parameters might very well vary significantly between grid nodes. Using the task-farm approach, together with use of parallel slackness, would make it reasonable to use measured values for g and l (suitably averaged) to predict cost.

3.5 An Example: Strassen's Algorithm

McColl [24] (see also [25]) proposed a synchronisation-efficient BSP Strassen matrix multiplication algorithm, which generates block multiplication subtasks recursively in a data-parallel fashion. When the number of tasks becomes sufficiently high (equal to the number of physical processors, or more if one needs parallel slackness), matrix data are redistributed and the computation is completed in task-parallel fashion.

In our model, the master will generate the first "root" task, which will request the data server to do data-parallel work (without communication), and then spawn some children tasks. The children will do the same recursively. All this can be done in the master processor, since the tasks do not need to download data from the data server, hence their cost is at this point negligible. When the number of spawned tasks is large enough, they are distributed across the workers, and enter the task-parallel phase of the computation (i.e. download the matrix data, synchronise, compute block products, upload them back to the data server, and synchronise again). As soon as the task-parallel part of the computation is finished, the workers can send the tasks back to the master. The children tasks now start to terminate, and the parents resume and combine the childrens' results by issuing data-parallel computation requests to the data server. Upon termination of the root task, the data server contains the final output.

4 Conclusions and Future Work

We have investigated the potential issues in implementation of the BSP model over the grid. We have reviewed some useful existing work in this context, and also proposed a new dynamic model. Our model builds on Vasilev's BSPGRID model, and retains some of its key elements: a dynamic task pool and a virtual shared memory. In contrast with BSPGRID, our model utilises the task-farm approach to implement supersteps, and allows the tasks to spawn an arbitrary number of subtasks within a superstep. We have also introduced into the model some capability of data-parallel computation, which can be performed by the tasks remotely via the data server. The flexibility of this approach has been demonstrated by the Strassen matrix multiplication example. Since computational tasks are decoupled from data, both BSPGRID and our approach require an efficient implementation of distributed/remore shared memory for the data server.

The next logical step is implementing our model and testing it on a real-life system. In addition to that, here are some issues that would be worthy of further consideration.

Improved fault-tolerance. Instead of timeouts, it might be possible to use more sensitive mechanisms, such as ping clients.

Security. Commercial enterprises have to be extremely careful about data security, and this tends to be the main barrier to the uptake of grid computing in industry. A BSP implementation offering data encryption could help to solve this problem.

Persistent data. Many computationally intensive algorithms in use today require local access to substantial databases, e.g. the Blast program for biological sequence similarity analysis [26]. We need to consider extending our protocols to allow external resources to be requested with special attributes such as this.

Economics. In real-life grid applications, there is likely to be a tradeoff between quality of service and price. Commercial service providers, such as [27], offer use of dedicated reliable homogeneous virtual clusters for a competitive fee, whereas it is also possible to harness idle cycles on workstations within an organisation at very little cost. Work [28] contains an analysis of some of the economic factors involved in running a supercomputing service. It could be possible to take these factors into account by making financial cost an integral part of the cost model. Vasilev's BSPGRID makes the first step in this direction: the time cost of a computation is appropriate for evaluation of an algorithm implemented using inexpensive idle cycles, whereas the work cost is more relevant to time hired on commercial processor warehouses.

Acknowledgements

We thank the anonymous referees for helpful comments.

References

[1] L. G. Valiant. A bridging model for parallel computation. *Communications of the ACM*, 33(8):103–111, August 1990.

[2] R. H. Bisseling. *Parallel Scientific Computation: A structured approach using BSP and MPI*. Oxford University Press, 2004.

[3] BSP machine parameters. http://www.bsp-worldwide.org/implmnts/oxtool/params.html.

[4] J. M. R. Martin and Y. Huddart. Parallel algorithms for deadlock and livelock analysis of concurrent systems. In *Proceedings of Communicating Process Architectures*, pages 1–14. IOS Press, 2000.

[5] I. Foster and C. Kesselman. *The Grid: Blueprint for a new computing infrastructure*. Morgan Kaufmann, second edition, 2004.

[6] J. M. R. Martin and A. V. Tiskin. BSP modelling of two-tiered parallel architectures. In B. M. Cook, editor, *Proceedings of WoTUG*, volume 57 of *Concurrent Systems Engineering Series*, pages 47–55, 1999.

[7] V. Vasilev. BSPGRID: Variable resources parallel computation and multiprogrammed parallelism. *Parallel Processing Letters*, 13(3):329–340, 2003.

[8] A. Tiskin. The bulk-synchronous parallel random access machine. *Theoretical Computer Science*, 196(1–2):109–130, April 1998.

[9] A. Goldchleger, C. A. Queiroz, F. Kon, and A. Goldman. Running highly-coupled parallel applications in a computational grid. In *Proceedings of Brazilian Symposium on Computer Networks*, 2004.

[10] A. Goldchleger, F. Kon, A. Goldman, M Finger, and C. C. Bezerra. InteGrade: object-oriented Grid middleware leveraging idle computing power of desktop machines. *Concurrency and Computation: Practice and Experience*, 16:449–454, 2004.

[11] J. M. D. Hill, W. F. McColl, D. C. Stefanescu, M. W. Goudreau, K. Lang, S. B. Rao, T. Suel, T. Tsantilas, and R. H. Bisseling. BSPlib: The BSP programming library. *Parallel Computing*, 24:1947–1980, 1998.

[12] H. Mattsson and C. W. Kessler. Towards a virtual shared memory programming environment for grids. In *Proceedings of PARA*, Lecture Notes in Computer Science. Springer-Verlag, 2004. To appear.

[13] A. Tiskin. A new way to divide and conquer. *Parallel Processing Letters*, 11(4):409–422, 2001.

[14] M. Nibhanupudi and B. Szymanski. Runtime support for virtual BSP computer. In *Proceedings of IIPS/SPDP*, volume 1388 of *Lecture Notes in Computer Science*, pages 147–158. Springer-Verlag, 1996.

[15] R. V. van Nieuwpoort, J. Maassen, G. Wrzesinska, T. Kielmann, and H. E. Bal. Satin: Simple and efficient Java-based Grid programming. *Journal of Parallel and Distributed Computing Practices*. To appear.

[16] A. L. Rosenberg. To BSP or not to BSP in heterogeneous NOWs. In *Proceedings of Workshop on Advances in Parallel and Distributed Computation Models*, 2003.

[17] M. Adler, Ying Gong, and A. L. Rosenberg. Optimal sharing of bags of tasks in heterogeneous clusters. In *Proceedings of ACM SPAA*, pages 1–10, 2003.

[18] E. K. Davies, M. Glick, K. N. Harrison, and W. G. Richards. Pattern recognition and massively distributed computing. *Journal of Computational Chemistry*, 23(16):1544–1550, 2002.

[19] J.-P. Goux, S. Kulkarni, M. Yoder, and J. Linderoth. Master-worker: An enabling framework for applications on the computational grid. *Cluster Computing*, 4:63–70, 2001.

[20] L. F. G. Sarmenta. An adaptive, fault-tolerant implementation of BSP for Java-based volunteer computing systems. In *Proceedings of IPPS Workshop on Java for Parallel and Distributed Computing*, volume 1586 of *Lecture Notes in Computer Science*, pages 763–780. Springer-Verlag, 1999.

[21] T. L. Williams and R. J. Parsons. The heterogeneous bulk synchronous parallel model. In J. Rolim et al., editors, *Proceedings of IPDPS Workshops*, volume 1800 of *Lecture Notes in Computer Science*, pages 102–108. Springer-Verlag, 2000.

[22] P. Morin. Coarse grained parallel computing on heterogeneous systems. In *Proceedings of ACM SAC*, pages 628–634, 2000.

[23] J. M. D. Hill, S. R. Donaldson, and T. Lanfear. Process migration and fault tolerance of BSPlib programs running on a network of workstations. In D. Pritchard and J. Reeve, editors, *Proceedings of Euro-Par*, volume 1470 of *Lecture Notes in Computer Science*, pages 80–91. Springer-Verlag, 1998.

[24] W. F. McColl. A BSP realisation of Strassen's algorithm. In M. Kara et al., editors, *Abstract Machine Models for Parallel and Distributed Computing*, pages 43–46. IOS Press, 1996.

[25] W. F. McColl and A. Tiskin. Memory-efficient matrix multiplication in the BSP model. *Algorithmica*, 24(3/4):287–297, 1999.

[26] S. F. Altschul, W. Gish, W. Miller, E. W. Myers, and D. J. Lipman. Basic local alignment search tool. *Journal of Molecular Biology*, 215(3):403–410, 1990.

[27] Sychron Inc. http://www.sychron.com.

[28] J. M. R. Martin K. M. Measures and R. C. F. McLatchie. Supercomputing resource management — experience with the SGI Cray Origin 2000. In *Proceedings of WoTUG*. IOS Press, 1999.

Communicating Process Architectures 2004
Ian East, Jeremy Martin, Peter Welch, David Duce, and Mark Green (Eds.)
IOS Press, 2004

227

CSP: The Best Concurrent-System Description Language in the World – Probably!

Extended Abstract

Michael GOLDSMITH

Formal Systems (Europe) Ltd, 26 Temple Street, Oxford OX4 1JS, UK

Worcester College, Oxford, UK

michael@fsel.com

Abstract. CSP, Hoare's *Communicating Sequential Processes*, [1, 2] is one of the formalisms that underpins the antecedents of CPA, and this year celebrates its Silver Jubilee [3]. Formal Systems' own FDR refinement checker [4] is among the most powerful explicit exhaustive finite-state exploration tools, and is tailored specifically to the CSP semantics. The CSP_M ASCII form of CSP, in which FDR scripts are expressed, is the de-facto standard for CSP tools. Recent work has experimentally extended the notation to include a probabilistic choice construct, and added function-ality into FDR to produce models suitable for analysis by the Birmingham University *PRISM* tool [5].

1 Introduction

The motivation for this work is provided by the increasing maturity of model-checking ap-proaches to probabilistic analysis of concurrent systems, and the desire to move beyond the black-and-white precision of pure CSP refinement to richer grey-scale measures of confi-dence. Such probabilistic analysis is appropriate to 'natural' interference with a system, but may have less application in the case where deliberate malevolence is potentially involved: but even in this case it may play a role in quantifying the effect of simplifying assumptions, such as the improbability of guessing nonces or keys, or where an assailant can himself take advantage of probabilistic analysis [6, for example].

A number of attempts have been made to extend the theory of CSP with probabilistic con-structs, from the original work of Lowe [7] to more recent efforts by Morgan *et al* [8]. There is an unfortunate tension between nondeterministic choice representing underspecification and probabilistic choice denoting some kind of run-time resolution. The classic refinement paradox of information-flow illustrates that these are very different concepts:

$$SECURE = high?\_ : \{0,1\} \rightarrow (low!0 \rightarrow SECURE \\ {}_{0.5}\boxplus_{0.5} \\ low!1 \rightarrow SECURE)$$

(where the ${}_{0.5}\boxplus_{0.5}$ operator represents a fair coin toss) is reasonably free of information flow (allowing only the detection of activity on the *high* channel, not what that activity is); but if we replace the probabilistic choice with a nondeterministic one, then the resulting process is refined by

$$INSECURE = high?x : \{0,1\} \rightarrow low!x \rightarrow INSECURE$$

which patently is not!

There has so far been no entirely satisfactory treatment for combining the two concepts: either probabilistic choice fails to distribute over nondeterminism, or else some other desirable laws have to be sacrificed: in [8], since all probabilistic choices can effectively be made at process initiation, we have that one can detect when different instances of a process exist. Thus in general we have that P strictly probabilistically-refines $P \sqcap P$. For example, if we define

$$P = a \rightarrow STOP\ _{0.5}\boxplus_{0.5}\ b \rightarrow STOP$$

by 'multiplying out' the choices we get

$$P \sqcap P = (a \rightarrow STOP\ _{0.5}\boxplus_{0.5}\ b \rightarrow STOP)\ _{0.5}\boxplus_{0.5}\ (a \rightarrow STOP \sqcap b \rightarrow STOP)$$

which has only a probability of 0.25 of behaving like $a \rightarrow STOP$, as compared with the 0.5 probability in P.

While this treatment does give a well defined meaning to refinement, if we recall that $P \sqsubseteq Q$ is normally characterised as $P \sqcap Q = P$, there is clearly something a little counterintuitive going on (and that equivalence cannot hold, if $\sqsubseteq$ is to be reflexive).

We largely sidestep these difficulties by restricting our attention to a particular idiom of probabilistic analysis, which should nevertheless be rich enough to provide interesting and useful results.

1.1 PRISM Language

PRISM supports a variety of probabilistic models: Discrete-Time Markov chains (DTMC), Continuous-Time Markov Chains (CTMC), and Markov Decision Processes (MDP). MDP support nondeterministic scheduling, but more importantly for our purposes, we need MDP for nondeterminism.

The *PRISM* language, like FDR's view of CSP, combines one or more 'modules' (leaf processes) using a variety of high-level process operators. The semantics of leaf processes are described in terms of 'Labelled Transition Systems', but these are rather dissimilar to the familiar event-labelled ones underlying the operational semantics of CSP_M: the nodes in the graph are particular assignments of values to state variables, and the arcs are labelled with probabilities. In fact, one should strictly distinguish two levels of arc: the first selecting nondeterministically between probability distributions, and then a partition of the probability space between the arcs within that distribution.

In an important extension to this scheme, the choice of distribution from any node may be constrained by labelling it with a named action. This makes that choice available only when it is also available in the zero or more other modules with which it must synchronise, according to the high-level system composition.

The tests that we support are to calculate the maximum and minimum probability, over all nondeterministic schedulers and environmental choice of events offered deterministically, that a counterexample state to some refinement query can be reached. In picking a path through these (internal and external) choices, the *PRISM* semantics allows the scheduling dæmon to take note of how any probabilistic choice is resolved, which the choice in question does not causally *happen-before* it (and which might therefore be scheduled to happen before it, in a non-causal sense).

This gives a quite different view of the world to that in [8], where the dæmon has to pick a path before any of the probabilistic choices is made. We recover idempotence of nondeterministic choice, but probabilistic choice still does not distribute over nondeterministic.

2 Extended Syntax

CSP_M is already endowed with two choice operators: '|~|' which represents internal (non-deterministic) choice, and ' [] ', which allows the environment to choose the initial event of the combined process and so control which of the two arguments proceeds to evolve; unless the event is common to both, in which case which 'wins' is nondeterministic.

The probabilistic choice operator '$_p\boxplus_{1-p}$' lies conceptually somewhere in between, so we have chosen a syntax reminiscent of both. When one considers the role that dot '.' plays in the formation of events and datatype values in CSP_M, it rapidly becomes clear that adding support for floating-point numerals is likely to be fraught with sorrow; so rather than probabilities directly, we allow probabilities of each branch to be expressed by an integer weight. Thus

$$P\ [m\widetilde{\ }n]\ Q$$

corresponds to what we have been writing

$$P\ _{\frac{m}{m+n}}\boxplus_{\frac{n}{m+n}}\ Q$$

and we can express $P\ _{0\cdot5}\boxplus_{0\cdot5}\ Q$ as

$$P\ [1\widetilde{\ }1]\ Q$$

or even

$$P\ [50\widetilde{\ }50]\ Q$$

as we might express it colloquially.

Both the choice operators have distributed forms:

$$|\widetilde{\ }|\ i:I\ @\ P(i)$$
$$[]\ i:I\ @\ P(i)$$

where in general an arbitrarily complex collection of generators and filter expressions can occur between the choice operator and the '@'.

For probabilistic choice, we have a similar construct:

$$\widetilde{\ }\ i:I\ @\ [w(i)]\ P(i)$$

where the weights $w(i)$ can also vary with the 'loop index' i. Here, as with nondeterministic choice, it doesn't make much sense if the generators and filters give rise to an empty construct. Otherwise the probability of each branch is its weight divided by the sum of the weights across all admitted values of the loop index.

Currently the bridge between CSP_M and *PRISM* is mediated by special forms of assertion in FDR:

```
assert Spec [T= Impl : [probabilistic translation]
```

```
assert Spec [F= Impl : [probabilistic translation]
```

Running such an assertion uses FDR's compiler and some of its other internal machinery to generate a *PRISM* model file, which can then be loaded manually into *PRISM* and checked against some supplied PCTL formulæ. It is clearly desirable in the longer term to automate this process, and to provide a route back for analysing any counterexample with the FDR debugger.

In both of these assertions, *Spec* must be a normal (in a nontechnical sense) nonprobabilistic process, while *Impl* is allowed to (and presumably does, as otherwise FDR would vastly outperform the route via *PRISM* to checking the refinement) contain probabilistic choices. The fact that *Spec* is nonprobabilistic means that it can unproblematically be normalised (in the technical sense of reducing it to a deterministic transition system, while retaining sufficient annotations to be able to reconstitute its nondeterministic behaviour), which is key to efficient refinement checking.

3 Translation

The translation of an individual leaf process into a *PRISM* module is relatively straightforward: as within FDR, we tabulate the transitions as between numbered states, and supply the resulting module with a program-counter variable which can be updated accordingly. (Each module requires its own distinct variable, as 'ownership' of a variable controls only which module can modify it, not its visibility, which is global.) Visible events correspond to transitions with a synchronisable action label; internal (τ-) transitions to anonymous, autonomous ones; and probabilistic choice gives rise to a probabilistic update of the state variable. For a variety of technical reasons, we forbid the (external) choice between a probabilistic choice and any other action.

The system section of a *PRISM* model now admits a rich enough set of operators to permit direct translation of the high-level operator tree, so we can simply enough create an overall model of the implementation *Impl*; but there is no direct way to compare that, within *PRISM*, with an analogous translation of *Spec*.

In fact we use a different strategy, based on another situation where we want to approach a refinement query indirectly.

3.1   Watchdog Transformation

It has long been known [9] that the hierarchical compression operators provided by FDR tend to work best when there is a lot of hidden activity that can be compressed away. One evident possible route towards maximising this is somehow to move the specification over to the right-hand-side of the refinement, in such a way that the resulting check is invariant under hiding; and then hide everything!

We have shown [10, 11] that this is indeed possible, and we have addressed the issue that it is not just hidden activity, but rather localised hidden activity, which is necessary in order to get real benefit from hierarchical compression. Unfortunately the simple execution of the watchdog transformation, where the specification is transformed into a monitor process which signals a failure of refinement either through an error-flag event or by deadlocking the system (in the traces and failures models respectively), yields a system where the hidden events are nearly all shared immediately below the outermost hiding, so that virtually no extra compression is obtained. We explain in the cited works how the syntax tree can be rebalanced to solve this problem, but CSP operators are generally not precisely associative and do not commute with one another, so the transformation is quite intricate.

More recently, to be reported in [3], we have been able to take advantage of another part of FDR's internal machinery, the supercompiler. Any CSP operator tree can be transformed, leaving the leaf processes untouched, into an equivalent one (unique up to reordering and choice of new event names) that uses only outward (inverse-functional) renaming at the leaves, 'natural' alphabetised parallel, and functional renaming and hiding at the outermost level. Using this transformation, which FDR already makes use of for efficient exploration of the operational semantics of the system, allows the system to be expressed in a form which can be reordered and rebracketed at relatively little cost in either CPU cycles or, more importantly, intellectual effort.

In the interests of code re-use, as much as anything else, exactly the same approach has been followed in performing a watchdog transformation on the specification for *PRISM*. The only real difference is that the global visibility of *PRISM* variables and the fact that the actual specification property in the *PRISM* analysis is a PCTL formula which is expressed in terms of them together allow a slight simplification in detecting failure of refinement. In particular, the use of the interrupt operator in [11, §4] can be avoided. Some quite neat encodings have been found of, for instance, the slices through the minimal acceptances in the failures-model watchdog, and the resulting *PRISM* code is quite compact (if not much more readable than most autogenerated code).

4 Conclusions and Further Work

Only limited amounts of experimentation have been performed at the time of writing, but the results are encouraging: a variety of small technical examples have been checked to validate the translation (successfully), and a version of the classic Alternating-Bit Protocol with probabilistic media has been shown to refine its specification (as a small buffer) with probability 1. By the time of the conference there should be substantial results from its application to ad-hoc routing protocol analysis within the *FORWARD* project [12].

As mentioned above, a more streamlined workflow is desirable, and a facility for back-annotation into the FDR debugger. But it is here that the fact that we have used the FDR supercompiler may come into its own: given a path in terms of the state variables of the *PRISM* model, all that is required is to drop the special control variables (marking the presence of a trace error, or controlling the minimal acceptances of the watchdog), and the result is *precisely* the path that FDR itself would have generated internally from a failed refinement check, and passed to the debugger.

One less attractive feature of this approach is that all regularity in the input process has been lost as a side-effect of the compilation process: neither state numbers nor event numbers reflect any symmetry or structure in the leaf processes. Since it is precisely this regularity which enables BDD-related technology to operate effectively on large problems (and *PRISM* is based on Multi-Terminal BDDs), this bodes ill for scaling the approach to significant examples; it remains to be seen how significant an issue this is in practice. It may be possible to address this likely problem by a symbolic compilation strategy, which can preserve the structure of process definitions and of the corresponding data components of events; a pilot version of such a tool is currently under development.

The purely CSP watchdog transformation scheme has difficulty handling the full failures-divergences model, since it is not possible for the watchdog to stop the implementation from diverging when the specification wants to allow it to (and so should stop it). It is also hardly worth adopting any of the rather more intrusive transformations that would allow this to be simulated, since there are no significant (fixed-specification) refinement queries in that model which are invariant under hiding, so the exercise would be more than a little academic. Neither of these considerations apply in the case of the *PRISM* models, however: it is easy for the watchdog to set a variable to inhibit any further action by the implementation, as part of its entry into a state corresponding to a divergent state of the implementation; and PCTL can express the necessary eventualities to capture livelock-freedom of the combination. So this is an enhancement to be anticipated.

However useful the bridge between the two tools proves in the long run, the transformation has a certain elegance of its own. It illustrates once more the unintended extra utility of some of the constructs within FDR, whose sole motivation were efficiency and robustness in refinement checking.

5 Acknowledgements

Much of the work in this paper was carried out as part of the DTI Next Wave Technologies and Markets project *FORWARD* [12], building upon research undertaken for QinetiQ Trusted Information Management System Assurance Group.

The assistance of the *PRISM* design team at Birmingham University, in particular Dave Parker, is gratefully acknowledged.

References

[1] C.A.R. Hoare. *Communicating Sequential Processes*. Prentice Hall International, 1985.

[2] A.W. Roscoe. *The Theory and Practice of Concurrency*. Prentice Hall, 1998. ISBN 0-13-6774409-5, pp. xv+565.

[3] Ali Abdullah, Cliff Jones, and Jeff Sanders, editors. *25 Years of CSP*. Springer Verlag, To appear, 2005? Workshop at Institute for Computing Research, London South Bank University, 7–8 July 2004, organised by Formal Aspects of Computing Science BCS Specialist Group.

[4] Formal Systems (Europe) Ltd. *Failures-Divergence Refinement: FDR 2 User Manual*, 1992-2004.

[5] PRobabilistIc Symbolic Model checker. http://www.cs.bham.ac.uk/~dxp/prism/.

[6] Vitaly Shmatikov. Probabilistic analysis of anonymity. In *IEEE Computer Security Foundations Workshop (CSFW)*, pages 119–128, 2002.

[7] Gavin Lowe. Pravda: A tool for verifying probabilistic processes. In *Proceedings of the Workshop on Process Algebra and Performance Modelling*, number CSR-2693, pages 57–64. Department of Computer Science, University of Edinburgh, 1993.

[8] Carroll Morgan, Annabelle McIver, Karen Seidel, and Jeff Sanders. Refinement-oriented probability for CSP. *Formal Aspects of Computing*, 3(1–000), 1995.

[9] A.W. Roscoe, P.H.B. Gardiner, M.H. Goldsmith, J.R. Hulance, D.M. Jackson, and J.B. Scattergood. Hierarchical compression for model-checking CSP *or* How to check 10^{20} dining philosophers for deadlock. In *Proceedings of TACAS Symposium, Aarhus, Denmark*, 1995.

[10] Irfan Zakiuddin, Nick Moffat, Michael Goldsmith, and Tim Whitworth. Property based compression strategies. In *Proceedings of Second Workshop on Automated Verification of Critical Systems (AVoCS 2002)*. University of Birmingham, April 2002.

[11] Michael Goldsmith, Nick Moffat, Bill Roscoe, Tim Whitworth, and Irfan Zakiuddin. Watchdog transformations for property-oriented model-checking. In Keijiro Araki, Stefania Gnesi, and Dino Mandrioli, editors, *FME 2003: Formal Methods*, pages 600–616, Pisa, September 2003. Formal Methods Europe.

[12] QinetiQ, Birmingham University, Formal Systems, and Oxford University. *FORWARD: A Future of Reliable Wireless Ad-hoc networks of Roaming Devices*. http://www.forward-project.org.uk.

Communicating Process Architectures 2004
Ian East, Jeremy Martin, Peter Welch, David Duce, and Mark Green (Eds.)
IOS Press, 2004

233

gCSP: A Graphical Tool for Designing CSP Systems[†]

Dusko S. JOVANOVIC, Bojan ORLIC, Geert K. LIET, Jan F. BROENINK
Twente Embedded Systems Initiative,
Drebbel Institute for Mechatronics and Control Engineering,
Faculty of EE-Math-CS, University of Twente,
P.O.Box 217, 7500 AE, Enschede, the Netherlands
d.s.jovanovic@utwente.nl

Abstract. For broad acceptance of an engineering paradigm, a graphical notation and a supporting design tool seem necessary. This paper discusses certain issues of developing a design environment for building systems based on CSP. Some of the issues discussed depend specifically on the underlying theory of CSP, while a number of them are common for any graphical notation and supporting tools, such as provisions for complexity management and design overview.

1. Introduction

In the last two decades of the 20th century the transputer [1], a processor specifically designed for simple parallel processing, was successfully applied in a number of engineering fields but eventually fell out of use. However, the occam language [3], designed for programming systems based on transputers, is still referred to in contemporary text books (for instance, [4]) because of its unique properties that do not yet have a match in industrial state-of-the-art languages. Much of the credit given to the occam language, transputers, and the overall design mindset stems from their foundation in the process algebra CSP (Communicating Sequential Processes) [5]. CSP provides a clear and simple approach for reasoning about concurrent systems. Thanks to its sound mathematical foundation, one of the most needed properties of modern system engineering – formal analysis – is incorporated in the paradigm inherently.

Research efforts have been pursued in both hardware and software application areas of CSP in the post-transputer era. Successful experiences composing complex distributed systems inspired development of several communication platforms and protocols [6-8]. On the software engineering side, CSP influenced the design of Ada and inspired development of occam-like libraries for Java, C and C++ [9-14]; although occam is now rarely used for programming transputers, research on extending the language is still active [15].

Before the proposal for graphical notation for CSP [16] by Hilderink, ways of drawing CSP designs were being adopted for each particular occasion in an ad-hoc manner. This, of course, brings difficulties in communication of ideas and concepts and easily introduces design ambiguities as well. A commonly accepted graphical notation would ease acceptance of CSP by a larger software community and provide great assistance for teaching the CSP notions as well.

[†] This research is supported by PROGRESS, the embedded system research program of the Dutch organization for Scientific Research, NWO, the Dutch Ministry of Economic Affairs and the Technology Foundation STW.

The proposed graphical notation has been used in practical applications at the Control laboratory of the University of Twente in the last couple of years. It has proved to be useful for transforming block diagrams to data flow models which can be further refined by introducing relationships describing concurrent aspects of both communication and process composition [17]. Block diagrams are well established for control applications and used in all recognized modelling and simulation tools, such as Matlab/Simulink [18], or – as reported in [17] – 20-SIM [19]. Moreover, CSP diagrams were successfully applied for accomplishing a more complicated task: describing mode switching among a set of control laws developed for different operational modes of a mechatronic system [20].

In [20], CSP diagrams were edited manually in general-purpose drawing tools. The absence of special tools for editing CSP diagrams hampers many other facilities a CSP-based paradigm could offer. Development of a specially crafted CSP design tool permits much more design freedom and reuse, managing complexity through process hierarchy, automatic code generation for concurrent networks, exporting designs to formal checkers and so forth.

In the original proposals of CSP diagrams [16, 21], the graphical CSP language is referred to as GML (Graphical Modelling Language); the tool discussed in this paper is named gCSP (graphical CSP). Basic language and tool elements are summarized in Sections 2, 3 and 4. Section 5 deals with managing complexity in CSP (graphical) designs. The tool's potentials for automatic code generation are presented in Section 6. Section 7 summarizes the status of the tool development and announces further points of attention.

2. General issues of modelling concurrent networks

Composition of any occam program and hence any program based on occam-like libraries is always shaped as a strict tree-like hierarchy of SEQ, (PRI)PAR and (PRI)ALT constructs as branches and user-defined processes as leaves. As such, it can be depicted easily and naturally using a tree hierarchy.

2.1 Tree-based modelling

This fact led to the development of a tree-based CSP design tool [2]. Although the modelling approach based on a strict hierarchical structure provided by the tree resembled the vital compositional aspect of the occam reasoning, the tool's design abilities exhibited two serious flaws.

Firstly, the communication patterns over channel nets were hardly readable from the processes' interfaces scattered over the branches of the tree. An additional view representing data flow was needed.

The second problem was much more serious. The primary aim of implementing such a tool was to assist in designing concurrent programs. A strict hierarchical view can only depict the design that is already shaped as a hierarchy of constructs and processes. But during the design, one starts with process blocks existing in isolation or connected only using data-flow diagrams. Modelling compositional structure in a tree hierarchy does not allow compositional ambiguities (i.e. underspecification) in the course of the design and, therefore, limits the design freedom. In further research, the tree concept was discarded.

Instead, development focused on the fact that during a design process constructs might not yet be formed while compositional relationships between some processes are known. In the follow-up research conducted by Hilderink and Volkerink, the initial idea of GML was conceived.

2.2 *GML design principles*

A construct can be seen as a set of processes with the same type of relationship between any two processes. In sequential, prioritized parallel, and prioritized alternative constructs, these relationships are not symmetrical and strict order must be maintained within a construct.

In GML, the recommended design process starts with a data flow model. This model is represented by the network of communicating processes. The concurrency structure is then added to this model by specifying compositional relationships between the processes involved. Some concurrency relationships between processes are known in advance and some are subject to various trade-offs. A tool that would allow one to make arbitrary compositional relationships (sequential, parallel, alternative) between any two processes would offer greater flexibility than a tool based solely on the tree compositional hierarchy. GML models can express designs that are not fully specified. Compared to tree views, GML views seem to be better suited for entering designs.

Refining the data flow model with compositional relationships expressing the concurrency structure can be done without changing the layout of the original data-flow model. This feature makes a prospective tool based on GML suitable for use in a chain of tools. In our research group, focus is on development of control systems; one possible predecessor to a GML-based tool in such a chain is 20-SIM [19].

20-SIM is a tool for modelling and simulation of control systems. It can generate code for specified controllers, but the code is generated *after* sequentialization of the data-flow models. It would be advantageous if one could import data-flow models from 20-SIM into a GML tool, extend them with compositional relationships specifying the concurrency structure, perform formal checking, and then automatically generate code free of unwanted concurrency phenomena such as deadlock and livelock.

It is expected that the combination of 20-SIM and gCSP will result in a tool chain that can support the design of control applications, whereas gCSP alone can serve as a graphical tool for using CSP.

3. Purpose of the tool and its specification

The most elaborate standard for describing software graphically, UML [22], is described as "a graphical language for visualizing, specifying, constructing, documenting and communicating the artefacts of a software-intensive system". The same goes for the general idea of GML. In short, the purpose of the language and the tool can be described as "supporting the building concurrent software based on the Communicating Sequential Processes algebra". In order to meet this goal, the development of the tool started with the following set of requirements. The tool should:

1. allow the modelling of concurrent systems using the Graphical Modelling Language (GML) for drawing CSP diagrams.
2. preserve notions of the CSP theory and its peculiarities, but bring it closer to implementation needs.
3. support means for managing complex CSP models – allowing hierarchical organisation by containment relations among parent (complex) and children (leaf or also complex) processes.
4. allow the expression of communication and compositional patterns of process networks, the latter not only in terms of an extended set of CSP constructs, but also in terms of compositional relationships (likewise communication relationships,

which represent CSP channels), as defined in the GML proposal.

5. transform the software models to a number of types of human- and machine-readable code.
6. allow semantic and integrity checks of the specified models.
7. allow visualization also in the domains of (formal) analysis and other imaginable CSP model processing.
8. generate CSP networks suitable for incorporation of operational code derived from other tools (for instance one-shot processes from 20-SIM, as reported in [17] and [20]).

The set of CSP constructs applied and extended in occam with prioritized variants, recently formally described in the work of Lawrence [23], is appended with one more construct for modelling exception handling, as described by Hilderink [16]. Table 3-1 summarizes the set of constructs used in the GML and the gCSP tool.

Table 3-1. Constructs in GML.

Construct symbols	Constructs
→	sequential (SEQ)
||	parallel (PAR)
→ ||	priparallel (PRIPAR)
□	alternative (ALT)
→ □	prialternative (PRIALT)
→ △	exception (EXCEPTION)

The following vocabulary was derived to describe some important terms for the gCSP tool development:

- *Processes* and *channels* are defined as in the CSP theory [5]. A process in a CSP diagram is depicted as a rectangle, while a channel is represented by an arrowed line.
- SEQ, (PRI)PAR, (PRI)ALT and EXCEPTION are called *constructs*. The occam WHILE loop is proposed in [16] to be represented as the SEQ of the μ primitive process (see Table 3-2) and the process whose repetition is required. Being an idiom of GML, the SEQuences with the μ primitive process are, in the tree of constructs (see discussion of the C-tree in Section 4), optimized to be presented with one repetition construct marked by the μ glyph.
- *Relationships* are represented as lines augmented with the construct symbols (see Table 3-1) that connect processes. Relationships are divided in two sets: *compositional*, that connect (ordered) pairs of a construct's children, and *communication*, channels that connect two or more processes (shared channels are allowed).
- A *CSP diagram* consists of processes and their relationships.
- A *view* on a CSP diagram displays processes and a set of relationships. gCSP can display three standard views: the *communication view* that shows processes and channels (communication relationships), the *compositional view* showing processes and compositional interrelationships, and the *full CSP view* with processes and both

compositional relationships and channels. The topology of the processes is preserved on all the views (compare Figures 4-1, 4-2 and 4-3).

Hilderink's GML proposal [16] includes also the following primitive processes:

Table 3-2. Primitive processes.

Symbol	Primitive processes
①	Writer
②	Reader
⊛	Barrier sync process
ⓜ	Repetition

Use of the µ primitive process is already mentioned in the context of repetitions. Writer and reader primitive processes denote points of communication among processes, as shown on the example in Figure 5-9. On notions of barrier and the use of the barrier synchronisation process the reader is referred to [16].

In the GML proposal grouping of processes into constructs is depicted by attaching indexed bubbles to compositional relationships tied to borders of newly created constructs. For detailed semantics of the grouping mechanism see Subsection 5.1.

4. Graphical user interface

gCSP has a standard windowed user interface (Figure 4-1) that consists of several panes, a menu and toolbars:

- The graphical editor (G-editor) consisting of:
  - *Communication view* and the corresponding toolbar.
  - *Compositional view* and the corresponding toolbar.
  - Full CSP view.
- Tree views:
  - *Compositional tree* that shows organization in constructs (C-tree).
  - *Graphical tree* that summarizes graphical elements in the G-editor (G-tree).
- The *Messages pane* intended for giving feedback to the user.
- A standard window application toolbar extended with a few specific icons for navigating through the model hierarchy in the G-editor (◐, ◑) and saving and retrieving submodels (⊟, ⊠).

Entering a design (inserting processes and relationships) is performed *exclusively* through the views of the graphical editor (G-editor). The full CSP view (as in Figure 4-3), anticipated already in the GML proposal, has been added upon suggestions of users. While the compositional and communication views are clearly suitable for focusing on one of the corresponding architectural aspects, users of the tool suggested that in the design phase it is also handy to have an overview of both compositional and communication relationships at the same time.

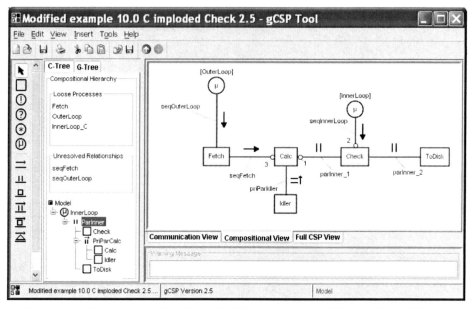

Figure 4-1. Graphical user interface of gCSP (with displayed Compositional View).

While the compositional view can be seen in Figure 4-1, the communication view and the full CSP view are shown in Figure 4-2 and Figure 4-3 respectively.

These figures reveal something that may look rather odd to an occam or a CSP person. The *Fetch* process is composed in sequence with the rest of the system on the right hand side; still, there is a channel in between (*chRawData*). This would certainly cause a deadlock in a CSP model. However, a GML communication relationship (i.e. channel) between processes that run in sequence is not a channel in the CSP sense. In occam it would be a variable. In the CT libraries, due to OOP data encapsulation, variables defined in a parent construct are not automatically visible in a child process. Therefore, in CT, type ChannelVar [20] is created as a non-blocking channel that passes variables between sequential processes.

The option to have a channel between sequential processes comes from the GML's intention to capture all interprocess communications by drawing them as channels. The tool is supposed to allow a control engineer to impose explicitly certain sequences of a system's component activations, i.e. in mode switching (see [20]). The sequentialisation in execution would anyway happen in practice if the two processes were composed in parallel – channel synchronization would automatically force them to run in a sequential order. While this is obvious for those familiar with CSP, the intention of the tool is to be receptive to a wider community.

In generating machine-readable CSP (CSP$_M$ scripts) this problem needs to be solved by detecting channels between sequentially composed processes and handling them in a proper way. Making an option for different visualization of the non-blocking channels in gCSP is under consideration.

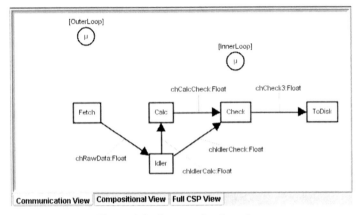

Figure 4-2. Communication view.

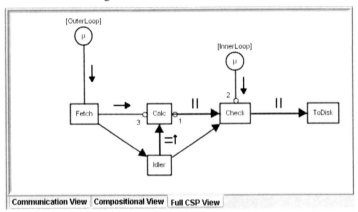

Figure 4-3. Full CSP view.

Trees have shown as the best means for navigation through a model hierarchy. The compositional tree (C-tree in Figure 4-4) also corresponds to a model representation that is most suitable for code generation.

The C-tree actually consists of three compartments:

- list of Loose processes
- list of Unresolved relationships
- trees representing emerging hierarchies of constructs and processes

The term *loose process* is used for a process whose parent construct in the compositional hierarchy is not yet determined. *Unresolved relationship* is a term used for a compositional relationship that connects two processes that are not yet composed in a construct. These issues are discussed in detail in Subsection 5.2.

The G-tree (Figure 4-5) allows inspection of the graphical objects and browsing through the hierarchy; furthermore it assists working with the full CSP view when compositional relationships and channels are overlapping.

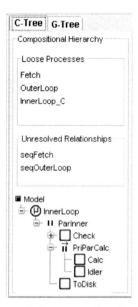

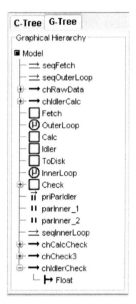

Figure 4-4. Compositional tree.   Figure 4-5. Graphical tree.

5. Managing a CSP model complexity

5.1 Representing compositional hierarchies in flat models

A bottom-up approach of building a complex CSP model starts by connecting processes with compositional relationships. Since any process can be connected with many others, some kind of grouping processes and relationships is necessary to establish a proper compositional hierarchy. Otherwise, the model would be compositionally ambiguous.

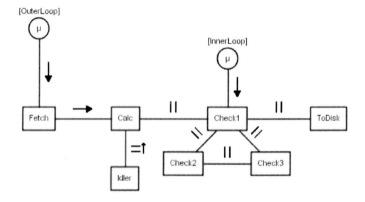

Figure 5-1. An ambiguous model.

Figure 5-1 depicts an example of a compositionally ambiguous model. For instance, it is ambiguous whether the sequence of *Fetch* and *Calc* is composed in a priparallel composition with *Idler*, or after the termination of *Fetch* the priparallel construct consisting of *Calc* and *Idler* takes place. The reader may spot many other ambiguities as well.

A construct in a compositional graphical view is represented by a *group* of processes connected with compositional relationships of the same kind. An intuitive representation of a construct (group) would be a rectangle ("box") embracing the grouped processes. One possible solution that eliminates compositional ambiguities turns the model from Figure 5-1 into the one depicted in Figure 5-2.

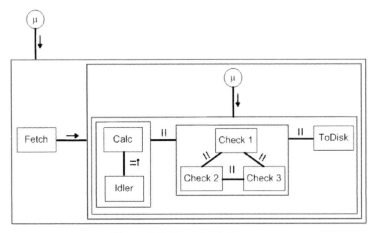

Figure 5-2. Boxed notation.

However, in a complex network, rectangles that mark nested structures take a lot of display space. Adapting this kind of diagram by rearranging the structure may result in a rather serious amount of editing work. Furthermore, maintaining the boundaries of the constructs may be very laborious for a proper GUI development.

In order to compensate for these drawbacks, GML has so-called "parentheses", little indexed bubbles at the end(s) of a composition relationship to indicate the nesting, as in Figure 5-4. An intermediate step between the boxed and parenthesized ("bubbled") representations is given in Figure 5-3. Only parts of rectangles intersecting relationships carry the nesting information.

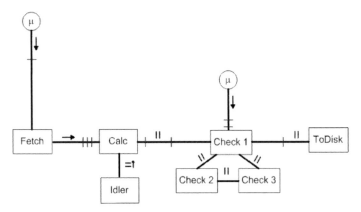

Figure 5-3. The intermediate step between the two grouping notations.

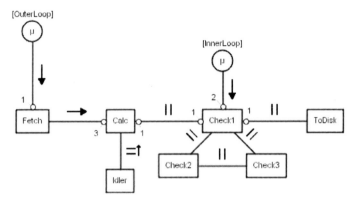

Figure 5-4. Compositional hierarchy shown by parenthesizing.

An index of a parenthesizing bubble is equal to the number of rectangles to be crossed going from a process to an external relationship in the boxed notation, as can be seen by comparing Figures 5-2, 5-3 and 5-4. It is quite obvious that parenthesis notation, although compact, demands practice to become readable.

5.2 C-tree as compositional hierarchy representation

It is not possible to generate code directly for the ambiguous model from Figure 5-1, but it becomes possible once compositional ambiguities are solved – for instance as depicted in Figure 5-4. In other words, one cannot generate an occam-like code in a unique way before a model is shaped as a strict hierarchy of constructs as branches and user defined processes as leaves.

A tool based on a strict tree hierarchy, as described in Subsection 2.1, is naturally suited for the generation of occam-like code. GML models, however, offer much more design freedom. The price to be paid is that a GML model which contains compositional ambiguities or conflicts cannot be uniquely displayed in a strict tree hierarchy. Therefore, a view based on a strict tree hierarchy and a view based on the GML model cannot be used together. One is forced to choose one or the other. In either case some valuable properties of the model are lost.

Possibly, in the design tool, an engine could be constructed that detects compositional underspecification by making queries to a model database. It would rely on some prescribed methods or perhaps built-in heuristics in resolving compositional ambiguities by deriving unspecified relationships, as suggested in the original GML proposal [16].

However, at this stage of the research these issues would put too much of a burden on the tool. Even the necessary minimal check whether a model is free of compositional conflicts would probably not scale well with the complexity of the design. Instead, a practical decision was made to share the responsibility of detecting compositional conflicts between the tool and the user. A supplementary view into the GML model is constructed that can give better insight in the hierarchy of models while keeping the design freedom of the GML modelling approach. The idea is to let the user build this alternative view gradually while creating a graphical design. A complex structure containing one or several tree views and two additional compartments can completely reflect the compositional side of the model at any moment of the design process. Two compartments contain flat lists of loose processes and unresolved relationships. The third compartment contains a set of tree hierarchies of which the roots and the branches represent constructs or complex processes while the leaves represent user-defined processes. This structure is the C-tree presented in

Figure 4-4 in Section 4. The C-tree view and G-editor view are always two views of the same GML model.

When someone adds a process or a relationship in the G-editor, they are automatically added in appropriate compartments of the C-tree. The ambiguous model from Figure 5-1 would be represented with all processes listed in the *Loose Processes* compartment, all relationships shown as unresolved, and with an empty third compartment. That model can be transformed to an unambiguous model from Figure 5-4 in several steps. One can start by grouping the *Check1*, *Check2* and *Check3* processes connected with parallel relationships into the parallel construct. The same can be done with the *Calc* and *Idler* processes.

When several processes connected via relationships of the same type are grouped to make one construct, this change will be reflected in the C-tree by the appearance of the construct as a root or a branch in the appropriate tree hierarchy. Processes that are grouped by a newly created construct have a parent process and cannot be classified as loose processes any more. Therefore they are moved from the first compartment to become leaves of a newly created branch representing their parent construct in the third compartment. Associated relationships contained in this construct are not unresolved further. For the given example this is illustrated in Figure 5-5. The next steps in resolving compositional ambiguities are shown in Figures 5-6 and 5-7.

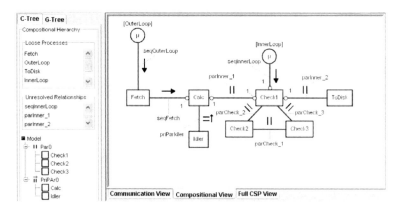

Figure 5-5. The model after creating two parallel constructs.

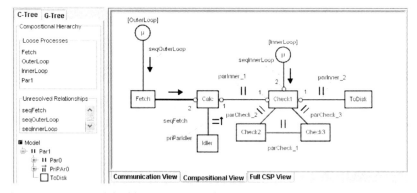

Figure 5-6. The model with *parInner* relationships resolved into *Par1* construct.

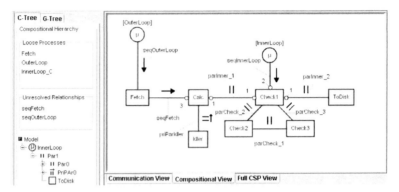

Figure 5-7. The model after creating the repetition construct.

The C-tree gives to a designer a better insight in the transient phases of hierarchy building. The designer can easily visually inspect a C-tree to determine how far the design is from a strict hierarchy. Code can be generated only after a strict tree hierarchy is obtained. More details about the role of the C-tree in code generation are given in Section 6.

A *complex process* is a process that contains other processes. By definition, every construct is a type of complex process. During a design one can have complex processes whose internals are not yet shaped as a strict hierarchy of constructs and user defined processes. Contents of complex processes can be encapsulated using containment; this is the subject of the next subsection.

5.3 Structuring compositional hierarchy by the parent-child containment

So far, flat models have been considered. With a growing process network, a G-editor view quickly becomes overpopulated. In order to manage complexity of a model, in gCSP one can partition a model in larger logical chunks by building complex processes.

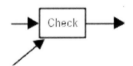

(a) Communication interface of the *Check* process.

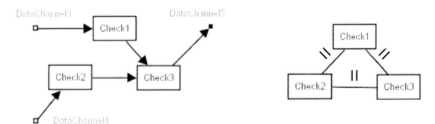

(b) Communication view of *Check*'s internals.   (c) *Check*'s internal composition.

Figure 5-8. Complex (parent) *Check* process.

At any moment the designer may decide to encapsulate several processes inside a separate process, which becomes the complex one. For example, the parallel composition of *Check1*, *Check2* and *Check3* (Figure 5-4) could be encapsulated inside the complex *Check* process (Figure 5-8a).

In turn, the body of the *Check3* process could be further refined as a sequence consisting of primitive input processes, output processes, and blocks for specification of the processing code (note that such blocks are not yet implemented in gCSP), as Figure 5-9 suggests.

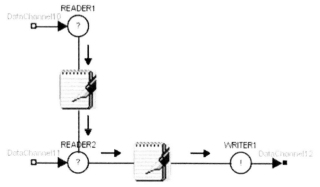

Figure 5-9. Possible representation for the body code place holders (for process *Check3*).

When building complex processes, channel interfaces to the next-higher level are indicated with symbols that are in line with the 20-SIM submodels notation: empty squares for input channel interfaces, and filled squares for output channel interfaces.

Note that one who prefers the top-down design approach would start with a smaller number of processes (as in the figures in Section 4, with the *Check* process capturing the functionality later distributed over three processes). When a global network of processes with well-defined interfaces is established, each of them can be further refined with subprocesses that fulfil the interface contract of the parent.

In the trees, the existence of hierarchical organization is indicated by means of the usual "+" and "−" (respectively expanding and collapsing) boxes in front of the complex processes and the constructs as well (Figure 5-10).

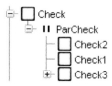

Figure 5-10. Containment hierarchy in the trees.

5.4 Containment hierarchy versus overview

Clearly, it is the user's decision to what extent to build complex compositions in a flat view and at which moment to "implode" some groups of processes into complex ones. Facilities for both building containment hierarchies based on complex processes made out of simpler ones *and* flat compositions with several constructs on the same visual level are implemented. Obviously, both are necessary to allow the user to find a proper balance between managing complexity of the design and providing sufficient overview.

Having both these facilities available, with a limited complexity of the subprocesses, the first disadvantage (inefficient space usage) of the boxed grouping notation discussed in 5.2 is no longer significant. The idea of adding the boxed notation along with the parenthesized one is not definitely abandoned and remains a subject for the future work.

While flat models at one visual level represent only the current abstraction level, the C-tree always represents the whole system. Of course, one can represent the whole system with one flat model as well, but this is not recommended for complex designs.

As is shown in Figure 5-10, the C-tree treats complex processes and constructs coherently. When a model is completely specified, every complex process contains exactly one (top) construct. The children of the top constructs are at the same time children of a complex process containing that construct.

6. Code generation

As stated on the list of the tool development requirements, converting the graphical (human-readable) models into machine-readable forms by automatic code generation is an essential feature.

The following targets are of interest:

- CSP$_M$ (machine-readable CSP), the input for the model checker FDR [24]. Analyses with FDR can be done directly to check the quality of a specification. Furthermore, using existing converters [25], the CSP$_M$ code can be translated to CTJ, JCSP or CCSP.
- Executable programs based on use of the CSP libraries like CTJ [11], [10], [26] or JCSP [27], or their C or C++ versions. Graphical CSP models directly correspond to process networks that are built with the CSP libraries. As discussed later, after filling in application-specific code, the programs can be compiled and run directly.
- occam, which can be executed on transputers, or by compiling with KRoC [15] on standard processors.

CSP is a notation and algebra that describes communication patterns in which different components interact. Parts of code that contain only pure computation are not of interest to CSP. Therefore this tool is also oriented towards generation of *network builders* - program files implementing concurrent networks that reflect the modelled concurrent structure, leaving empty place holders for the application-specific code. Filling this part of operational code can be done in different ways. One way is to do that also within the tool by using code blocks as sketched in Figure 5-9. The other option is importing code produced by other tools, for instance automatically coded control laws from 20-SIM, as described in [17] and [20].

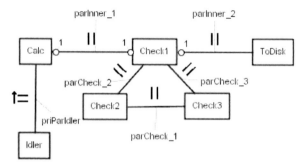

(a) Compositional view.

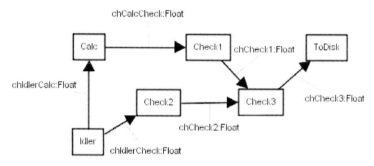

(b) Communication view.

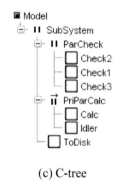

(c) C-tree

Figure 6-1. Example model for code generation.

For an example of code generation, a submodel of the previous example is shown in Figure 6-1. The C-tree structure gives a good starting point for any kind of code generation. Code can be generated whenever the state of strict hierarchy is reached. This state is reached when two conditions are met:

☐ there must not exist any unresolved relationship.
☐ only loose process that can exist is the top level construct.

Verifying whether code can be generated or not is therefore straightforward and also intuitively clear to the user (it is visual) - there is no need for a complex parsing algorithm. This does not yet mean that such a code is free of deadlocks, livelocks, etc. For this purpose a CSP_M script will be generated.

Listing 6-1. CSP$_M$ code generated by gCSP.

```
channel   chCheck3
channel   chIdlerCheck
channel   chCheck2
channel   chCalcCheck
channel   chCheck1
channel   chIdlerCalc


SubSystem = ParCheck [| {| chCheck3 |} |] (PriParCalc [| {| chIdlerCheck,
chCalcCheck |} |] (ToDisk))
ParCheck = Check2 [| {| chCheck2 |} |] (Check1 [| {| chCheck1 |} |]
(Check3))
PriParCalc = Calc [| {| chIdlerCalc |} |] Idler


Calc = Calc
Idler = Idler
ToDisk = ToDisk
Check1 = chCalcCheck?x -> chCheck1!x -> Check1
Check2 = chIdlerCheck?x -> chCheck2!x -> Check2
Check3 = chCheck1?x -> chCheck2?x -> Check3
```

The CSP$_M$ script for the model in Figure 6-1 is shown in Listing 6-1. Note that the channel communication for *Check1*, *Check2* and *Check3* is added manually after the network is generated by gCSP.

It has been decided to model the interleaving parallel construct (|||) in the graphical models in the same way as the sharing parallel construct. Firstly, the tool easily checks whether a channel is present between any two processes composed in parallel, and consequently decides to generate an interleaving or a shared parallel operator in the CSP$_M$ code as appropriate. Secondly, insisting on appearance of the interleaving operator (|||) in the CSP$_M$ code would complicate the code generation in some situations. For instance, a human would probably describe the *ParCheck* process as

```
(Check1 ||| Check2) [| {|chCheck1, chCheck2|} |] Check3
```

since *Check1* and *Check2* do not synchronise with each other. However, the tool, by parsing the C-tree, generates an equivalent composition that does not exhibit the interleaving explicitly.

An executable C++ code generated for use with the CTC++ library consists of pairs of .h and .cpp source files for each defined process and one .cpp file for the network builder as well. The structure of the network builder clearly corresponds to the compositional structure captured by the C-tree, as shown in Listing 6-2.

Listing 6-2. Network builder in CTC++.

```
/** Auto Generated - gCSP **/

//-- Includes
#include ...

int main (void) {

//-- Channel allocations
Channel<float> *chCheck3 = new Channel<float>();
Channel<float> *chIdlerCheck = new Channel<float>();
Channel<float> *chCheck2 = new Channel<float>();
Channel<float> *chCalcCheck = new Channel<float>();
Channel<float> *chCheck1 = new Channel<float>();
Channel<float> *chIdlerCalc = new Channel<float>();

//-- Process allocations
Calc *Calc_1 = new Calc(chCalcCheck, chIdlerCalc);
Idler *Idler_1 = new Idler(chIdlerCheck, chIdlerCalc);
ToDisk *ToDisk_1 = new ToDisk(chCheck3);
Check1 *Check1_1 = new Check1(chCalcCheck, chCheck1);
Check2 *Check2_1 = new Check2(chIdlerCheck, chCheck2);
Check3 *Check3_1 = new Check3(chCheck3, chCheck2, chCheck1);

//-- Network builder
Parallel *ParCheck = new Parallel(
      Check2_1,
      Check1_1,
      Check3_1,
NULL);

PriParallel *PriParCalc = new PriParallel(
      Calc_1,
      Idler_1,
NULL);

Parallel *SubSystem = new Parallel(
      ParCheck,
      PriParCalc,
      ToDisk_1,
NULL);

SubSystem->run();

//delete's...

return 0;
}
```

7. Conclusions and future work

A basic version of a graphical CSP editor and code generator has been built. The first tests, as shown in this paper, indicate that the tool has the potential to meet its initial requirements, and can help proliferate the ideas and usage of CSP.

The idea of the C-tree view can also be generalized and applied to similar problems where an additional view is needed to visualize the process of forming the hierarchy rather than the hierarchy itself.

Building a usable graphical tool is a laborious process; many interesting features can be thought of. The following features are recognized as vital for acceptance in a somewhat broader audience that could supply the tool and methodology developers with valuable feedback:

1. Further improvement of managing complex models; imploding a group of processes to a complex one; exploding complex processes by bringing their children higher up in the hierarchy with proper handling of the network topology.
2. Reassessing the benefits and drawbacks of the boxed and bubbled grouping notations.
3. Extending reusability of developed CSP models. At this moment reuse is possible only by saving and retrieving submodels (complex processes).
4. Letting the user enter the body (operational code) of the processes via code blocks or import external program files.
5. Allowing for diagrams partly populated – as desired by the user – with the processes and relationships from the model.
6. Enabling layered organization of complex models; for instance, a user may choose different ensembles of coexisting networks reflecting a control application layer, safety components layer, and hardware deployment layer to be displayed in various combinations. The preserving topology of the processes in different views with the layered compositions comes to its full effect.
7. Facilitating the tool with event trace analyses by mimicking the network interaction with the environment, as in ProBE [24]. This could lead to executable specification of CSP concurrent designs.
8. Bidirectional collaboration with model checkers and visualization of concurrency phenomena.
9. Allowing use of the C-tree for entering design as well. The manipulation of large structures (merging constructs or dragging and dropping processes) would be easily done in the tree.

8. Acknowledgements

The contribution of Gerald Hilderink to this project is substantial. Beside the fact that the tool is based on the GML modelling principles that he has established, Gerald has also supervised the development of a significant part of the GUI for gCSP during the internship project of Marvin Rumnit.

The authors are also grateful to the reviewers who carefully pointed out potentially weak points of the paper. Furthermore, we are grateful to Dyke Stiles for special diligence in correcting the English.

References

[1]   INMOS, "INMOS Website" www.inmos.com, 2004.

[2]   H. J. Volkerink, G. H. Hilderink, J. F. Broenink, W. A. Vervoort, and A. W. P. Bakkers, "CSP Design Model and Tool Support", *Communicating Process Architectures 2000, WoTUG-23*. Canterbury, United Kingdom 2000.

[3]   INMOS, *occam 2 Reference Manual*: Prentice Hall, 1988.

[4]   A. Burns and A. Wellings, *Real-TIme Systems and Programming Languages*, 3rd ed: Pearson Education, 2001.

[5]   A. W. Roscoe, *The Theory and Practice of Concurrency*: Prentice Hall, 1997.

[6]   S. Triger, B. C. O'Neill, and J. Clark, "Adapted OS Link / DS Link Protocols for Use in Multiprocessor Routing Networks", In A. Chalmers, M. Mirmehdi, and H. Muller, Eds., *Communicating Process Architectures 2001*. Bristol, UK, 2001.

[7]   R. Peel, "A Reconfigurable Host Interconnection Scheme for occam-Based Field Programmable Gate Arrays", In A. Chalmers, M. Mirmehdi, and H. Muller, Eds., *Communicating Process Architectures 2001*. Bristol, UK, 2001.

[8]   R. Mosely, "Reconnectics: A system for the Dynamic Implementation of Mobile Hardware Processes in FPGAs", In J. Pascoe, P. H. Welch, R. Loader, and V. Sunderam, Eds., *Communication Process Architectures 2002*. Reading, UK, 2002.

[9]   G. H. Hilderink, "JavaPP project at UT: http://www.ce.utwente.nl/JavaPP", 2002.

[10]   G. H. Hilderink, A. W. P. Bakkers, and J. F. Broenink, "A Distributed Real-Time Java System Based on CSP", *The third IEEE International Symposium on Object-Oriented Real-Time Distributed Computing ISORC 2000*. Newport Beach, CA, 2000.

[11]   G. H. Hilderink, J. F. Broenink, W. A. Vervoort, and A. W. P. Bakkers, "Communicating Java Threads", *Proc. WoTUG-20 on Parallel programming and Java*. Enschede, Netherlands, 1997.

[12]   P. H. Welch, "Process Oriented Design for Java: Concurrency for All", *ICCS 2002*. Amsterdam, 2002.

[13]   J. Moores, "CCSP - A portable CSP-based run-time system supporting C and occam", In B. M. Cook, Ed., *Architectures, Languages and Techniques - WoTUG-22*. Keele, UK, 1999.

[14]   N. C. C. Brown and P. H. Welch, "An Introduction to the Kent C++CSP Library", In J. F. Broenink and G. H. Hilderink, Eds., *Communicating Process Architectures 2003*. Enschede, 2003.

[15]   P. H. Welch and D. C. Wood, "The Kent Retargetable occam Compiler", *Parallel Processing Developments -- Proceedings of WoTUG 19*. Nottingham, UK, 1996.

[16]   G. H. Hilderink, "Graphical modelling language for specifying concurrency based on CSP," *IEE Proceedings: Software*, vol. 150, pp. 108-120, 2003.

[17]   D. Jovanovic, G. H. Hilderink, and J. F. Broenink, "A communicating Threads -CT- case study: JIWY", In J. Pascoe, P. H. Welch, R. Loader, and V. Sunderam, Eds., *Communicating Process Architectures 2002*. Reading UK, 2002.

[18]   Mathworks, "Matlab, Simulink" http://www.mathworks.com: Mathworks, 2002.

[19]   CLP, "20-SIM" http://www.20sim.com: Controllab Products, 2002.

[20]   G. H. Hilderink, D. S. Jovanovic, and J. F. Broenink, "A multimodal robotic control law modelled and implemented with the CSP/CT framework", In J. F. Broenink and G. H. Hilderink, Eds., *Communicating Process Architectures 2003*. Enschede, Netherlands, 2003.

[21]   G. H. Hilderink, "A graphical Specification Language for Modeling Concurrency based on CSP", In P. W. James Pascoe, Roger Loader, Vaidy Sunderam, Ed., *Communicating Process Architectures 2002*. Reading UK, 2002.

[22]   G. Booch, J. Rumbaugh, and I. Jacobson, *The Unified Modeling Language, User Guide*: Addison Wesley, 1999.

[23]   A. L. Lawrence, "CSPP and Event Priority", In A. Chalmers, M. Mirmehdi, and H. Muller, Eds., *Communicating Process Architectures 2001*. Bristol, UK, 2001.

[24]   FormalSystems, "FDR2 Refinement checker for CSP models" http://www.fsel.com, 2004.

[25]   V. Raju, L. Rong, and G. S. Stiles, "Automatic Conversion of CSP to CTJ, JCSP, and CCSP", In J. F. Broenink and G. H. Hilderink, Eds., *Communicating Process Architectures 2003*. Enschede, Netherlands, 2003.

[26]   G. H. Hilderink, "Communicating Threads home page: www.ce.utwente.nl/JavaPP,", 2002.

[27]   P. H. Welch, "Java Threads in the Light of occam / CSP", In P. H. Welch and A. W. P. Bakkers, Eds., *Architectures, Languages and Patterns for Parallel and Distributed Applications, WoTUG-21*. Canterbury, UK, 1998.

Communicating Process Architectures 2004
Ian East, Jeremy Martin, Peter Welch, David Duce, and Mark Green (Eds.)
IOS Press, 2004

Towards a Semantics for Prioritised Alternation

Ian EAST

Dept. for Computing, Oxford Brookes University, Oxford OX33 1HX, England.

ireast@brookes.ac.uk

Abstract. A new prioritised alternation programming construct and CSP operator have previously been suggested by the author to express behaviour that arises with machine-level prioritised vectored interruption. The semantics of each is considered, though that of prioritisation is deferred given the current lack of consensus regarding a suitable domain. Defining axioms for the operator are tentatively proposed, along with possible laws regarding behaviour. Lastly, the issue of controlled termination of component and construct is explored. This is intended as only a first step towards a complete semantics.

1 Introduction

Reactive behaviour has traditionally been regarded as the province of the operating system alone. Systems programmers were required to have additional programming skill, an understanding of concurrency, and knowledge of hardware. It was accepted that they would fall back on assembly language. The vast majority of applications could be designed and programmed with less capability, and using a purely sequential language. For the unavoidable concurrent and reactive behaviour within the system and with the the environment, they would defer to the operating system.

Such an approach is frequently no longer adequate for the engineering of software. First, the need for an operating system to satisfy the needs of every application has led it to become bloated, expensive, and unreliable. Second, the market for software application has moved away from the desktop and into the consumer product, as a result of a dramatic decrease in hardware cost. Embedded applications are themselves typically both concurrent and reactive, yet must be both cheap and reliable. A method is needed by which they can be engineered rapidly, but with high integrity and low cost, by people who can readily be hired.

Honeysuckle [1] is intended to provide the means to implement concurrent and reactive systems, secure against pathology such as deadlock and priority inversion. Static verification of formal design rules guarantees security against many errors, without the additional skill, cost, and delay, usually associated with the use of formal methods.

A *service* is a protocol between two processes that identifies a strict sequence of communications. The idea is derived from the master/servant protocol of Per Brinch-Hansen [2]. It may be drawn as a directed arc connecting two nodes within a *service digraph*. A design rule, denying any circuit in such a graph, has been proven to guarantee deadlock-freedom [3]. A companion paper shows how the protocol may be recast as statically verifiable conditions separably defining service and service network [4]. The addition of mutual exclusion and dependency between services proves necessary for compositionality, ensuring every system is a valid component and *vice versa*.

Like occam before it, Honeysuckle is a derivative of Hoare's Communicating Sequential Processes (CSP) [5]. Unlike occam, it models prioritisation as the ability of one process to interrupt another. An interrupting process is often cyclic. An interrupted process resumes only when a cycle is complete or when its interruptor terminates. A new CSP operator has been proposed which captures such behaviour, along with a programming construct (when) that provides mechanisms for components to asynchronously communicate and precipitate the termination of (disable) each other [6].

The purpose of this paper is to take a first step towards establishing the semantics of both operator and construct by discussing desirable behaviour and resolving certain issues that arise. The aforementioned companion paper also extends service architecture to incorporate prioritised service provision and shows how *a priori* deadlock-freedom may be retained, along with immunity to priority conflict and inversion.

2 Prioritised Alternation

2.1 Indirect Expression

Because reactive behaviour is unavoidable in practice, processor design typically includes a mechanism by which normal control flow can be interrupted. Since there is usually a number of distinct events that cause interruption, the mechanism often allows for the provision of a *vector* to direct control to the appropriate subroutine. *Interrupt service routines* may or may not be re-entrant and sometimes may pre-empt one another according to some recorded prioritisation. It is thus possible to *alternate* behaviour according to prioritised events (internal or external) by programming such hardware directly. This is commonly done using assembly language, but becomes tiresome and error-prone when the system is other than trivial.

When using a high-level programming language (one permitting a measure of abstraction), it is common to portray a set of alternating processes as concurrent. Some pre-emptive scheduler, outside application program control, is then relied upon to deliver alternation. This can be expressed directly, for example, using occam:

```
PRI PAR i=0 for n
   WHILE running
      SEQ
         input[i] ? request
         ... respond to request
```

Since, by definition, *no two responses may execute concurrently*, this is hardly ideal. Concurrency implies equivalence among all interleavings, but in an alternation each interleaving has meaning and therefore should be distinguished. There is also the issue of resumption. The solution above allows an interrupted process to resume when its interruptor is blocked. Prioritised vectored interruption (PVI) provides no mechanism for this but imposes the minimum overhead on latency. Disallowing resumption until completion is arguably simpler, both in abstraction and in implementation, though less efficient, in the sense that the alternation as a whole is blocked where otherwise it need not be. It might also be argued that a programming language should provide abstraction of *all* patterns of control flow offered by hardware, including PVI.

Pre-emptive scheduling offers a worsening solution as interaction between responses increases. Ultimately, some central process will be required to maintain state, communicating with every other process after each response. Scheduling will incur (possibly unacceptable) overheads on both performance and latency. Abstraction becomes complicated and obscure.

Although it is now common practice to simply rely on excess performance available, sometimes even discarding pre-emption, it surely remains sensible to pursue efficiency and the lowest possible latency. It is surely also sensible to provide direct abstraction, and thus transparent and efficient expression of the behaviour of any event-driven system.

2.2 Interrupts and Alternation in CSP

In his seminal book, Hoare accounts for both interruption and alternation [5, #5.4], but not priority. He denotes a process P_1, interruptible by P_2, by

$$P_1 \hat{} P_2 \tag{1}$$

The process thus formed starts and continues behaving as specified by P_1 until some event with which P_2 can start occurs. It then behaves as P_2. P_1 is never resumed.

He adds two qualifications. "To avoid problems", termination must not lie in the alphabet of P_1, αP_1. This means that P_1 is not in fact a sequential process at all, since it cannot be combined with another via the sequence operator ';'. (One obvious problem would be the interpretation following termination of P_1.) This permits the description of processes which can cease only via interruption. In fact, it's worse than that. If we compound the (associative, non-commutative) operator

$$(P_1 \hat{} P_2) \hat{} P_3 = P_1 \hat{} (P_2 \hat{} P_3) \tag{2}$$

we see that, in a string of interruptible processes, none may terminate save the last. In practice, we do not wish to be restricted in this way.

In order to preserve determinism and simplify reasoning about operators, Hoare further requires any interrupting event to lie outside the alphabet of the interrupted process:

$$P_2^0 \cap \alpha P_1 = \emptyset \tag{3}$$

(P^0 refers to the set of events with which P is willing to start. The function $initials(P)$ is used in later CSP texts.) In contrast, this is entirely acceptable. Only the environment can trigger interruption. The interruptible process is blind to the interrupting event.

Hoare goes on to provide abstraction for the class of events which prevent a process continuing (cause 'catastrophe') and for processes which subsequently restart. *Checkpoints* provide for the preservation of a state, upon an event denoted by 'ⓒ', to which a process may return upon catastrophe, instead of restarting. A third interrupting event is defined, denoted by '⊗', which causes two processes to alternate. (A circumflex is introduced here to distinguish event and operator.)

$$P_1 \hat{\otimes} P_2 \tag{4}$$

Hoare's second stipulation means that $\otimes$ lies in the alphabet of neither P_1 nor P_2, but in that of the process produced by the operator. $\otimes$ also secures a checkpoint. The state of the interrupted process is preserved.

2.3 Prioritised Alternation in CSP

A simple, but useful, interpretation of the term 'prioritisation' has been previously proposed by the author, together with a new *prioritised alternation* CSP operator [6]. A brief summary follows.

Consider a process composed via interruption, as described by Hoare [5, p. 180]. (The notation used by Roscoe is now preferred [7, p. 235].)

$$\Pi = ((P_1 \bigtriangleup P_2) \bigtriangleup P_3) \ldots \bigtriangleup P_n \tag{5}$$

It would only be natural to interpret the order in which processes appear, indexed by i, as a form of prioritization. Other interpretations of the term remain possible but surely this one is useful for describing the behaviour (desired or actual) of reactive systems.

Following interruption, no process resumes, and only the last of the given list may terminate. In practice, we usually wish no response to any interruption to disappear after completion. The solution is to allow any such process to be *cyclic* about interruption but also require it to be non–re-entrant. Thus P_2 starts with interruption of P_1. Instead of a single switching event, the new operator adds a dedicated event for each clause, marking the *completion* of a response. Upon completion, P_1 resumes, while P_2 awaits further interruption. Such behaviour might be denoted by a new operator '↩' with which to compose processes.

$$\Pi = ((P_1 \hookleftarrow P_2) \hookleftarrow P_3) \ldots P_n \tag{6}$$

A serial operator, concisely denoting a list of alternating processes, could also be defined, subject to an enumerating index.

A number of semantic issues surround prioritised alternation. For example, when process P_2 interrupts P_1, one must consider the possibility that P_1 is blocked awaiting synchronization with the environment. P_1 may also comprise multiple concurrent processes, each of which may be blocked. Upon interruption, all offers of communication must be withdrawn, pending completion of the response, whereupon they are re-established.

2.4   The Honeysuckle when Construct

The Honeysuckle programming language [1] introduces a dedicated prioritized alternation construct – when. For example:

```
when
    transfer draft to publisher
        ... celebrate
    acquire draft from editor
        ... check
    idle
        sleep
```

Each guard initiates a service. At least two clauses must be given and are listed in order of priority. The lowest priority clause may employ the symbol idle to indicate that it is unguarded. No clause is re-entrant. Part of each response may be to disable further interruption by either the same, or any other, event. Note that an alternation does not terminate until *all* interruption is disabled.

The order in which clauses may appear is constrained by an explicit process interface in Honeysuckle. A guard may be compounded by selection, allowing interruption by any member of a designated set of services, known as a *bunch* (see next section). This is supported by admitting a selection construct in place of a single guard.

Clauses may share memory, which should immediately raise concern regarding the possibility of interference. Each visible object (variable) may be assigned value within at most one clause (component), which is said to *own* it. One form of interference, commonly cited in textbooks on concurrency, is where interruption of (read or write) access leads to an outcome (final state) different to that given no interruption. Honeysuckle might protect against this by disabling interruption during every access. Assignment would be atomic, as is any procedure encapsulated within an object. (Shared objects may then be modelled using CSP. See Section 4.) The price paid for such security is in the form of extended latency when large objects are shared. Achieving security and adequate performance is then the responsibility of the designer, who must understand the issue, as indeed existing practitioners must, when using PVI explicitly.

Interference can only be defined with regard to the intended function of each component, specified, for example, by pre- and post-assertions. Interference-freedom between concurrent processes requires that every interleaving thereof yields precisely the same outcome. It remains a serious general issue in programming concurrency. (Because processes can model variables, distributing memory does *not* automatically confer a solution [8].)

Components of an alternation are *not* concurrent. Indeed, the interleaving that actually occurs *has meaning* and may thus legitimately affect outcome. It remains to prove that each interleaving has only the desired outcome. This is not a simple issue, nor one which currently knows a solution. Increasing atomicity according to granularity (disabling interruption longer when accessing larger objects) does not confer a complete solution for an alternation [8, #1.6]. It is not difficult to contrive an example where an interruption between two related accesses interferes with the outcome.

All that is claimed here is that the situation is no worse than it would be using pre-emptive scheduling (*e.g.* PRI PAR in occam) to address the same problem.

3 Regarding the Semantics of Prioritised Alternation

Viewed from the outside, an alternation consists of an enumerated list of server *bunches*. (A 'server' is the providing end of a service, *i.e.* a connection, not a process. A "server bunch" refers to a set of servers providing mutually exclusive services.) For the sake of simplicity, we shall consider only cases where there is just a single server per bunch.

Termination will be addressed in the next section and only briefly discussed here.

3.1 Alphabet

Rather like a parallel composition, the alphabet of an alternation is the union of that of its components:

$$\alpha(P_1 \hookleftarrow P_2) = \alpha P_1 \cup \alpha P_2 \tag{7}$$

On the other hand, component alphabets are disjoint. In an alternation, components do *not* communicate directly. While interleaving common events might be useful, we choose here the simpler option.

$$\alpha P_1 \cap \alpha P_2 = \emptyset \tag{8}$$

Each component P_i is characterised by its guards g_i^j, and a *completion* event h_i which marks the resumption of any interrupted process. The initial event set of the alternation is just the union of the initials of both components:

$$initials(P_i \hookleftarrow P_j) = initials(P_i) \cup initials(P_j) \tag{9}$$

Completion cannot force actual resumption, compelling the interrupted process to engage in its next event. There is no sense of *urgency* in our definition. Completion merely denotes the granting of *permission* to proceed. If further interruption occurs before it resumes then, well, it had the chance. As Hoare noted [5, p. 80], any requirement to take advantage of opportunity, and not be "infinitely overtaken", must be met in implementation, which in practice should not be difficult.

On the other hand, in practice, we *do* require that the operator guarantees acceptance of any offer of a guard by the environment, and according to the defined prioritization. Without introducing timing, we cannot however stipulate the delay. That must also be a matter for implementation.

It may be that the lowest priority process is required to run continuously without awaiting any particular event. In other words, it may be unguarded. This is identified with a *null* guard. occam employed *skip* as a null guard in an alt (alternative) construction. However, *skip* is a *process*, not an event – a distinction which proves necessary in a consistent algebra. Rather than introduce a null event, we shall simply allow a component to be unguarded. This is the interpretation place upon the notation *idle*, used in Honeysuckle. There seems no reason to restrict this possibility to the component with lower priority. One law is suggested as a direct consequence, at least in the traces domain. If the interrupting process is unguarded and non-terminating, an alternation is indistinguishable from that process alone:

$$initials(P_2) = \{\tau\} \land \checkmark \notin \alpha P_2 \Rightarrow (P_1 \hookleftarrow P_2) = P_2 \qquad (10)$$

P_2 may only engage in internal events and not communicate with the environment. Note that much depends upon whether or not a component terminates. It is often easier to understand alternation with cyclic, non-terminating, components.

3.2   Traces

Once again, an alternation may be compared with parallel composition. Every trace of each component is also a trace of the alternation. To these must be added those formed as a result of interruption:

$$traces(P_1 \hookleftarrow P_2) = traces(P_1) \cup traces(P_2) \cup$$
$$\{s = p \,^\frown u \,^\frown q \mid u \in traces(P_2)), \; h \in \lfloor u \rfloor, \; p \,^\frown q \in traces(P_1)\} \cup \qquad (11)$$
$$\{s = p \,^\frown u \,^\frown q \,^\frown v \,^\frown r \mid u, v \in traces(P_2), \; h \in \lfloor u \rfloor, \; h \in \lfloor v \rfloor,$$
$$p \,^\frown q \,^\frown r \in traces(P_1)\} \cup$$

$$\ldots$$

Note that we take care to ensure that any interruption is followed by a completed response. After g_2, no further progress by P_1 is allowed until completion h_2. There can be no interleaving.

3.3   An Axiom

It is useful here to define a Boolean operator to infer event precedence. We shall denote "x precedes y in trace s" by $x \overset{s}{\leadsto} y$[1], so that:

$$x \overset{s}{\leadsto} y \iff 1 \geqslant |s \downarrow x - s \downarrow y| \geqslant 0 \qquad (12)$$

assuming both x and y occur just once within any cycle – a condition fulfilled by both guard and completion of any clause. Note that the condition remains appropriate even if the clause concerned is not cyclic, and simply terminates.

A prioritised alternation may be understood as something which guarantees completion of a higher priority service before one of lower priority. To be more precise:

Condition 1. *If a higher priority event precedes the completion of a response to one of lower priority then the completion of its own response does also:*

$$\forall s \in traces(P_1 \hookleftarrow P_2). \; g_2 \overset{s}{\leadsto} h_1 \implies h_2 \overset{s}{\leadsto} h_1 \qquad (13)$$

---

[1]Not to be confused with use of the same symbol by Schneider to denote an *evolution* — a state transition over time [9, p. 270].

3.4 Prioritisation

Equation 13 is still not quite enough to guarantee the desired behaviour. Suppose the environment offers interruption simultaneously with the next communication of the current process. Having deprived it of the liberty to interleave high and low priority responses (Eq. 11), we must somehow compel interruption:

Condition 2. *If a higher priority guard is ever offered then it will be immediately accepted.*

Unfortunately, neither traces nor failures provide an adequate domain in which to express this precisely. Proof of some of the laws suggested in the next section would also require an adequate domain. Both are left for future publication. However, a brief review follows of the issue and existing literature on the issue.

Any "denotational semantics" rests on establishing a meaning for operators such as equivalence ('='). Deciding equivalence, for example, reduces to establishing whether or not two processes share a common value for some function (or set of functions) of their description. One possible attribute of a process P is the set of traces, $traces(P)$. If another process Q shares a common set of traces with P we can say that $P = Q$ "in the trace domain".

Two processes might exhibit identical trace sets but may behave quite differently under the same circumstances. It would be valuable to know what a process will do when presented with a set of offers of communication by its environment. An *acceptance set* circumscribes those events in which process would agree to engage, following a particular trace. Its complement, the *refusal set*, may be combined with the trace to form a *failure*. A set of failures may then be attributed to the process concerned (which subsumes a description of its traces). Equivalence in the failure domain tells a great deal more than one in the domain of traces, and allows many more deductions.

At this point, it is worth considering how a process is defined. It is usual to establish a list of conditions. (For example, see [5, #3.9].) When defining a language by which one can express process composition, it is essential to include a demonstration that all constituent operators are *well–defined*. By this we mean that each process produced by each operator itself obeys the same conditions. Furthermore, in order to employ recursion, one must show that each operator is *continuous* over some complete partial order (CPO). One process may then be said to *refine* another.

Failures still tell us nothing of process *preference*. If the environment offers two communications, it is possible to assert only that a process is 'willing' to engage in just one or either. In the latter case, the semantics of general choice reduces to that of a non-deterministic *internal* choice. It is not possible to describe a process that would repeatedly *prefer* one action over another. Neither is it then possible to decide, say, equivalence in this sense. Some process attribute is needed that would always expose such preference. Only then could the precise meaning of any *biased*, or *asymmetric*, operator on processes be defined.

Over a decade ago, Colin Fidge took an approach similar to the use of refusal sets to discriminate between responses to the environment a process might make following each trace. He established an attribute $preferences(P)$ that described a relation between each pair of events in the process alphabet [10]. Technically, each attribute is a function of the process description. In this case, it returns a set of ordered pairs. For example, $a \rightarrow b \in preferences(P)$ implies that, should both a and b be offered by the environment, the process will accept b.

Fidge goes as far as defining a set of operators in terms of traces and preferences. However, as far as the author is aware, he did not show they were either well-defined or continuous. Hence, their semantics remain undefined.

At around the same time as Fidge, Gavin Lowe also provided a semantics for prioritisation. However, its relation to *timed* CSP makes it more complicated and less relevant to the subject discussed here. In Lowe's model, a process offers a set of bags of events at each time-step. Like Fidge, a relation (a set of ordered pairs) is used to describe preference (bias). He shows that the language thus formed is entirely deterministic after the removal of non-deterministic choice and then proceeds to develop a probabalistic model on top of the prioritised one.

More recently, Adrian Lawrence has developed an alternative approach whereby bias may be expressed via the 'response' of a process Y to an offer X made by the environment following a trace s [11]. A domain of *triples* $\{(s, X, Y)\}$ is thus established [12]. Each response defines what a process is willing to do in a particular circumstance. It may be simply to terminate ($Y = \checkmark$) or even to do nothing at all ($Y = \{\ \}$).

Lawrence is thus able to distinguish 'soft' and 'hard' priority. In the former case, some means of arbitration is found when priorities conflict. Hard priority may result in deadlock. This contrasts with the approach taken here, where the means is sought to eliminate the possibility of priority conflict [4]. It may be argued to be at least risky to contrive a language where any such conflict may be directly expressed – a liberty surely better denied. However, a form of "prioritised interleaving" can be formulated that would seem to yield the same behaviour as prioritised alternation, though it is arguably much less transparent.

Overall, much progress has been made to introduce a semantic domain in which prioritisation can be defined, but it remains to achieve academic consensus. An appropriate operator, or set of operators, is a secondary issue, of greater concern here, where a single operator is preferred that abstracts prioritisation uniquely as interruptibility.

3.5   Laws

The following laws are suggested but not proven over any domain.

3.5.1   Unit and Zero

There appears to be no zero of of an alternation. *Stop*, however, suggests a unit:

$$P \hookleftarrow Stop \ = \ Stop \hookleftarrow P \ = \ P \qquad\qquad (14)$$

The first equality is self-evident. The second is valid only if we disregard termination, and thus whether an alternation may be regarded as a sequential process (*i. e.* can be composed via the ';' operator). To the outside observer, behaviour will otherwise be identical.

Skip also suggests a unit, but again we must be mindful of termination:

$$P \hookleftarrow Skip \ = \ P$$

The reverse, $Skip \hookleftarrow P$, requires clarification. A definition must be sought so that the alternation itself either terminates or continues as P. The latter would be simpler and arguably would more commonly correspond with intuition and requirements. It should hold even when P itself terminates and thus affords termination of the alternation also.

$$P \hookleftarrow Skip \ = \ Skip \hookleftarrow P \ = \ P \qquad\qquad (15)$$

Any law should hold over the entire process domain. Equation 15 seems to do this. Equation 14 clearly does not, and therefore lacks the status of law.

3.5.2 Association and Commutation

Alternation would seem associative:

$$(P_1 \hookleftrightarrow P_2) \hookleftrightarrow P_3 \;=\; P_1 \hookleftrightarrow (P_2 \hookleftrightarrow P_3) \tag{16}$$

but not generally commutative:

$$(P_1 = Skip) \vee (P_2 = Skip) \iff P_1 \hookleftrightarrow P_2 \;=\; P_2 \hookleftrightarrow P_1 \tag{17}$$

3.5.3 Distribution

Neither sequential nor parallel composition distribute through an alternation. Though it might be appealing to suggest:

$$P \hookleftarrow (Q;\ R) \;=\; (P \hookleftarrow Q);\ (P \hookleftarrow R)$$

Equation 15 quickly denies it. (Consider $P = Q = Skip$.) Clearly, an alternation does not distribute through parallel or sequence either.

The *after* operator $(/s)$ is expected to distribute through an alternation, exactly as it does a parallel composition:

$$(P_1 \hookleftrightarrow P_2)\,/s \;=\; (P_1/(s \upharpoonright \alpha P_1)) \hookleftrightarrow (P_2/(s \upharpoonright \alpha P_2)) \tag{18}$$

3.6 Specification

The axiomatic specification of a particular alternation looks very much like that of a parallel composition [5, p.90]:

$$\forall\, r \in traces(P_1),\ \forall\, s \in traces(P_2).\ P_1\ \textbf{sat}\ C_1(r) \wedge P_2\ \textbf{sat}\ C_2(s) \;\Rightarrow$$
$$\forall\, t \in traces(P_1 \hookleftrightarrow P_2).\ (P_1 \hookleftrightarrow P_2)\ \textbf{sat}\ (C_1(t \upharpoonright \alpha P_1) \wedge C_2(t \upharpoonright \alpha P_2)) \tag{19}$$

Many reactive systems may be specified by requiring pre-emptive responses to occur to certain events (guards) according to a given prioritisation. Response latency can arguably be computed by the compiler, given adequate information regarding the platform, affording the satisfaction of certain timed requirements.

4 Termination

It becomes apparent early, as in Equation 10, that an alternation can be understood differently according to whether or not components are capable of terminating. If P is non-terminating (not a sequential process), Equation 14 is correct as it stands, at least with regard to traces observed, but not otherwise. Such equivalence might well be useful in some applications.

It may be worthwhile to consider an alternation at distinct epochs, according to whether each component is cyclic or terminating. According to Equation 15, once a component terminates, its clause may be considered deleted, and a new epoch begins.

This is precisely how a prioritised vectored interrupt system is commonly regarded. A response to some event may be to *disable* further response to the same event, some other event, or even *all* events. As noted in the earlier summary, the Honeysuckle when construct allows for this, and will terminate only when all interruption is disabled.

On considering how this may be modelled in CSP, one qualification regarding completion is first necessary. When an interrupting process terminates it must first have completed its response, allowing the interrupted process to resume. Completion cannot follow termination; clearly, nothing can. Termination must follow completion.

Component termination obviously requires an assurance that the environment will never again offer the corresponding guard. An interface must therefore convey information regarding when any given service becomes available and ceases to be available. The design of Honeysuckle will address this.

A *disable* command might be implemented via a shared variable, which in CSP can be regarded as a process D_i composed in parallel with an alternation:

$$D_i = send.d_i \rightarrow receive.d_i \tag{20}$$

One such process is required for each component P_i of an alternation.

A when clause might then be expressed generically (in normal form):

$$P_i = ((g_i \rightarrow R_i); \ P_i) \ \Box \ (receive.d_i \rightarrow Skip) \tag{21}$$

One possibility is that a response includes disabling of further interruption, in which case R_i communicates $send.d_i$. After completion (the final event of R_i), P_i should terminate. Here, again we appear to face the need for bias. It is desirable that, should both initial events, g_i and $receive.d_i$, be offered, that the latter is always chosen. However, this circumstance should never arise. It would expose a design flaw that could (should?) lead to deadlock. A component of an alternation should never be disabled when another occurrence of its guard event might occur.

Some applications might call for more than one component to have the capacity to disable a peer. Later attempts to disable an already disabled component could be accommodated via a slightly more complicated "shared variable" process. However, its recursion must then be terminated somehow. Alternatively, the ability to disable each component might be limited to the same or just one other and required to occur just once. This would be statically verifiable but may narrow the application domain. Because it represents the simpler path, this will be the rule for when in Honeysuckle.

It has always been the intention to explicitly share variables between components of when, as discussed earlier in Section 2.4. These might be modelled in a similar manner. Further work is needed here with regard to interference.

5 Conclusion

While the semantics of both prioritised alternation ($\leftrightarrow$) and the when programming construct remain incomplete, some progress has been made. An axiom has been proposed, along with various laws that characterize behaviour. Some key issues have been explored, such as the behaviour desired when components terminate and how termination might be brought about. Further work is needed with regard to interference and communication within a when construct.

Prioritisation in alternation has been shown to reduce to the same issue as with other 'asymmetric' operators, such as biased choice. An appropriate semantic domain still needs to gain consensus, though strong candidates exist. Further work is needed in order to secure a complete semantics of both operator and programming construct. Once that has been achieved, proof can then be sought of freedom from both deadlock and priority conflict in systems with *prioritised service architecture*.

It is hoped soon to complete the definition of the Honeysuckle programming language, and implement a compiler. A demonstration of the complete methodology will then become possible.

Acknowledgements

I am very grateful for a number of conversations with Mark Green, Jeremy Martin, and Adrian Lawrence with regard to this work.

References

[1] Ian R. East. The Honeysuckle programming language: An overview. *IEE Software*, 150(2):95–107, 2003.

[2] Per Brinch Hansen. *Operating System Principles*. Automatic Computation. Prentice Hall, 1973.

[3] Jeremy M. R. Martin. *The Design and Construction of Deadlock-Free Concurrent Systems*. PhD thesis, University of Buckingham, Hunter Street, Buckingham, MK18 1EG, UK, 1996.

[4] Ian R. East. Prioritised service architecture. In East and Martin et al., editors, *Communicating Process Architectures 2004*, Series in Concurrent Systems Engineering, pages 55–69. IOS Press, 2004.

[5] C. A. R. Hoare. *Communicating Sequential Processes*. Series in Computer Science. Prentice Hall International, 1985.

[6] Ian R. East. Programming prioritized alternation. In H. R. Arabnia, editor, *Parallel and Distributed Processing: Techniques and Applications 2002*, pages 531–537, Las Vegas, Nevada, USA, 2002. CSREA Press.

[7] A. W. Roscoe. *The Theory and Practice of Concurrency*. Series in Computer Science. Prentice-Hall, 1998.

[8] C. B. Jones. Wanted: A compositional model for concurrency. In Annabelle McIver and Carroll Morgan, editors, *Programming Methodology*, Monographs in Computer Science, pages 1–15. Springer-Verlag, 2003.

[9] Steve Schneider. *Concurrent and Real-Time Systems: The CSP Approach*. Wiley, 2000.

[10] Colin J. Fidge. A formal definition of priority in CSP. *ACM Transactions on Programming Languages and Systems*, 15(4):681–705, 1993.

[11] Adrian E. Lawrence. Hard and soft priority in CSP. In Barry Cook, editor, *Architectures, Languages and Techniques for Concurrent Systems*, Series in Concurrent Systems Engineering, pages 169–195. IOS Press, 1999.

[12] Adrian E. Lawrence. Triples. In East and Martin et al., editors, *Proceedings of Communicating Process Architectures 2004*, Series in Concurrent Systems Engineering, pages 157–184. IOS Press, 2004.

Communicating Process Architectures 2004
Ian East, Jeremy Martin, Peter Welch, David Duce, and Mark Green (Eds.)
IOS Press, 2004

A Calculated Implementation of a Control System

Alistair A. McEWAN

Computing Laboratory, University of Kent at Canterbury, UK

Abstract. In this paper, a case study consisting of a plant, and associated control laws, is presented. An abstract specification of the control system is given in Hoare's Communicating Sequential Processes (CSP). Via a series of calculated refinements, an implementation is developed, and translated into a simulation in a Java-based library for CSP, JCSP. Verification of the development process is performed using the model-checker for CSP, FDR. The result is a complete, verified implementation of the control system.

"**Control** (*n*): The apparatus by means of which a machine, as an aeroplane or motor vehicle, is controlled during operation; also, any of the mechanisms of a control apparatus, or collectively for the complete apparatus. " *Oxford English Dictionary, 2nd edition*

1 Introduction

In this paper, a case study consisting of a plant, and control laws, is investigated. An executable simulation of the control system is developed via a full, verified, top down procedure from an existing abstract specification. Proof obligations are discharged using FDR. The case study in question is a steam boiler—a device which accepts water input from a set of pumps, boils the water, and allows steam to escape through sets of valves. The boiler can be seen as analogous to, for instance, a cooling system in a nuclear reactor. An instantiation of the abstract control system is developed, and its correctness verified. This instantiation is then transformed into an executable refinement, and from this, a simulation is produced by translating this model into a Java-based library for CSP, JCSP.

Development of the new device is done in a top-down manner. The existing abstract specification of the device is refined in several stages into models where the implementation is exposed gradually. It is our belief that, by taking an abstract specification, and using a calculational approach to refining it into a concrete model, a high level of confidence can be achieved in the correctness of the implementation. The contribution of this paper, therefore, can be summarised as a demonstration of a full top-down development technique, from a high level specification to a dependable, verified, executable program.

The paper begins by presenting some relevant background material, including the case study in question. This is followed by a detailed description of the control laws in section 2. In section 3, a refinement of this model is produced, involving concrete instantiations of the processes necessary to implement the laws, and is further refined into an executable model in section 4. The executable model is translated into JCSP in section 5, resulting in a verified implementation of the abstract model. Some conclusions are drawn in section 6.

1.1 CSP and FDR

The process algebra Communicating Sequential Processes (CSP)[3, 11] is a mathematical approach to the study of concurrency and communication. It is suited to the specification, design, and implementation of systems that continuously act and interact with their environment. CSP is a state-based approach to modelling, where systems are characterised by the events in which they are willing to participate in their lifetime. The collection and interaction of these events form processes, which can be combined using the operators of CSP, to describe more complex systems. *Failures Divergences Refinement* (FDR) [4] is a tool for model-checking networks of CSP processes, checking the containment of processes, and allowing the proving or refuting of assertions about those processes.

1.2   Multi-way Synchronisations

The term *multi-way synchronisation* refers to the situation where three or more processes simultaneously engage in a common event. In CSP, this situation arises from synchronising processes in a network on a single event, and can be used, for instance, as a technique for composing different units of a specification [7], even thought the designer may never intend to implement the specification in this manner. Another use is for modelling common events in a system: for instance a system clock [13], or a quiescent, stable system state [12, 14]. Concurrent programming languages such as *Handel-C*[2] and occam[5] support one-to-one communication between processes: only two processes may read to, or write from, a channel. There is no direct support for implementing multi-way synchronisations. To produce executable code multi-way synchronisations must be replaced with constructs supported by these languages; and a family of protocols allowing this is presented in [6].

1.3   JCSP

JCSP[9, 10] is a Java class library providing a CSP-style interface to concurrent Java programming. A JCSP program consists of a network of communicating, independent processes, interacting with each other via synchronous channel communications. Although JCSP offers several constructs that do not have a direct, one-to-one correspondence with CSP primitives, the code developed in this case study utilises only those that do.

The JCSP model of concurrent programming corresponds to that of occam: processes interact via synchronous channel communication. The same communication constraints that are expected of a *Handel-C* or occam program exist: channel communications are one-to-one, and a process may not have an output on a channel as a possibility in a guard. Simple synchronisations do not exist—as in *Handel-C* and occam, these are implemented by passing arbitrary values across typed channels. Several extensions to classical occam exist: for instance, processes can be created and destroyed dynamically; and object-oriented concepts such as inheritance are commonly exploited in a JCSP program.

1.4   The Steam Boiler

The steam boiler case study is formally presented in [1], and is an example of a class of system where control in the presence of non-manifest failures is a fundamental issue. The boiler itself consists of a tank of water, a set of pumps that supply water to the tank, a valve allowing steam to escape, an emergency outlet, and sensors reporting the water level in the tank (table 1).

Pumps can be either open or closed—an open pump supplies water to the boiler. Four water levels are pre-defined: levels $N1$ and $N2$ depict the minimum and maximum normal, safe, operating levels respectively; while $M1$ and $M2$ represent minimum and maximum critical levels. If there is too much water in the boiler, the emergency overflow may be opened; and if pressure is too great, the steam outlet may be opened. Figure 1 shows a boiler

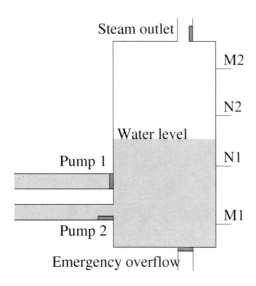

Figure 1: The steam boiler

Sense	Meaning
*LtM*1	Water level critically low
*LtN*1	Water level dropped below safe level
*BetweenN*1*N*2	Water level is between normal operating parameters
*GtN*2	Water level above safe level
*GtM*2	Water level critically high

Table 1: Senses in the system

state in which the water level lies between $N1$ and $N2$, the steam outlet is open, the overflow is closed, and one pump is open and the other closed.

Definition 1.1 *Basic control system requirements*

- *If the water level falls below N1, open closed pumps;*

- *If the water level rises above N2, close open pumps.*

It is the job of the control system to ensure that the quantity of water in the boiler remains at a safe level, summarised by definition 1.1. In the full model of the boiler, the control system may shut down the boiler if the water level becomes critical. Additionally, failures may occur non-deterministically in any of the components, and these failures must be mitigated. In this paper, only the normal operating mode is considered. Laws for initialisation, shut down, and failure mitigation exist, but as the derivation technique for their implementation is identical, they are not considered in this paper.

In [8], an *inference engine* is presented, which takes this set of rules, and instantiates a control system. The model of the inference engine uses an idiom that relies on concurrency and synchronisation, but not on data flow. For this reason, it is highly suitable to implementation in *Handel-C* on an FPGA, as concurrency can be exploited without the additional

$$rule_0 \triangleq Normal \wedge Level.LtN1 \wedge ClosePump.Pump1 \Rightarrow Disable.ClosePump.Pump1$$
$$rule_1 \triangleq Normal \wedge Level.LtN1 \wedge ClosePump.Pump2 \Rightarrow Disable.ClosePump.Pump2$$
$$rule_2 \triangleq Normal \wedge Level.GtN2 \wedge OpenPump.Pump1 \Rightarrow Disable.OpenPump.Pump1$$
$$rule_3 \triangleq Normal \wedge Level.GtN2 \wedge OpenPump.Pump2 \Rightarrow Disable.OpenPump.Pump2$$

Table 2: Assertion disablers

overhead of complex abstract data types being implemented directly into hardware. Each rule is declared as a CSP channel; and processes monitoring senses, inferring facts, and effecting actuates by synchronising on these channels are declared. These processes are given in the following sections.

2 The Control System

The control laws governing operation of the steam boiler are represented as a set of rules. In normal operating mode, rules can be divided into two distinct categories: those that react to senses, and those that infer facts about the plant—some of which are actuates to be performed on the plant. Rules are expressed as implications: the hypothesis of a rule is the conjunction of a set of facts which imply the conclusion—when all the facts in the hypothesis have been asserted, the conclusion can be inferred. All the rules used in this paper are taken from [8].

Definition 2.1 *The structure of a rule*

$$hypothesis \triangleq fact_1 \wedge fact2 \wedge ... \wedge fact_n$$

$$rule \triangleq hypothesis \Rightarrow conclusion$$

2.1 Assertion Disablers

An *assertion disabler* is a rule that prevents the control system from inferring facts that are incorrect, or from repeatedly asserting a known fact. The complete set of assertion disablers for normal, unfailed operating mode is given in table 2. In, for instance, $rule_0$, if the boiler is in *Normal* operating mode, and the level is below $N1$ and $Pump1$ is closed, then it is inferred that the ability to close $Pump1$ should be disabled.

In the case of a process monitoring a sense, when that sense is detected, the process attempts to synchronise on the channels corresponding to rules containing that sense in the hypothesis. This is shown in figure 2. This process monitors the occurrence of sense x; and when detected, it offers to synchronise on two different channels.

The CSP model of this is given in definition 2.2. The process *YetToSense* is initially willing to either engage in a *tock*—an event that delimits units of time in the boiler, after which it returns to its initial state. Alternatively, it may engage in a specific sense. If the sense occurs, subsequent behaviour is the process *Sensed*.

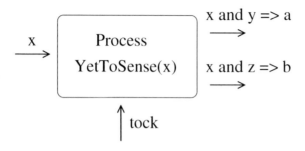

Figure 2: A sense process

Definition 2.2 *YetToSense and Sensed*

$YetToSense(i) \; \hat{=}$
   $i \rightarrow Sensed(i)$
   $\Box$
   $tock \rightarrow YetToSense(i)$

$Sensed(i) \; \hat{=}$
   let
      $use\_i\_to\_infer \; \hat{=} \; \{(A, b) \mid (A, b) \leftarrow deductions \cup ddeductions, i \in A)\}$
   within
      $\Box(H, c) : use\_i\_to\_infer \bullet infer.(H, c) \rightarrow Sensed(i)$
      $\Box$
      $tock \rightarrow YetToSense(i)$

The set *use_i_to_infer* in the process *Sensed* consists of all of the rules in the system where the sense event *i* appears in the hypothesis. Initially, this process is willing to synchronise on all of the channels corresponding to rules in this set. Alternatively, the time-slice may end with a *tock* event, and subsequent behaviour is the process *YetToSense*. The consequence of this is that the sense is no longer current and it is forgotten that it had been received—none of the rules requiring its assertion in the hypothesis are enabled.

2.2 Inference Assertions

Complementary to the assertion disablers are the rules for inferring assertions, given in table 3. In, for instance, $rule_4$, if it asserted that closing $Pump1$ has been disabled, and $Pump1$ is closed, then it can be inferred that $Pump1$ should be opened. In this way, it can be seen how these rules are complementary: $rule_0$ asserted, that when the water level is critically low, closing the pump should be disabled; and $rule_4$ asserted that if the pump were closed, and the ability to close the pump were disabled, then it should be opened—the fact that this is because of the water level dropping is left implicit.

The CSP model of this is given in definition 2.3. The set *i_inferred_from* corresponds to all the rules concluding the fact *i*, and initially, the process is willing to synchronise on any of the channels corresponding to these rules. Should one such synchronisation occur, then it must be the case that all processes attempting to assert a fact in the hypothesis of that rule have been successful. If its consequent is an actuation event, this can be performed, and subsequent behaviour is the process *Inferred*.

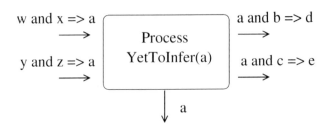

Figure 3: Inferring a fact from two possible hypothesis

$rule_4 \;\hat{=}\; Disable.ClosePump.Pump1 \wedge ClosePump.Pump1 \Rightarrow OpenPump.Pump1$	
$rule_5 \;\hat{=}\; Disable.ClosePump.Pump2 \wedge ClosePump.Pump2 \Rightarrow OpenPump.Pump2$	
$rule_6 \;\hat{=}\; Disable.OpenPump.Pump1 \wedge OpenPump.Pump1 \Rightarrow ClosePump.Pump1$	
$rule_7 \;\hat{=}\; Disable.OpenPump.Pump2 \wedge OpenPump.Pump2 \Rightarrow ClosePump.Pump2$	

Table 3: Performing actuates

Definition 2.3 *YetToInfer*

$YetToInfer(i) \;\hat{=}$
     let
         $i\_inferred\_from = \{(A, b) \mid (A, b) \leftarrow deductions \cup ddeductions, b = i\}$
     within
         $\Box(H, c) : i\_inferred\_from \bullet infer.(H, c) \rightarrow ($
             $i \in Actuate \;\&\; c \rightarrow Inferred(i)$
             $\Box$
             $i \notin Actuate \;\&\; Inferred(i)$
         $)$

$Inferred(i) \;\hat{=}$
     let
         $Applicable \;\hat{=}\; \{(A, b) \mid (A, b) \leftarrow deductions, i \in A\}$
         $Forget \;\hat{=}\; \{(A, b) \mid (A, b) \leftarrow ddeductions, i \in A\}$
     within
         $\Box(H, c) : Applicable \bullet infer.(H, c) \rightarrow Inferred(i)$
         $\Box$
         $\Box(H, c) : Forget \bullet infer.(H, c) \rightarrow YetToInfer(i)$

In the process *Inferred*, the set *Applicable* comprises all of the assertion disablers where the event i appears in the hypothesis. Similarly, the set *Forget* consists of all the inference assertions where the event i appears in the hypothesis. Initially, *Inferred* is willing to synchronise on any channel in these sets. Should a synchronisation drawn from *Forget* occur, the process returns to a state where it needs to assert the hypothesis once more.

     The complete control system is the instantiation of these processes, synchronising on the channels corresponding to rules. By constructing the system in this way there is no explicit data flow in the system: processes do not contain any data structures recording system state. Knowledge is implicitly held in the overall state of the system.

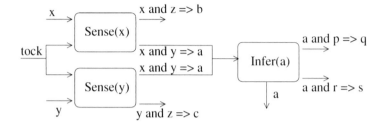

Figure 4: Connecting senses and inference

$rule_0 \triangleq Level.LtN1 \wedge ClosePump.Pump1 \Rightarrow Disable.ClosePump.Pump1$
$rule_1 \triangleq Level.LtN1 \wedge ClosePump.Pump2 \Rightarrow Disable.ClosePump.Pump2$
$rule_2 \triangleq Level.GtN2 \wedge OpenPump.Pump1 \Rightarrow Disable.OpenPump.Pump1$
$rule_3 \triangleq Level.GtN2 \wedge OpenPump.Pump2 \Rightarrow Disable.OpenPump.Pump2$

Table 4: Simplified assertion disablers

3 Calculating Process Instantiations

In this section, the network of processes corresponding to the concrete instantiation of the inference engine is given. In doing so, several possible observations and optimisations are made, and operators used in the abstract description, but not available in the target programming environment, are removed.

3.1 Sense Dependencies

In the previous section, it was stated that only the rules for normal operating mode were being considered. Therefore, by propositional logic, a simpler set of assertion disablers may be used (table 4). Consequently, a process attempting to establish *Normal* is redundant, thereby reducing the costs of implementation.

Five instantiations of the process *YetToSense* are required, drawn from table 1. A static analysis of the rules reveals the set *use_i_to_infer* in each; the results are given in table 5— only $LtN1$ and $GtN2$ have consequences. Two parameterised versions of this process can be specified to reflect this, given in definition 3.2 and definition 3.1. When there are no consequents, the only possibility in the process *Sensed* is that the clock ticks after the sense has been received. In the case of two consequents, wither may fire. The complete network of senses are these instantiations, all synchronising on clock ticks.

Sense	$use\_i\_to\_infer$
$LtM1$	$\emptyset$
$LtN1$	$rule_0, rule_1$
$BetweenN1N2$	$\emptyset$
$GtN2$	$rule_2, rule_3$
$GtM2$	$\emptyset$

Table 5: Sense dependencies

Actuate fact	$i\_inferred\_from$	$Applicable$	$Forget$
$OpenPump.Pump1$	$rule_4$	$rule_6$	$rule_2$
$OpenPump.Pump2$	$rule_5$	$rule_7$	$rule_3$
$ClosePump.Pump1$	$rule_6$	$rule_4$	$rule_0$
$ClosePump.Pump2$	$rule_7$	$rule_5$	$rule_1$
Non-actuate fact	$i\_inferred\_from$	$Applicable$	$Forget$
$Disable.OpenPump.Pump1$	$rule_2$	$\emptyset$	$rule_6$
$Disable.OpenPump.Pump2$	$rule_3$	$\emptyset$	$rule_7$
$Disable.ClosePump.Pump1$	$rule_0$	$\emptyset$	$rule_4$
$Disable.ClosePump.Pump2$	$rule_1$	$\emptyset$	$rule_5$

Table 6: Inference dependencies

Definition 3.1 *A sense with two consequents, A and B.*

$$YetToSense(i, A, B) \;\hat{=}$$
$$\qquad i \rightarrow Sensed(i, A, B)$$
$$\qquad \Box$$
$$\qquad tock \rightarrow YetToSense(i, A, B)$$

$$Sensed(i, A, B) \;\hat{=}$$
$$\qquad A \rightarrow Sensed(i, A, B)$$
$$\qquad \Box$$
$$\qquad B \rightarrow Sensed(i, A, B)$$
$$\qquad \Box$$
$$\qquad tock \rightarrow YetToSense(i, A, B)$$

Definition 3.2 *A sense with no consequents*

$$Sense'(i) \;\hat{=}$$
$$\qquad i \rightarrow tock \rightarrow Sense'(i)$$
$$\qquad \Box$$
$$\qquad tock \rightarrow Sense'(i)$$

3.2   Assertion Dependencies

A similar analysis can be performed for the eight facts involving assertion enablers (table 6). The first four facts correspond to actuates, the second four do not, meaning that two different versions of *YetToInfer* are required. Furthermore, a static analysis of the rules reveals that each of these facts appears precisely once in the hypothesis of the other rules—the set $i\_inferred\_from$ can be calculated for each process; the results of this calculation are given in table 6 and the concrete, parameterised versions of the processes given in definition 3.3 and definition 3.4 respectively.

Definition 3.3 *An inference with an actuate*

$$YetToInfer(i, A, B, C) \;\hat{=}$$
$$\qquad A \rightarrow i \rightarrow Inferred(i, A, B, C)$$

$$Inferred(i, A, B, C) \;\hat{=}$$
$$\qquad B \rightarrow Inferred(i, A, B, C)$$
$$\qquad \Box$$
$$\qquad C \rightarrow YetToInfer(i, A, B, C)$$

Definition 3.4 *An inference without an actuate*

$$YetToInfer'(A, B) \triangleq$$
$$A \rightarrow B \rightarrow YetToInfer'(A, B)$$

Further analysis reveals that each actuate assertion has precisely one rule in *Applicable*, and one in *Forget*, while non-actuate assertions only have a single rule in *Forget* (table 6).This gives rise to two versions of the process *YetToInfer*. In definition 3.3, the process offers either of the consequent rules, while in definition 3.4 there is no choice, and laws of CSP permit this simpler representation.

Definition 3.5 *The network of actuate assertions*

$$ActuateAssertions \triangleq$$
$$(YetToInfer(OpenPump.Pump1, rule4, rule2, rule6)$$
$$\|\{rule4, rule6\}\|$$
$$YetToInfer(ClosePump.Pump1, rule6, rule0, rule4))$$
$$\|\|$$
$$(YetToInfer(OpenPump.Pump2, rule5, rule3, rule7)$$
$$\|\{rule5, rule7\}\|$$
$$YetToInfer(ClosePump.Pump2, rule7, rule1, rule5))$$

Definition 3.6 *The network of non-actuate assertions*

$$NonActuateAssertions \triangleq$$
$$(YetToInfer'(rule0, rule4) \|\| YetToInfer'(rule1, rule5)$$
$$\|\| YetToInfer'(rule2, rule6) \|\| YetToInfer'(rule3, rule7))$$

The system of assertion dependencies is given by the parallel composition of the processes in each of definition 3.5 and definition 3.6, synchronising on the full set of rules. A full instantiation of the control system is this resulting process, in parallel with the sense dependencies, synchronising on the clock event and the set of rules. Rules are internal to the system, and are then hidden. The resulting system of processes can be verified equivalent to the original abstract model by model-checking using FDR. [1]

Theorem 3.1 *The instantiation is equivalent to the abstract model in section 2.*

Proof Model-check using FDR □

---

[1]This implementation assumes the boiler has initialised—establishing pumps are closed. Therefore this fact must be established manually: processes parameterised by *ClosePump.Pump1* and *ClosePump.Pump2* must be prefixed with their inferences firing: ($rule0 \rightarrow YetToInfer(ClosePump.Pump1, ...)$) and $rule1 \rightarrow$ *YetToInfer(ClosePump.Pump2, ...)* respectively.

4   Implementing Rules as Multi-way Synchronisations

As discussed in the previous section, each rule is a implemented as a channel. Further inspection of the complete system reveals that, for each rule, there are three processes whose agreement is required to enable any one given rule—this can be seen from table 5 and table 6. For instance, each of the processes $YetToSense(GtN2)$, $YetToInfer(OpenPump.Pump1, ...)$, and $YetToInfer'(Disable.OpenPump.Pump1, ...)$ all synchronise on $rule_2$. Furthermore, the clock ticking is a synchronisation between all of the sense processes and the boiler. To derive an executable implementation, these multi-way synchronisations must be removed. A straight application of the protocol presented in [6] is used to eliminate these multi-way synchronisations.

The elimination involves introducing a controller process, and set of channels to implement each multi-way synchronisation. As each controller is independent, they are interleaved. The protocol is applied to all of the processes developed in the previous section for each rule. The correctness of this development step is assured through the verification of the protocol in [6]; it is also possible, although unnecessary, to model check the resulting network using FDR. The CSP produced as a result of applying the protocol is rather long, and is included in appendix A. [2]

Theorem 4.1 *Removing the multi-way synchronisations has produced an equivalent system.*

Proof By the correctness of the multi-way synchronisation protocol. □

5   A JCSP Implementation

In this section, a description of the translation into an executable JCSP program is given. This simulation is only a demonstration of the derivation to executable code: while every step in the derivation to the executable model has been verified, the JCSP interface has not. No claims are made, therefore, about the behaviour of the JCSP library. JCSP was chosen to allow demonstrations of the results of this case study to be run on commodity personal computer environments.

Each channel in the CSP is declared as a JCSP channel. Many channels in the CSP specification utilise a process index and the value to be communicated. In the executable code, these indexes are statically determined by tagging the name of each process onto the channel name. For instance, example 5.1 gives the JCSP declaration of the channels corresponding to pumps in the original specification; all channels are declared in this manner.

Example 5.1 *Declaring the pump channels*

```
private static final int pumps = 2;
private static final int WIDTH = 2;
private One2OneChannelInt[] [] open =
   new One2OneChannelInt [pumps] [WIDTH];
private One2OneChannelInt[] [] close =
   new One2OneChannelInt [pumps] [WIDTH];
```

JCSP processes are classes that implement the library interface CSProcess. Each process instantiation in the complete CSP system is declared to implement this interface. Local private state, corresponding to the process parameters and the channels upon which that process

---

[2]For details of the protocol, the reader is referred to [6].

synchronises, are declared; and references to these passed to the object constructor. For instance, definition 5.1 contains the definition of a JCSP process implementing a non-actuate assertion disabler of definition 3.4. In this definition, local state corresponding to the channels used in the multi-way synchronisation (and the processes index in the synchronisation) are declared, and references to the global channels supplied on construction. From this example, it can be seen that the translation from a CSP process definition to a JCSP process definition is relatively straightforward, providing the specification has been refined to an executable subset.

Definition 5.1 *A process class for an inference without an actuate*

```
public class NonActuateAssertion implements CSProcess {

    ChannelOutputInt toA, toB;
    ChannelInputInt fromA, fromB;
    int a, b;
    Fact fact;

    public NonActuateAssertion (
        ChannelOutputInt toA, ChannelInputInt fromA, int a,
        ChannelOutputInt toB, ChannelInputInt fromB, int b,
        Fact fact
    ) {
        this.toA = toA;  this.fromA = fromA;  this.a = a;
        ...  etc
    }
}
```

Every process must implement the abstract method run, which is analogous to a main method in a program, and specifies what the process does when it is given a thread of control. In the run method for the non-actuate inference of definition 5.2, the process enters an infinite loop, engaging in the multi-way synchronisation corresponding to establishing its fact, and then the multi-way synchronisation corresponding to alerting other processes of the truth of this fact.

Definition 5.2 *The run method for an inference without an actuate*

```
public void run () {
    while (true) {

        toA.write (a);
        do {
            fromA.read ();
            toA.write (a);
        } while (fromA.read () != 1);

        toB.write (b);
        do {
            fromB.read ();
            toB.write (b);
        } while (fromB.read () != 1);

    }
}
```

A full JCSP program consists of a network of processes, grouped together in an array structure allowing for their parallel instantiation and execution, along with the relevant global declarations of common channels. Instruction as to how this is implemented is covered in the documentation for JCSP, and is omitted from this paper for brevity. However, a complete JCSP implementation of the steam boiler, the control system, and a graphical interface depicting the state of the system, has been developed and can be run on commodity personal computers.

6   Summary

In this paper, a full, top down derivation of an executable program was calculated from an abstract CSP specification. The result was a simulation of a control system, and associated plant, in a Java library for CSP that compiled, and ran without apparent error, and without need for an experiment/test cycle normally expected for a highly concurrent program.

Despite this notable success, there are several limitations. Firstly, the final stage of development, in moving from CSP to JCSP, is largely an approximation. There was no direct application of a refinement calculus to guide the translation from CSP to JCSP, so it cannot be completely justified. However, the library offering implementations of the primitives used has a clear one-to-one correspondence, so confidence can be earned from the simplicity of the process.

Secondly, although the JCSP library claims to implement these primitives, the majority of library itself has not been verified—therefore it cannot be guaranteed that the executable code behaves precisely as the specification intended. For instance, a non-terminating, mutually (infinitely) recursive pair of processes is a common appearance in CSP; but if translated directly into JCSP, stack overflow errors occur, leading to programs crashing. Such an error is not readily detectable by model-checking in FDR as it is a property of the implementation of the target executable language that does not exist in the mathematical model. Areas such as this need to be addressed if justified claims that the executable JCSP code was equivalent to the abstract CSP specification are to be made.

Despite these limitations, the production of the simulation is a definite success. The intention was to demonstrate that techniques exist allowing for the accurate, calculated production of executable concurrent code; and to produce a simple example of this which could be run on commodity personal computers for demonstration purposes—and this has been achieved. However, clearly, for the production of real control systems, applying the refinement calculus to a verified subset of, for instance, *Handel-C* on an FPGA, is necessary.

Acknowledgements

The author wishes to thank QinetiQ Malvern and Bedford for their role in funding this work, and Jim Woodcock and Peter Welch for extensive technical discussion and assistance.

References

[1] J. R. Abrial, E. Borger, and H. Laangmack, editors. *Formal methods for industrial applications: specifying and programming the steam boiler control*, volume 1165 of *LNCS*. Springer–Verlag, 1996.

[2] Celoxica. Handel-C reference manual. Technical report, Celoxica, 1999.

[3] C. A. R. Hoare. *Communicating Sequential Processes*. Prentice-Hall International Series in Computer Science. Prentice-Hall, 1985.

[4] Formal Systems (Europe) Ltd. FDR: User manual and tutorial, version 2.28. Technical report, Formal Systems (Europe) Ltd., 1999.

[5] INMOS Ltd. occam *Programming manual*. International Series In Computer Science. Prentice-Hall, 1984.

[6] Alistair A. McEwan. *Concurrent Program Development*. DPhil thesis, The University of Oxford, Submitted Trinity Term, 2004.

[7] Carroll Morgan and J. C. P Woodcock. What is a specification? In Dan Craigen and Karen Summerskill, editors, *Formal Methods for Trustworthy Computer Systems*, Workshops in Computing, pages 38–43. Springer-Verlag, 1989.

[8] Colin O'Halloran. Identifying critical requirements. Internal report of work in progress, Qinetiq, 2003.

[9] P.H.Welch. Process Oriented Design for Java: Concurrency for All. In H.R.Arabnia, editor, *Proceedings of the International Conference on Parallel and Distributed Processing Techniques and Applications (PDPTA'2000)*, volume 1, pages 51–57. CSREA, CSREA Press, June 2000.

[10] P.H.Welch, J.R.Aldous, and J.Foster. CSP networking for java (JCSP.net). In P.M.A.Sloot, C.J.K.Tan, J.J.Dongarra, and A.G.Hoekstra, editors, *Computational Science - ICCS 2002*, volume 2330 of *Lecture Notes in Computer Science*, pages 695–708. Springer-Verlag, April 2002.

[11] A. W. Roscoe. *The theory and practice of concurrency*. Prentice Hall Series in Computer Science. Prentice Hall, 1998.

[12] J. C. P. Woodcock. Montigel's Dwarf, a treatment of the Dwarf Signal problem using CSP/FDR. In *Proceedings of the 5th FMERail Workshop*, Toulouse, France, 1999.

[13] J. C. P Woodcock and Alistair A. McEwan. An overview of the verification of a *Handel-C* program. In *Proceedings of the International Conference on Parallel and Distributed Processing Techniques and Applications*, volume V, page 3003. CSREA Press, 2000.

[14] J. C. P. Woodcock and Alistair A. McEwan. Verifying the safety of a railway signalling device. In H. Ehrig, B. J. Kramer, and A. Ertas, editors, *Proceedings of IDPT 2002*, volume 1. The 6th Biennial World Conference on Integrated Design and Process Technology, Society for Design and Process Science, 2002. Winner of the best paper award.

A   Control system processes implementations

Auxiliary definitions

Definition A.1 *Withdrawing from a synchronisation*

$$Withdraw(to, from, i) \; \widehat{=}$$
$$(to!flip(i) \; \rightarrow \; SKIP)$$
$$\|\|$$
$$(from?invite \; \rightarrow \; invite \; \& \; from?any \; \rightarrow \; SKIP \; \Box \; \neg \; invite \; \& \; SKIP)$$

Definition A.2 *A guaranteed synchronisation*

$$GSync(to, from, i) \; \widehat{=} \qquad\qquad GSync' \; \widehat{=}$$
$$to!i \; \rightarrow \; GSync' \qquad\qquad\qquad from?any \; \rightarrow$$
$$to!i \; \rightarrow \; from?sync \; \rightarrow$$
$$(sync \; \& \; SKIP \; \Box \; \neg \; sync \; \& \; GSync')$$

Sense inferences

Definition A.3 *Senses not in a hypothesis, with multi-way synchronisations removed*

$$Sense'(to, from, i, s) \; \widehat{=}$$
$$to!i \; \rightarrow \; Sense''(to, from, i, s)$$

$$Sense''(to, from, i, s) \; \widehat{=}$$
$$s \; \rightarrow \; Withdraw(to, from, i);$$
$$GSync(to, from, i);$$
$$Sense'(to, from, i, s)$$
$$\Box$$
$$from?any \; \rightarrow$$
$$to!i \; \rightarrow$$
$$from?sync \; \rightarrow$$
$$sync \; \& \; Sense'(to, from, i, s)$$
$$\Box$$
$$\neg \; sync \; \& \; Sense''(to, from, i, s)$$

Definition A.4 *Senses in a hypothesis, with multi-way synchronisations removed*

$$Sense(to, from, i, toA, fromA, a, toB, fromB, b, s) \; \widehat{=}$$
$$to!i \; \rightarrow \; Sense'(to, from, i, toA, fromA, a, toB, fromB, b, s)$$

$$Sense'(to, from, i, toA, fromA, a, toB, fromB, b, s) \; \widehat{=}$$
$$sense \; \rightarrow \; Withdraw(to, from, i);$$
$$Sensed(to, from, i, toA, fromA, a, toB, fromB, b, s)$$
$$\Box$$
$$from?any \; \rightarrow$$
$$to!i \; \rightarrow$$
$$from?sync \; \rightarrow$$
$$sync \; \& \; Sense(to, from, i, toA, fromA, a, toB, fromB, b, s)$$
$$\Box$$
$$\neg \; sync \; \& \; Sense'(to, from, i, toA, fromA, a, toB, fromB, b, s)$$

$Sensed(to, from, i, toA, fromA, a, toB, fromB, b, s) \ \widehat{=}$
   $(to!i \rightarrow SKIP \ ||| \ toA!a \rightarrow SKIP \ ||| \ toB!b \rightarrow SKIP);$
      $Sensed'(to, from, i, toA, fromA, a, toB, fromB, b, s)$

$Sensed'(to, from, i, toA, fromA, a, toB, fromB, b, s) \ \widehat{=}$
   $from?any \rightarrow$
     $to!i \rightarrow$
       $from?sync \rightarrow$
         $sync \ \& \ (Withdraw(toA, fromA, a) \ ||| \ Withdraw(toB, fromB, b));$
           $YetToSense(to, from, i, toA, fromA, a, toB, fromB, b, s)$
         $\square$
         $\neg \ sync \ \& \ Sensed'(to, from, i, toA, fromA, a, toB, fromB, b, s)$
   $\square$
   $fromA?any \rightarrow$
     $toA!a \rightarrow$
       $fromA?sync \rightarrow$
         $sync \ \& \ (Withdraw(to, from, i) \ ||| \ Withdraw(toB, fromB, b));$
           $Sensed(to, from, i, toA, fromA, a, toB, fromB, b, s)$
         $\square$
         $\neg \ sync \ \& \ Sensed'(to, from, i, toA, fromA, a, toB, fromB, b, s)$
   $\square$
   $fromB?any \rightarrow$
     $toB!a \rightarrow$
       $fromB?sync \rightarrow$
         $sync \ \& \ (Withdraw(to, from, i) \ ||| \ Withdraw(toA, fromA, a));$
           $Sensed(to, from, i, toA, fromA, a, toB, fromB, b, s)$
         $\square$
         $\neg \ sync \ \& \ Sensed'(to, from, i, toA, fromA, a, toB, fromB, b, s)$

Assertion inferences

Definition A.5 *An inference without an actuate, with multi-way synchronisations removed*

$YetToInfer'(toA, fromA, a, toB, fromB, b) \ \widehat{=}$
   $GSync(toA, fromA, a);$
     $GSync(toB, fromB, b);$
       $YetToInfer'(toA, fromA, a, toB, fromB, b)$

Definition A.6 *An inference with an actuate, with multi-way synchronisations removed*

$YetToInfer(toA, fromA, a, toB, fromB, b, toC, fromC, c, i) \ \widehat{=}$
   $GSync(toA, fromA, a);$
     $i \rightarrow Inferred(toA, fromA, a, toB, fromB, b, toC, fromC, c, i)$

$Inferred(toA, fromA, a, toB, fromB, b, toC, fromC, c, i) \ \widehat{=}$
   $(toB!b \rightarrow SKIP \ ||| \ toC!c \rightarrow SKIP);$
     $Inferred'(toA, fromA, a, toB, fromB, b, toC, fromC, c, i)$

$Inferred'(toA, fromA, a, toB, fromB, b, toC, fromC, c, i) \;\widehat{=}$
    $fromB?any \rightarrow$
           $toB!a \rightarrow$
                $fromB?sync \rightarrow$
                    $sync$ & $Withdraw(toC, fromC, c);$
                            $Inferred(toA, fromA, a, toB, fromB, b, toC, fromC, c, i)$
                    $\square$
                    $\neg\ sync$ &
                            $Inferred'(toA, fromA, a, toB, fromB, b, toC, fromC, c, i)$
    $\square$
    $fromC?any \rightarrow$
        $toC!a \rightarrow$
                $fromC?sync \rightarrow$
                    $sync$ & $Withdraw(toB, fromB, b);$
                      $YetToInfer(toA, fromA, a, toB, fromB, b, toC, fromC, c, i)$
                  $\square$
                  $\neg\ sync$ & $Inferred'(toA, fromA, a, toB, fromB, b, toC, fromC, c, i)$

Communicating Process Architectures 2004
Ian East, Jeremy Martin, Peter Welch, David Duce, and Mark Green (Eds.)
IOS Press, 2004

Refining Industrial Scale Systems in Circus

Marcel OLIVEIRA, Ana CAVALCANTI, and Jim WOODCOCK

Computing Laboratory, University of Kent, Canterbury, CT2 7NF, England

Abstract. *Circus* is a new notation that may be used to specify both data and behaviour aspects of a system, and has an associated refinement calculus. Although a few case studies are already available in the literature, the industrial fire control system presented in this paper is, as far as we know, the largest case study on the *Circus* refinement strategy. We describe the refinement and present some new laws that were needed. Our case study makes extensive use of mutual recursion; a simplified notation for specifying such systems and proving their refinements is proposed here.

1 Introduction

Circus (Concurrent Integrated Refinement CalculUS) [1, 2] characterises systems as processes that combine constructs that describe data and control behaviour. The Z notation [3, 4] is used to define most of the data aspects, and CSP [5] and Dijkstra's guarded-command language are used to define behaviour. The semantics of *Circus* is based on unifying theories of programming [6], a framework that unifies the science of programming across many different computational paradigms. *Circus*, unlike other combinations of data and behavioural aspects, such as CCS-Z [7, 8], CSP-Z [9], and CSP-OZ [10], supports refinement in a calculational style similar to that presented in [11].

A refinement strategy for *Circus* is presented in [2], with the complete development of a reactive buffer into a distributed implementation as an example. Refinement notions and many refinement laws are also presented. In the current paper, we provide a more significant case study on the *Circus* refinement calculus: a safety-critical fire protection system. As far as we know, it is the largest case study on the *Circus* refinement calculus.

Throughout the development of our case study there were some problems; we present the solutions for some of them in this paper. First, the set of laws presented in [2] was not sufficient; we propose new refinement laws. For instance, we require some laws for inserting and distributing assumptions, and a new process refinement law. In total, more than fifty new laws have been identified during the development of our case study.

In [2], the refinement of mutual recursive actions is not considered; our case study, however, includes mutually recursive definitions. We present here a notation used to prove refinement of such systems; this results in more concise and modular proofs. The necessary theorems that justify the notation have been proved in [12].

The main objective of this paper is to illustrate an application of the refinement strategy in an existing industrial application [13]. We believe that, with the results in this paper, we provide empirical evidence of the power of expression of *Circus* and, principally, that the strategy presented in [2] is applicable to large industrial systems.

In Section 2, we present an introduction to refinement in *Circus*: we describe *Circus* and the refinement notions for processes and their constituent actions. Section 3 presents our case study. Finally, we present our conclusions and discuss future work in Section 4.

2 Refinement in *Circus*

In what follows, we summarise the *Circus* notation and its refinement technique. More details can be found in [1, 2], and an example is presented in Section 3.

2.1 *Circus*

Circus programs are sequences of paragraphs: channel declarations, channel set definitions, Z paragraphs, or process definitions. A system is defined as a process that encapsulates some state and communicates through channels.

A channel declaration declares its name and type; if the channel is used purely for synchronisation, then no type is needed. The generic channel declaration **channel** $[T]$ c : T declares a family of channels c. In this declaration, $[T]$ is a parameter used to determine the type of the values that are communicated through channel c. We may introduce sets of channels in a **chanset** paragraph.

Processes may be defined explicitly or in terms of other processes (compound processes). An explicit process definition is delimited by the keywords **begin** and **end**: it is formed by a state definition, a sequence of paragraphs, and a nameless action, which defines its behaviour. In [2], we have introduced the keyword **state** before the state declaration in order to make it clear which schema represents a process state.

Compound processes are defined using the CSP operators of sequence, external (occam ALT) and internal choice, parallelism and interleaving, or their corresponding iterated operators, event hiding, or indexed operators, which are particular to *Circus* specifications. The parallelism follows the alphabetised approach adopted by [5], instead of that adopted by [14].

An action can be a schema, a guarded command, an invocation of another action, or a combination of these constructs using CSP operators. Three primitive actions are available: *Skip*, *Stop*, and *Chaos*. The prefixing operator is standard, but a guard construction may be associated with it. For instance, given a Z predicate p, if the condition p is *true*, the action p & $c?x \rightarrow A$ inputs a value through channel c and assigns it to the variable x, and then behaves like A, which has the variable x in scope. If, however, the condition p is *false*, the same action blocks. Such enabling conditions like p may be associated with any action.

The CSP operators of sequence, external and internal choice, parallelism, interleaving, their corresponding iterated operators, and hiding may also be used to compose actions. Communications and recursive definitions are also available.

To avoid conflicts in the access to the variables in scope, parallelism and interleaving of actions declare a synchronisation channel set and two sets that partition all the variables. In the parallelism $A_1 \llbracket ns_1 \mid cs \mid ns_2 \rrbracket A_2$, the actions A_1 and A_2 synchronise on the channels in set cs (unlike in occam, where the synchronisation channel set is implicit). Both A_1 and A_2 have access to the initial values of all variables in both ns_1 and ns_2. However, A_1 and A_2 may modify only the values of the variables in ns_1 and ns_2, respectively. The changes made by A_1 in variables in ns_1 are not seen by A_2, and *vice-versa*.

Finally, an action may also be a variable block. Further operators are available in *Circus* [1]; only those that are used in this paper are described here.

2.2 Refinement Strategy

A refinement strategy for *Circus* is presented [2]. It is based on laws of simulation, a technique used to prove data refinement in Z, and action and process refinement; some of them are presented in Appendix A. We present further simulation and refinement laws in Appendix B.

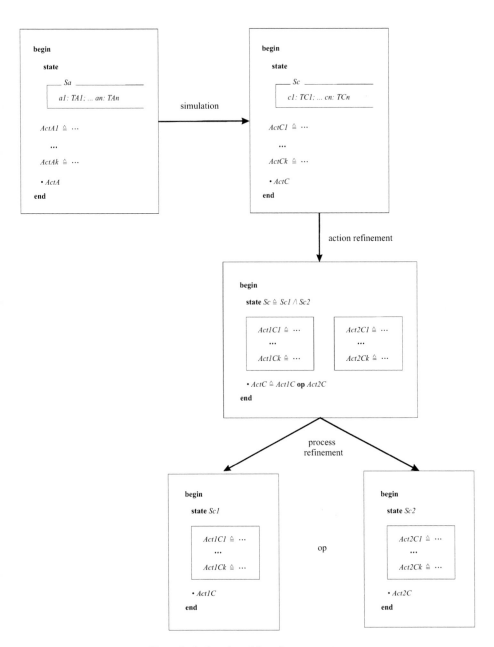

Figure 1: An iteration of the refinement strategy

Table 1: The System States and Corresponding Actions

System State	Abstract FC Action	Concrete FC Action	Concrete Area Action
fireSysStart$_s$	*AbstractFireSysStart*	*FireSysStart*	*StartArea*
fireSys$_s$	*AbstractFireSys*	*FireSys*	*AreaCycle*
manual$_s$	*AbstractManual*	*Manual*	*ManualArea*
auto$_s$	*AbstractAuto*	*Auto*	*AutoArea*
reset$_s$	*AbstractReset*	*Reset*	*ResetArea*
countdown$_s$	*AbstractCountdown*	*Countdown*	*WaitingDischarge*
discharge$_s$	*AbstractDischarge*	*Discharge*	*WaitingDischarge*
fireSysD$_s$	*AbstractFireSysD*	*FireSysD*	*AreaD*
disabled$_s$	*AbstractDisabled*	*Disabled*	*DisabledArea*

The strategy aims at refining an abstract centralised specification to a distributed *Circus* program, which involves only executable constructs. The strategy consists of possibly many iterations involving simulation, actions, and process refinement; in each iteration a process is split as presented in Figure 1. In this figure, each process is represented as a box. For instance, before the simulation, we have a process with an internal state Sa, and actions $ActA1, \cdots, ActAk$; its behaviour is determined by the main action $ActA$. First, elements of the concrete system state are included using simulation; next, the state space and actions are partitioned in such a way that each partition, represented in the figure by internal boxes, groups some state components and the actions which access these components; and, finally, all these partitions become individual processes, which are combined in the same way as their main actions were in the previous process.

The semantics of *Circus* is defined using Hoare and He's unifying theories of programming. In [2], we have a definition for action refinement; process refinement amounts to refinement of the main action, with the state components taken as local variables. Backwards and forwards simulation are also defined and proved sound in [2]. Here, we do not use the definitions in [2], but simulation and refinement laws.

3   Case Study

Our case study consists of a fire control system that covers two separate areas. Each area is divided into two zones; two different zones cannot be covered by two different areas. Two extra zones are used for detection only. Fire detection happens in a zone, and, in consequence, a gas discharge may occur in the area that contains that zone.

The system includes a display panel composed of lamps that indicates whether the system is on or off, whether there are system faults, or a fire has been detected, whether the alarm has been silenced or not, the need to replace the actuators of the system, and gas discharges.

The system can be in one of three modes: manual, automatic, or disabled. In manual mode, an alarm sounds when a fire is detected, and the corresponding detection lamp is lit on the display. The alarm can be silenced, and, when the reset button is pressed, the system returns to normal. In manual mode, gas discharge is manually initiated.

In automatic mode, a fire detection is also followed by the alarm being sounded; however, if a fire is detected in the second zone of the same area, the second stage alarm is sounded, and a countdown starts. When the countdown finishes, the gas is discharged and the circuit fault lamp is illuminated in the display; the system mode is switched to disabled.

In disabled mode, the system can only have the actuators replaced, identify relevant faults within the system, and be reset. The system is back to its normal mode after the actuators are

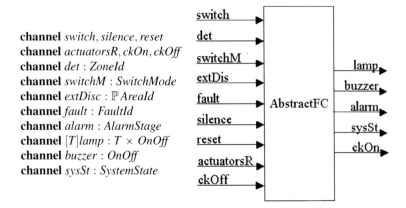

channel *switch, silence, reset*
channel *actuatorsR, ckOn, ckOff*
channel *det* : *ZoneId*
channel *switchM* : *SwitchMode*
channel *extDisc* : $\mathbb{P}$ *AreaId*
channel *fault* : *FaultId*
channel *alarm* : *AlarmStage*
channel [*T*]*lamp* : *T* × *OnOff*
channel *buzzer* : *OnOff*
channel *sysSt* : *SystemState*

Figure 2: System External Channels

replaced and the reset button is pressed.

The system may be in one of the states presented in Table 1. Initially, the system is on *fireSysStart$_s$* state. After being switched on, its state is changed to *fireSys$_s$*; in this state, a fire detection yields to the state being changed to *manual$_s$* or *auto$_s$* depending on the system mode. In the state *reset$_s$* the system is waiting to be reset; in *countdown$_s$*, it is waiting for the clock to finish the countdown. During gas discharge, the system is on the *discharge$_s$* state, after which, the state is changed to *fireSysD$_s$*. Finally, if a fire is detected on *fireSysD$_s$*, the system state is changed to *disabled$_s$*.

Some further requirements should also be satisfied: the system must be started with a *switch* event, and, afterwards, the system *on* lamp should be illuminated; the system mode can be switched between manual and automatic mode provided no detection happens. Also, when the system is reset, all fire detection lamps must be switched off; if a gas discharge occurred, the actuators need to be replaced, and the system mode is switched to automatic. Following a fire detection, the corresponding lamp must be lit. After a gas discharge, no subsequent discharge may happen before the actuators are replaced.

The external channels of the fire control system are presented in Figure 2. Fire detection is indicated through channel *det*, which inputs the zone where it happened. The system mode can be manually switched using channel *switch*. In manual mode, when the conditions that lead to a gas discharge are met, gas can be manually discharged using the channel *extDisc*. Faults are reported to the system through the channel *fault*. The channel *alarm* can be used to sound the alarm, which can be silenced through *silence*. Channel *reset* resets the system. The channel *actuatorsR* indicates that the actuators have been replaced. The system indicates that a lamp must be switched using the generic channel *lamp*; it provides the type of lamp and the new lamp mode. The buzzer is controlled using channel *buzzer*. After each state change, the system reports its current state using channel *sysSt*. The fire control system may request a clock to execute the countdown using channel *ckOn*; the clock indicates that the countdown is finished using channel *ckOff*.

The display is composed of the lamps and the buzzer. The lamps can be of three different types; however, the three types of lamps are instances of the same generic process *GenericLamp*, which has a component *status* : *OnOff*. Initially, all the lamps are switched *off*; they can be switched *on* using an appropriate instance of channel *lamp*.

$Areald ::= 0 \mid 1$
$Zoneld ::= 0 \mid 1 \mid 2 \mid 3 \mid 4 \mid 5$
$Mode ::= automatic \mid manual \mid disabled$
$SwitchMode == Mode \setminus \{disabled\}$
$OnOff ::= on \mid off$
$AlarmStage ::= alarmOff \mid firstStage \mid secondStage$
$LampId ::= zoneFaultL \mid earthFaultL \mid sounderLineFaultL \mid powerFaultL \mid sysOnL$
$\qquad \mid remoteSignalL \mid actuatorLineFaultL \mid circuitFaultL \mid alarmSilencedL$
$FaultId ::= ZoneF \mid earthF \mid sounderLineF \mid powerF \mid remoteSignal \mid actuatorLineF$
$SystemState ::= fireSysStart_s \mid fireSys_s \mid fireSysD_s \mid auto_s$
$\qquad \mid countdown_s \mid discharge_s \mid reset_s \mid manual_s \mid disabled_s$

Figure 3: System Types

3.1 Abstract Fire Control System

The basic types used within the system are presented in Figure 3. The areas and zones are identified by the types $Areald$ and $Zoneld$; the system modes are represented by the type $Mode$; the type $SwitchMode$, is a subset of type $Mode$. All the lamps and the buzzer of the display can be either on or off, which are represented by the type $OnOff$. The alarm states are represented by the type $AlarmStage$. The type $LampId$ contains identifiers for all the lamps in the system's display. Faults are represented by the type $FaultId$. Finally, the system can be in one of the states of the type $SystemState$.

Process $AbstractFC$ formalises the requirements previously described. Throughout this paper we omit some formal definitions for the sake of conciseness; they can be found in [12]. The abstract state is defined by the Z schema named $AbstractFCSt$ presented below. Z schemas can either be represented as boxes, as $AbstractFCSt$, or in a horizontal notation as we shall see later in this paper. $AbstractFCSt$ is composed of five components, which are declared in the declaration part of the schema: $mode$ indicates the mode in which the fire control is running; $controlZns$ is a total function that maps the areas to a set that contains their controlled zones; $actZns$ maps the areas to the zones in which a fire detection has occurred; $discharge$ indicates in which areas a gas discharged happened; finally, $active$ contains the active areas identifications.

process $AbstractFC \mathrel{\widehat{=}}$ **begin**
state $\underline{\quad AbstractFCSt \quad\rule{3cm}{0pt}}$
$\quad mode : Mode$
$\quad controlZns, actZns : Areald \rightarrow \mathbb{P}\, Zoneld$
$\quad discharge, active : \mathbb{P}\, Areald$
$\underline{\rule{6cm}{0pt}}$
$\quad \forall\, a : Areald \bullet$
$\qquad (mode = manual) \Rightarrow a \in active \Leftrightarrow \#actZns\, a \geq 1$
$\qquad \wedge\ (mode = automatic) \Rightarrow a \in active \Leftrightarrow \#actZns\, a \geq 2$
$\qquad \wedge\ actZns\, a \subseteq controlZns\, a \wedge controlZns\, a = getZones\, a$

The state invariant is declared in the predicate part of the schema; it determines that, if the system is running in *manual* mode (predicate *mode = manual*), an area is *active* if, and only if, some zone controlled by it is active. On the other hand, if the mode is *automatic*, an area is active if, and only if, there is more than one active zone controlled by it. Finally, for each area, its controlled zones are defined by the function *getZones*, whose definition we omit.

Initially, the system is in *automatic* mode, there is no active zone, and no discharge occurred in any area. The state invariant guarantees that there is no active area.

$$
\begin{array}{l}
\_InitAbstractFC _____ \\
AbstractFCSt' \\
\hline
mode' = automatic \wedge discharge' = \emptyset \wedge actZns' = \{a : AreaId \bullet a \mapsto \emptyset\}
\end{array}
$$

Undashed variables represent the variable values before the execution of an operation; on the other hand, dashed variables represent the variable values after the execution of an operation. The decoration of a schema $Schema \ \hat{=}\ [x_1 : T_1 \dots x_n : T_n \mid p]$, is defined as the decoration of all the components of the schema, and the modification of the predicate part of the schema to reflect the new names of these components. For instance, we have that $Schema' \ \hat{=}\ [x_1' : T_1 \dots x_n' : T_n \mid p[x_1'/x_1, \dots, x_n'/x_n]]$. Finally, the inclusion of the schema $AbstractFCSt'$ in the declaration part of $InitAbstractFC$, merges the declarations of both schemas, and conjoins their predicates.

Three operations are used to switch the system mode; they leave the other components unchanged. The first operation receives the new mode as argument. For any schema $State$ that describes the state of a system, $\Delta\ State$ is a schema that includes both $Schema$ and $Schema'$. Furthermore, the name of input components must end with a query (?) and the name of output components must end with a shriek (!).

$$
\begin{array}{l}
\_SwitchAbstractFCMode _____ \\
\Delta AbstractFCSt;\ nm? : Mode \\
\hline
mode' = nm? \wedge actZns' = actZns \wedge discharge' = discharge
\end{array}
$$

$SwitchAbstractFC2Auto$ and $SwitchAbstractFC2Dis$ do not receive arguments; they switch the mode to *automatic* and *disabled*, respectively.

The schema $AbstractActivateZone$ receives a zone $nz?$ and changes $actZns$ by including $nz?$ in the set of active zones of the area that controls it; *active* may also be changed to maintain the state invariant. All other state components are left unchanged.

$$
\begin{array}{l}
\_AbstractActivateZone _____ \\
\Delta AbstractFCSt;\ nz? : ZoneId \\
\hline
mode' = mode \wedge discharge' = discharge \\
actZns' = actZns \oplus \{a : AreaId \mid nz? \in controlZns\ a \bullet \\
\qquad\qquad\qquad a \mapsto actZns\ a \cup \{nz?\}\}
\end{array}
$$

The schema $AbstractAutomaticDischarge$ activates the discharge in the active areas, only *discharge* is changed. Finally, $AbstractManualDischarge$ receives the areas in which the user wants to discharge the gas, but discharges only in those that are *active*.

All the other actions are defined using CSP operators. Basically, we have one action for each possible state within the system as described in Table 1.

The action $AbstractFireSysStart$ starts by communicating the current system state. Then, it waits for the system to be switched on through channel *switch*, switches on the lamp $SysOnL$, initialises the system state and, finally, behaves like action $AbstractFireSys$.

$$
AbstractFireSysStart \ \hat{=}\ sysSt!fireSysStart_s \rightarrow switch \rightarrow
$$
$$
lamp[LampId].sysOnL!on \rightarrow InitAbstractFC;\ AbstractFireSys
$$

In action $AbstractFireSys$, after communicating the system state, the mode can be manu-

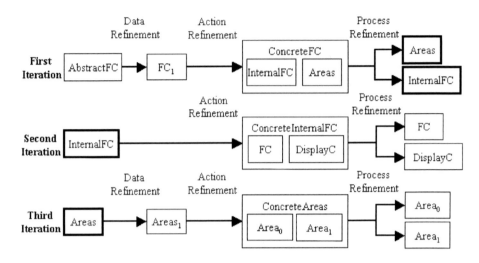

Figure 4: Refinement Strategy for the Fire Control System

ally switched between *automatic* and *manual*. Furthermore, if any detection occurs, the zone in which the detection occurred is activated, the corresponding lamp is lit, the alarm sounds in *firstStage*, and then, the system behaves like *AbstractManual* or *AbstractAuto*, depending on the current system mode. If the actuators are replaced, the *circFaultL* is switched off, the system is set to *automatic* mode, and waits to be *reset*. Finally, if any *fault* is identified, the corresponding *lamp* is lit, and the buzzer is switched *on*.

$$AbstractFireSys \,\widehat{=}$$
$$\quad sysSt!fireSys_s \,\rightarrow$$
$$\qquad switchM?nm \rightarrow SwitchAbstractFCMode;\; AbstractFireSys$$
$$\qquad \square\; det?nz \rightarrow AbstractActivateZone;\; lamp[ZoneId].nz!on \rightarrow$$
$$\qquad\qquad alarm!firstStage \rightarrow$$
$$\qquad\qquad\qquad (mode = manual)\; \&\; AbstractManual$$
$$\qquad\qquad\qquad \square\; (mode = automatic)\; \&\; AbstractAuto$$
$$\qquad \square\; actuatorsR \rightarrow lamp[LampId].circFaultL!off \rightarrow$$
$$\qquad\qquad SwitchAbstractFC2Auto;\; AbstractReset$$
$$\qquad \square\; fault?faultId \rightarrow lamp[LampId].(getLampId\,faultId)!on \rightarrow$$
$$\qquad\qquad buzzer!on \rightarrow AbstractFireSys$$

The function *getLampId* maps fault identifications to their corresponding lamp in the display.

Throughout this paper, we illustrate the refinement of the fire control system using these two actions only. For this reason, we omit the definitions of the remaining actions.

The main action of process *AbstractFireSys* is defined below.

- *AbstractFireSysStart* **end**

In the next section, we refine *AbstractFC* to a concrete distributed system.

3.2 Refinement

The motivation for the fire control system refinement is the distribution of the areas, in order to increase efficienct. Section 3.2.1 presents the target of our refinement, the concrete

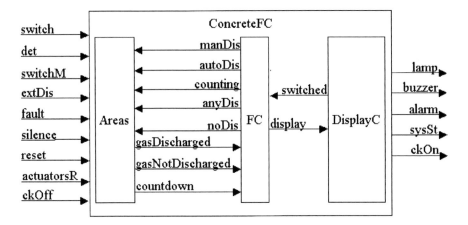

Figure 5: Concrete Fire Control

fire control system. In the following sections, we present the refinement steps summarised graphically in Figure 4.

In the first iteration, we split *AbstractFC* into two process *Areas* and *InternalFC*. The first models the areas of the system, and is split into two interleaved *Area* processes in interleaving in the last iteration. The second is the core of the system, which is split into a display controller *DisplayC* and the system controller *FC* in the second iteration.

3.2.1 Concrete Fire Control System

The concrete fire control system has three components: the controller, the display, and the detection system. They communicate through the channels below.

> **channel** *display, manDis* : $\mathbb{P}$ *AreaId*
> **channel** *switched, autoDis, anyDis, noDis, countdown, counting*
> **channel** *gasDischarged, gasNotDischarged* : *AreaId*

The controller indicates discharges to the display through *display*. The display acknowledges this communication through channel *switched*. The controller request gas discharges to the detection process through *manDis* and *autoDis*. The detection process may reply to these requests indicating if the gas has been discharged (*anyDis*) or not (*noDis*); it may request a *countdown*, if it is *automatic* mode and the conditions for a gas discharge are met. The controller indicates that it started counting through *counting*. In Figure 5, we summarise the internal communications of the concrete fire control system.

Controller The process *FC* is similar to the abstract specification. However, all the state components and events related to the detection areas and to the display are removed. For conciseness, some schemas, as the system state presented below, are presented in their horizontal form *name* $\hat{=}$ [*declaration* | *predicate*].

> **process** *FC* $\hat{=}$ **begin state** *FCSt* $\hat{=}$ [*mode*$_1$: *Mode*]
> *InitFC* $\hat{=}$ [*FCSt'* | *mode*$_1$ = *automatic*]

The state of the concrete fire control is composed of only one component, *mode*$_1$, which indicates the mode in which the system is running. This mode is initialised to *automatic*.

Three operations can be used to switch the system mode. The first one receives the new mode as argument.

$$SwitchFCMode \; \widehat{=} \; [\,\Delta FCSt; \; nm? : Mode \mid mode_1 = nm?\,]$$

The second and third operations do not receive any argument; they simply switch the system mode to *automatic* or *disabled*.

The fire control system is responsible for communicating the current system state. After being switched on, the fire control initialises its state and behaves like action *FireSys*. Where a lamp was switched *on* in the abstract specification, an acknowledgment event *switched* is received from the the display controller.

$$FireSysStart \; \widehat{=} \; sysSt!fireSysStart_s \to switch \to switched \to InitFC; \; FireSys$$

Similar to the abstract system, all the other actions corresponds to a possible state within the system as described in Table 1.

In action *FireSys*, after communicating the system state, the mode can be switched. Furthermore, if any detection occurs, the controller waits for a *switched* signal, sets the alarm to *firstStage*, and behaves like *Manual* or *Auto*, depending on the current system mode. Since the areas are the processes which have the area-zone information, following a *det* communication, the zone activation is not part of the controller behaviour. If the actuators are replaced, the system is set to *automatic* mode, and waits to be *reset*. Finally, all the faults are ignored by this process, except that it waits for a *switched* signal from the display.

$$FireSys \; \widehat{=} \; sysSt!fireSys_s \to \left(\begin{array}{l} switchM?nm \to SwitchFCMode; \; FireSys \\ \Box \; det?nz \to switched \to alarm!firstStage \to \\ \quad (mode_1 = manual) \; \& \; Manual \\ \quad \Box \; (mode_1 = automatic) \; \& \; Auto \\ \Box \; actuatorsR \to switched \to SwitchFC2Auto; \; Reset \\ \Box \; fault?faultId \to switched \to FireSys \end{array} \right)$$

• *FireSysStart* **end**

As for the abstract system, we omit the definition of the remaining actions. The main action of process *FC* is *FireSysStart* presented above.

Display Controller This process models the display controller requests for the lamps to be switched *on* or *off* after the occurrence of the relevant events. It waits for the system to be *switched* on, switches the lamp *sysOnL* on, and indicates this to *FC* through *switched*. A gas discharge is indicated by *FC* to this process through *display*. If the system is *reset*, the display switches *off* the buzzer and all the lamps, except the lamps *circFaultL* and *sysOnL*.

Areas The process *Area* is parametrised by the area identifier.

process *Area* $\widehat{=}$ (*id* : *AreaId* • **begin**

The state of an area is composed of the mode in which it is running, its controlled zones, the active zones in which a fire detection occurred, a boolean *discharge* that records whether a gas discharge has occurred or not, and a boolean *active* that records whether the area is willing to discharge gas or not.

state

$\underline{\quad AreaState\ \underline{\hspace{7cm}}}$
$mode : Mode$
$controlZns, actZns : \mathbb{P}\, ZoneId$
$discharge, active : Bool$
$\underline{\hspace{5cm}}$
$controlZns = getZones\ id \wedge actZns \subseteq controlZns$
$(mode = automatic) \Rightarrow active = true \Leftrightarrow \#actZns \geq 2$
$(mode = manual) \Rightarrow active = true \Leftrightarrow \#actZns \geq 1$

The invariant establishes that the component $actZns$ is a subset of the controlled zones of this area, which is defined by $getZones$. Besides, if running in *automatic* mode, an area is active if, and only if, all controlled zone are *active*. On the other hand, if running in *manual* mode, an area is *active* if, and only if, any controlled zone is active.

Each area is initialised as follows: there is no active zone; no discharge occurred; and it is in *automatic* mode. The state invariant guarantees that it is not *active*.

$$InitArea \;\widehat{=}\; [\,AreaState' \mid actZns' = \emptyset \wedge discharge' = false \wedge mode' = automatic\,]$$

The schema *SwitchAreaMode* receives the new mode and sets the area mode. Schemas *SwitchArea2Auto* and *SwitchArea2Dis* set the are *mode* to *automatic* and *disabled*. All other state components are left unchanged. A zone can be activated using the operation *ActivateZone*. If the given zone is controlled by the area, it is included in the *actZns*.

Initially, an area synchronises in the *switch* event, initialises its state, and starts its cycle.

$$StartArea \;\widehat{=}\; switch \rightarrow InitArea; AreaCycle$$

During its cycle, if the *actuatorsR* event occurs, the mode is switched to *automatic* and the area waits to be *reset*. If the system mode is switched, so is the area mode. Finally, any detection may activate a zone, if it is controlled by this area; after this, the area behaves like either *AutoArea* or *ManualArea*, depending on its current mode.

$$
\begin{aligned}
AreaCycle \;\widehat{=}\; & actuatorsR \rightarrow SwitchArea2Auto; ResetArea \\
& \square\ switchM?nm \rightarrow SwitchAreaMode; AreaCycle \\
& \square\ det?nz \rightarrow ActivateZone;\ (mode = automatic)\ \&\ AutoArea \\
& \qquad\qquad\qquad \square\ (mode = manual)\ \&\ ManualArea
\end{aligned}
$$
$\bullet\ StartArea\ \mathbf{end})$

The main action of the process *Area* is the action *StartArea*.

The process *ConcreteAreas* represents all the areas within the system. Basically, it is a parallel composition of all areas. They synchronise on the channel set Σ_{areas}.

chanset $\Sigma_{areas}\ ==\ \{\!|\ switch, reset, switchM, det, silence, actuatorsR,$
$autoDis, manDis, anyDis, noDis, counting\ |\!\}$
process $ConcreteAreas \;\widehat{=}\; \|\ id : AreaId \|\ \Sigma_{areas}\|\ \bullet\ Area(id)$

The internal system is defined as the parallel composition of the fire control *FC* and the display controller *DisplayC*. All the communications between them are hidden.

chanset $DisplaySync\ ==\ \{\!|\ display, switched\ |\!\}$
chanset $\Sigma_1\ ==\ \{\!|\ switch, reset, det, display, silence, actuatorsR, fault\ |\!\}$
process $ConcreteInternalFC \;\widehat{=}\; FC\ \|\,\Sigma_1\,\|\ DisplayC \setminus DisplaySync$

The concrete fire control is the parallel combination of *ConcreteInternalFC* and *Areas*.

Internal communications are again hidden.

> **chanset** $GSync == \{| manDis, autoDis, countdown, counting,$
> $gasDischarged, gasNotDischarged, anyDis, noDis |\}$
> **chanset** $\Sigma_2 == \{| switch, reset, det, switchM, silence, actuatorsR |\} \cup GSync$
> **process** $ConcreteFC \triangleq (ConcreteInternalFC \| \Sigma_2 \| Areas) \setminus GSync$

In the following sections, we prove that $AbstractFC$ is refined by $ConcreteFC$, or rather, $AbstractFC \sqsubseteq ConcreteFC$.

3.2.2   First Iteration: splitting the AbstractFC into InternalFC and Areas

Data refinement   In this step we make a data refinement in order to introduce a state component that is used by the areas. The new $mode_A$ component indicates the mode in which the areas are running. The process $AbstractFC$ is refined to the process FC_1 presented below.

> **process** $FC_1 \triangleq$ **begin**
> **state**

$$
\begin{array}{l}
\hline
FCSt_1 \\
\hline
mode_1, mode_A : Mode \\
controlZns_1, actZns_1 : AreaId \rightarrow \mathbb{P}\,ZoneId \\
discharge_1, active_1 : \mathbb{P}\,AreaId \\
\hline
\forall\, a : AreaId \bullet \\
(mode_1 = automatic) \Rightarrow a \in active_1 \Leftrightarrow \#actZns_1\, a \geq 2 \\
\wedge\, (mode_1 = manual) \Rightarrow a \in active_1 \Leftrightarrow \#actZns_1\, a \geq 1 \\
\wedge\, actZns_1\, a \subseteq controlZns_1\, a \wedge controlZns_1\, a = getZones\, a \\
\hline
\end{array}
$$

The state $FCSt_1$ is the same as that of $AbstractFC$, except that it includes an extra component $mode_A$. In order to prove that the FC_1 is a refinement of the $AbstractFC$, we have to prove that there exists a forwards simulation between the main actions of FC_1 and $AbstractFC$. The retrieve relation $RetrFC$ relates each component in the $AbstractFCSt$ to one in $FCSt_1$.

$$
\begin{array}{l}
\hline
RetrFC \\
\hline
AbstractFCSt;\ FCSt_1 \\
\hline
mode_1 = mode \wedge mode_A = mode \wedge controlZns_1 = controlZns \\
actZns_1 = actZns \wedge discharge_1 = discharge \wedge active_1 = active \\
\hline
\end{array}
$$

The laws of *Circus* establish that simulation distributes through the structure of an action. The laws used here are in Appendices A and B; we refine each schema using Law A.1. In the concrete initialisation, the new state component $mode_A$ is initialised in *automatic* mode.

$$
\begin{array}{l}
\hline
InitFC_1 \\
\hline
FCSt_1' \\
\hline
mode_1' = automatic \wedge mode_A' = automatic \wedge discharge_1' = \emptyset \\
actZns_1' = \{a : AreaId \bullet a \mapsto \emptyset\} \\
\hline
\end{array}
$$

The following lemma states that this is actually a simulation of the abstract initialisation. The symbol $\preceq$ represents the simulation relation.

Lemma 3.1 *InitAbstractFC $\preceq$ InitFC$_1$*

Proof. The application of Law A.1 raises two proof obligations. The first one concerns the preconditions of both schemas.

$$\forall \, AbstractFCSt; \ FCSt_1 \bullet RetrFC \wedge \text{pre } InitAbstractFC \Rightarrow \text{pre } InitFC_1$$

It is easily proved because the preconditions of both schemas are *true*. The second proof obligation concerns the postcondition of both operations.

$$\forall \, AbstractFCSt; \ FCSt_1; \ FCSt'_1 \bullet RetrFC \wedge \text{pre } InitAbstractFC \wedge InitFC_1 \Rightarrow$$
$$\exists \, AbstractFCSt' \bullet RetrFC' \wedge InitAbstractFC$$

This proof obligation can also be easily discarded using the one-point rule. When this rule is applied, we remove the universal quantifier, and then, we are left with an implication in which the consequent is present in the antecedent. $\square$

There is no special rule to handle initialisation operations. This is because the behaviour of a process is defined by its main action; there is no implicit initialisation. An initialisation schema is just a simplified way of specifying an operation like any other.

All other schema expressions are refined in pretty much the same way. Their definitions are very similar to the corresponding abstract operations except that the value assigned to $mode_1$ is also assigned to the new state component $mode_A$.

For the remaining actions, we rely on distribution of simulation. The new actions have the same structure as the original ones, but use the new schemas. By way of illustration, we present the action *FireSysStart$_1$* that simulates *AbstractFireSysStart*.

$$FireSysStart_1 \ \widehat{=} \ sysSt!fireSysStart_s \rightarrow switch \rightarrow lamp[LampId].sysOnL!on \rightarrow$$
$$InitFC_1; \ FireSys_1$$

To establish the simulation, we need Laws A.2 and A.3. Since all the output and input values, and guards are not changed, only their second proviso must be proved. They follow from Lemma 3.1 and *FireSys $\preceq$ FireSys$_1$*.

FireSysStart$_1$ is the main action of *FC$_1$*, and we have just proved that it simulates the main action of *AbstractFC*.

> $\bullet$ *FireSysStart$_1$* **end**

This concludes this data refinement step.

Action Refinement In this step we change *FC$_1$* so that its state is composed of two partitions: one that models the internal system and another that models the areas. We also change the actions so that the state partitions are handled separately.

> **process** *ConcreteFC* $\widehat{=}$ **begin**

The internal system state is composed only by its mode.

> *InternalFCSt* $\widehat{=}$ $[\, mode_1 : Mode \,]$

The remaining components are declared as components of the areas partition of the state.

$$
\begin{array}{|l}
\hline
\_AreasSt_____ \\
mode_A : Mode \\
controlZns_1, actZns_1 : AreaId \to \mathbb{P}\,ZoneId \\
discharge_1, active_1 : \mathbb{P}\,AreaId \\
\hline
\forall\, a : AreaId \;\bullet \\
\quad (mode_A = automatic) \Rightarrow a \in active_1 \Leftrightarrow \#actZns_1\, a \ge 2 \\
\quad \wedge\ (mode_A = manual) \Rightarrow a \in active_1 \Leftrightarrow \#actZns_1\, a \ge 1 \\
\quad \wedge\ actZns_1\, a \subseteq controlZns_1\, a \wedge controlZns_1\, a = getZones\, a \\
\hline
\end{array}
$$

The state of $FCSt_1$ is declared as the conjunction of the two previously defined schemas.

state $FCSt_1 \;\hat{=}\; InternalFCSt \wedge AreasSt$

The first group of paragraphs access only $mode_1$. It is initialised to *automatic*.

$InitInternalFC \;\hat{=}\; [\,InternalFCSt';\ AreasSt'\ |\ mode'_1 = automatic\,]$

Another convention is used in the definitions that follow: for any schema Sch, ΞSch represents the schema that includes both Sch and Sch' and leaves the components values unchanged. The notation θSch denotes the bindings of components from Sch.

$$
\begin{array}{|l}
\hline
\_\Xi Schema_____ \\
Sch \\
Sch' \\
\hline
\theta Sch = \theta Sch' \\
\hline
\end{array}
$$

The schema *SwitchInternalFCMode* receives the new mode as argument, and switches the *InternalFC* mode.

$SwitchInternalFCMode \;\hat{=}\; [\,\Delta InternalFCSt;\ \Xi AreasSt;\ nm? : Mode\ |\ mode'_1 = nm?\,]$

Similarly, *SwitchInternalFC2Auto* and *SwitchInternalFC2Dis* set the *InternalFC* mode to *automatic* and *disabled*, respectively.

The behaviour of this internal system is very similar to that of the abstract one (Table 1); however, after being switched on, it initialises only $mode_1$ and behaves like action $FireSys_2$. All the operations related to the areas are no longer controlled by the internal system actions, but by the areas actions. For instance, consider the action $FireSysStart_2$ below.

$$FireSysStart_2 \;\hat{=}\; sysSt!fireSysStart_s \to switch \to lamp[LampId].sysOnL!on \to$$
$$InitInternalFC;\ FireSys_2$$

When a synchronisation on *switchM* happens, only the *InternalFC* mode is switched by action $FireSys_2$. Furthermore, since the information about the areas are no longer part of this partition, following a *det* communication, this action does not activate the area in which the detection occurred. If the actuators are replaced, this action switches the corresponding lamp *on*, switches only $mode_1$ to *automatic*, and waits to be *reset*. The behaviour, if any *fault* happens, is not changed.

$$FireSys_2 \mathrel{\widehat{=}} sysSt!fireSys_s \rightarrow$$
$$switchM?nm \rightarrow SwitchInternalFCMode; FireSys_2$$
$$\Box \ det?nz \rightarrow lamp[ZoneId].nz!on \rightarrow alarm!firstStage \rightarrow$$
$$(mode_1 = manual) \ \& \ Manual_2$$
$$\Box \ (mode_1 = automatic) \ \& \ Auto_2$$
$$\Box \ actuatorsR \rightarrow lamp[LampId].circFaultL!off \rightarrow$$
$$SwitchInternalFC2Auto; Reset_2$$
$$\Box \ fault?faultId \rightarrow lamp[LampId].(getLampId \ faultId)!on \rightarrow$$
$$buzzer!on \rightarrow FireSys_2$$

The second group of paragraphs is concerned with the areas. They are initialised in *automatic* mode; furthermore, there are no active zones, no *discharge* has occurred, and no area is *active*.

$$\begin{array}{|l}
\hline
\_InitAreas \underline{\hspace{6cm}} \\
AreasSt'; \ InternalFCSt' \\
\hline
mode'_A = automatic \wedge discharge'_1 = \emptyset \\
actZns'_1 = \{a : AreaId \bullet a \mapsto \emptyset\} \\
\hline
\end{array}$$

The areas mode can be switched to a given mode with schema *SwitchAreasMode*. The areas mode can also be switched to *automatic* or *disabled* mode with the schema operations *SwitchAreas2Auto* and *SwitchAreas2Dis*, respectively.

$$\begin{array}{|l}
\hline
\_SwitchAreasMode \underline{\hspace{5cm}} \\
\Delta AreasSt; \ \Xi InternalFCSt; \ nm? : Mode \\
\hline
mode'_A = nm? \wedge actZns'_1 = actZns_1 \wedge discharge'_1 = discharge_1 \\
\hline
\end{array}$$

The schema *ActivateZoneAS* includes a given zone $nz?$ in the set of active zones of the area that controls $nz?$.

$$\begin{array}{|l}
\hline
\_ActivateZoneAS \underline{\hspace{5cm}} \\
\Delta AreasSt; \ \Xi InternalFCSt; \ nz? : ZoneId \\
\hline
mode'_A = mode_A \wedge discharge'_1 = discharge_1 \\
actZns'_1 = actZns_1 \oplus \{a : AreaId \mid nz? \in controlZns_1 \ a \bullet \\
\qquad\qquad\qquad\qquad a \mapsto actZns_1 \ a \cup \{nz?\}\} \\
\hline
\end{array}$$

Initially, the areas synchronise on *switch*, initialise the state, and start their cycle.

$$StartAreas \mathrel{\widehat{=}} switch \rightarrow InitAreas; \ AreasCycle$$

In *AreasCycle*, the actuators can be replaced, setting the mode to *automatic*, and the areas wait to be *reset*. If the system mode is switched, so is the areas mode. Any detection in a zone nz leads to the activation of nz; the behaviour afterwards depends on the *Areas* mode.

$$AreasCycle \mathrel{\widehat{=}} actuatorsR \rightarrow SwitchAreas2Auto; ResetAreas$$
$$\Box \ switchM?nm \rightarrow SwitchAreasMode; AreasCycle$$
$$\Box \ det?nz \rightarrow ActivateZoneAS; (mode_A = automatic) \ \& \ AutoAreas$$
$$\Box \ (mode_A = manual) \ \& \ ManualAreas$$

As for the paragraphs of the internal system, the areas have an action corresponding to each action in the abstract system (Table 1); the remaining actions are omitted here.

The main action of *ConcreteFC* is the parallel composition of the actions *FireSysStart$_2$* and *StartAreas*. These actions actually represent the initial actions of each partition within the process. They synchronise on the channel set Σ_2. All the synchronisation events between the internal system and the areas are hidden in the main action.

- $(FireSysStart_2 \parallel \alpha(InternalFCSt) \mid \Sigma_2 \mid \alpha(AreasSt) \parallel StartAreas) \setminus GSync$ **end**

Action *FireSysStart$_2$* may modify only the components of *InternalFCSt*, and *StartAreas* may modify only the components of *AreasSt*.

Despite the fact that this is a significant refinement step, it involves no change of data representation. In order to prove that this is a valid refinement, we must prove that the main action of process *ConcreteFC* refines the main action of process FC_1; however, they are defined using mutual recursion, and for this reason, we use the result below in the proof. The symbol $\sqsubseteq_A$ represents the action refinement relation.

Theorem 3.1 (Refinement on Mutual Recursive Actions) *For a given vector of actions S_S defined in the form $S_S \triangleq [N_0, \dots, N_n]$, where $N_i \triangleq F_i(N_0, \dots, N_n)$, we have that:*

$$S_S \sqsubseteq_A [Y_0, \dots, Y_n] \Leftarrow \left(\begin{array}{l} F_0[Y_0, \dots, Y_n/N_0, \dots, N_n] \sqsubseteq_A Y_0, \\ \dots, \\ F_n[Y_0, \dots, Y_n/N_0, \dots, N_n] \sqsubseteq_A Y_n \end{array} \right)$$

In order to prove that a vector of actions S_S as defined above is refined by a vector of actions $[Y_0, \dots, Y_n]$, it is enough to show that, for each action N_i in S_S, we can prove that its definition F_i, if we replace $N_0, \dots, N_n$ with $Y_0, \dots, Y_n$ in F_i, is refined by Y_i. This result is proved in [12].

We want to prove that *FireSysStart$_1$* $\sqsubseteq_A$ *(FireSysStart$_2$* $\parallel$ *StartAreas)* $\setminus$ *GSync*, where $\parallel$ stands for $\parallel\alpha(InternalFCSt) \mid \Sigma_2 \mid \alpha(AreasSt)\parallel$. As *FireSysStart$_1$* is defined using mutual recursion, we use the Theorem 3.1, with S_S as the vector including all actions involved in the definition of *FireSysStart$_1$*, $S_S = [FireSysStart_1, FireSys_1, \dots]$, to prove this refinement. The vector $[Y_0, \dots, Y_n]$ includes *(FireSysStart$_2$* $\parallel$ *StartAreas)* $\setminus$ *GSync* and all the refinements of each action in S_S as a parallel composition of the same form: with the same partition, the same synchronisation set, and the same hiding.

To prove this refinement, however, using Theorem 3.1, we need a modified S_S, in which some actions are preceded by an assumption. We introduce these assumptions using Law B.8.

$$[FireSysStart_1, FireSys_1, \dots]$$
$$\sqsubseteq_A [B.8]$$
$$[FireSysStart_1, \{mode_1 = mode_A\}; FireSys_1, \dots]$$

Although long, the proof obligation raised by this law application is trivial; we omit it here, for the sake of conciseness. Using Theorem 3.1 we get the following result.

$$\left[\begin{array}{l} FireSysStart_1, \\ \{mode_1 = mode_A\}; FireSys_1, \dots \end{array} \right] \sqsubseteq_A \left[\begin{array}{l} (FireSysStart_2 \parallel StartAreas) \setminus GSync, \\ (FireSys_2 \parallel AreasCycle) \setminus GSync, \dots \end{array} \right]$$

$$\Leftarrow \left(\begin{array}{ll} FireSysStart_1[subst] \sqsubseteq_A (FireSysStart_2 \parallel StartAreas) \setminus GSync, & (1) \\ FireSys_1[subst] \sqsubseteq_A (FireSys_2 \parallel AreasCycle) \setminus GSync, \dots & (2) \end{array} \right)$$

Here, *subst* corresponds to the following substitution.

$$subst = \left(\begin{array}{l} (FireSysStart_2 \parallel StartAreas) \setminus GSync, \\ (FireSys_2 \parallel AreasCycle) \setminus GSync, \dots \end{array} \right) / \left(\begin{array}{l} FireSysStart_1, \\ FireSys_1, \dots \end{array} \right)$$

Below, $A_1 \sqsubseteq_A [law_1, \dots, law_n]\{op_1\} \dots \{op_n\} A_2$ denotes that A_1 may be refined to A_2 using laws $law_1, \ldots, law_n$, if $op_1, \ldots, op_n$ holds. Lemmas 3.2 and 3.3 prove refinements (1) and (2), respectively.

Lemma 3.2 (1) $FireSysStart_1[subst] \sqsubseteq_A (FireSysStart_2 \parallel StartAreas) \setminus GSync$

Proof. We start the refinement using the definitions of $FireSysStart_1$ and substitution.

$FireSysStart_1[subst]$
$=$ [Definition of $FireSysStart_1$, Definition of Substitution]
$sysSt!fireSysStart_s \rightarrow switch \rightarrow lamp[LampId].sysOnL!on \rightarrow$
$\quad InitFC_1; (FireSys_2 \parallel AreasCycle) \setminus GSync$

First, we may expand the hiding since the channels *lamp*, *switch*, and *sysSt* are not in *GSync*.

$= [A.15] \{\{lamp, switch, sysSt\} \cap GSync = \emptyset\}$
$\left(\begin{array}{c} sysSt!fireSysStart_s \rightarrow switch \rightarrow lamp[LampId].sysOnL!on \rightarrow \\ InitFC_1; (FireSys_2 \parallel AreasCycle) \end{array} \right) \setminus GSync$

The schema $InitFC_1$ can be written as the sequential composition of two other schemas as follows. In [2], a refinement law is provided to introduce a schema sequence; however, in our case, we have a initialisation schema that has no reference to the initial state. For this reason, we use a new law that is similar to the one in [2]. Some trivial proof obligations are omitted.

$= [B.3] \left(\begin{array}{c} sysSt!fireSysStart_s \rightarrow switch \rightarrow lamp[LampId].sysOnL!on \rightarrow \\ InitInternalFC; InitAreas; (FireSys_2 \parallel AreasCycle) \end{array} \right) \setminus GSync$

Each one of the new inserted schema operations writes in a different partition of the parallelism that follows them. For this reason, we may distribute them over the parallelism. Again, two new laws are used: the first moves a (guarded) schema expression to one side of the parallelism; commutativity of parallelism is also provided as a new law.

$= [B.13, B.14]$
$\left(\begin{array}{c} sysSt!fireSysStart_s \rightarrow switch \rightarrow lamp[LampId].sysOnL!on \rightarrow \\ ((InitInternalFC; FireSys_2) \parallel (InitAreas; AreasCycle)) \end{array} \right) \setminus GSync$

Next, we move the *lamp* event to the internal system side of the parallelism. This step is valid because all the initial channels of *AreasCycle* are in Σ_2, and *lamp* is not.

$= [A.11] \{initials(AreasCycle) \subseteq \Sigma_2\} \{lamp \notin \Sigma_2\}$
$\left(sysSt!fireSysStart_s \rightarrow switch \rightarrow \left(\left(\begin{array}{c} lamp[LampId].sysOnL!on \rightarrow \\ InitInternalFC; FireSys_2 \end{array} \right) \parallel (InitAreas; AreasCycle) \right) \right) \setminus GSync$

Now, *switch* may be distributed over the parallelism because it is in Σ_2.

$= [A.14] \{switch \in \Sigma_2\}$
$\left(\left(\left(\begin{array}{c} sysSt!fireSysStart_s \rightarrow \\ switch \rightarrow \\ \quad lamp[LampId].sysOnL!on \rightarrow \\ \quad InitInternalFC; FireSys_2 \end{array} \right) \parallel \left(\begin{array}{c} switch \rightarrow InitAreas; \\ AreasCycle \end{array} \right) \right) \right)$
$\setminus GSync$

Since it is not in Σ_2, *sysSt* may be moved to the internal system side of the parallelism.

$$= [B.1, A.11] \{sysSt \notin \Sigma_2\}$$

$$\left(\left(\begin{array}{c} sysSt!fireSysStart_s \rightarrow switch \rightarrow \\ lamp[LampId].sysOnL!on \rightarrow \\ InitInternalFC; FireSys_2 \end{array} \right) \| \left(\begin{array}{c} switch \rightarrow InitAreas; \\ AreasCycle \end{array} \right) \right) \setminus GSync$$

Finally, using the definitions of $FireSysStart_2$ and $StartAreas$ we conclude this proof.

$$= [\text{Definition of } FireSysStart_2 \text{ and } StartAreas]$$
$$(FireSysStart_2 \| StartAreas) \setminus GSync \qquad \qquad \qquad \square$$

The next lemma we present is the refinement of the action $FireSys_1$.

Lemma 3.3 (2) $\{mode_1 = mode_A\}; FireSys_1[subst] \sqsubseteq_A (FireSys_2 \| AreasCycle) \setminus GSync$

Proof. We start the proof using the definitions of $FireSys_1$ and substitution.

$$\{mode_1 = mode_A\}; FireSys_1[subst]$$
$$= [\text{Definition of } FireSys_1, \text{Definition of Substitution}]$$
$$\{mode_1 = mode_A\};$$
$$sysSt!fireSys_s \rightarrow$$
$$\qquad switchM?nm \rightarrow SwitchFCMode_1; (FireSys_2 \| AreasCycle) \setminus GSync$$
$$\qquad \square \; det?nz \rightarrow ActivateZone_1; lamp[ZoneId].nz!on \rightarrow alarm!firstStage \rightarrow$$
$$\qquad\qquad (mode_1 = manual) \; \& \; (Manual_2 \| ManualAreas) \setminus GSync$$
$$\qquad\qquad \square \; (mode_1 = automatic) \; \& \; (Auto_2 \| AutoAreas) \setminus GSync$$
$$\qquad \square \; actuatorsR \rightarrow lamp[LampId].circFaultL!off \rightarrow$$
$$\qquad\qquad SwitchFC2Auto_1; (Reset_2 \| ResetAreas) \setminus GSync$$
$$\qquad \square \; fault?faultId \rightarrow lamp[LampId].(getLampId \, faultId)!on \rightarrow$$
$$\qquad\qquad buzzer!on \rightarrow (FireSys_2 \| AreasCycle) \setminus GSync$$

Next, we expand the hiding to the whole action. This is valid because all the events involved in the expansion are not in the hidden set of channels.

$$= [A.15] \{GSync \cap \{sysSt, switchM, det, lamp, alarm, fault, buzzer, reset\} = \emptyset\}$$

$$\left(\begin{array}{ll} \{mode_1 = mode_A\}; & \\ sysSt!fireSys_s \rightarrow & \\ \quad switchM?nm \rightarrow SwitchFCMode_1; (FireSys_2 \| AreasCycle) & (3) \\ \quad \square \; det?nz \rightarrow ActivateZone_1; lamp[ZoneId].nz!on \rightarrow alarm!firstStage \rightarrow & (4) \\ \qquad (mode_1 = manual) \; \& \; (Manual_2 \| ManualAreas) & \\ \qquad \square \; (mode_1 = automatic) \; \& \; (Auto_2 \| AutoAreas) & \\ \quad \square \; actuatorsR \rightarrow lamp[LampId].circFaultL!off \rightarrow & (5) \\ \qquad SwitchFC2Auto_1; (Reset_2 \| ResetAreas) & \\ \quad \square \; fault?faultId \rightarrow lamp[LampId].(getLampId \, faultId)!on \rightarrow & (6) \\ \qquad buzzer!on \rightarrow (FireSys_2 \| AreasCycle) & \end{array} \right)$$
$$\setminus GSync$$

Next, we aim at the refinement of each branch to a parallelism in order to be able to apply the exchange Law A.12. First, we refine (3) as follows: the schema $SwitchFCMode_1$ can be written as the sequential composition of $SwitchInternalFCMode$ and $SwitchAreasMode$.

$$(3) = [A.17] \; switchM?nm \rightarrow SwitchInternalFCMode; SwitchAreasMode;$$
$$\qquad\qquad (FireSys_2 \| AreasCycle)$$

Both schemas can be moved to different sides of the parallelism.

$$= [B.14, B.13]$$
$$switchM?nm \rightarrow$$
$$\qquad ((SwitchInternalFCMode; FireSys_2) \| (SwitchAreasMode; AreasCycle))$$

Finally, as $switchM$ is in Σ_2, we may distribute this event over the parallelism. Here, a new law (distribution of input channels over parallelism) is used.

$$= [B.2] \{ switchM \in \Sigma_2 \}$$
$$\left(\begin{array}{c} switchM?nm \rightarrow \\ SwitchInternalFCMode; FireSys_2 \end{array} \right) \| \left(\begin{array}{c} switchM?nm \rightarrow \\ SwitchAreasMode; AreasCycle \end{array} \right)$$

For (4), we first use the assumption laws in order to move the assumption into the action.

$$(4) \sqsubseteq_A [B.9, A.7, A.10, A.16, B.10, B.12]$$
$$det?nz \rightarrow ActivateZone_1; lamp[ZoneId].nz!on \rightarrow alarm!firstStage \rightarrow$$
$$\{ mode_1 = mode_A \}; (mode_1 = manual) \& (Manual_2 \| ManualAreas)$$
$$\Box \{ mode_1 = mode_A \}; (mode_1 = automatic) \& (Auto_2 \| AutoAreas)$$

Next, we use the assumption to change the guards.

$$= [A.8]$$
$$det?nz \rightarrow ActivateZone_1; lamp[ZoneId].nz!on \rightarrow alarm!firstStage \rightarrow$$
$$\{ mode_1 = mode_A \};$$
$$(mode_1 = manual \wedge mode_A = manual) \& (Manual_2 \| ManualAreas)$$
$$\Box \{ mode_1 = mode_A \};$$
$$(mode_1 = automatic \wedge mode_A = automatic) \& (Auto_2 \| AutoAreas)$$

The assumptions can then be absorbed by the guards.

$$= [A.4, A.5, A.10, A.16]$$
$$det?nz \rightarrow ActivateZone_1; lamp[ZoneId].nz!on \rightarrow alarm!firstStage \rightarrow$$
$$(mode_1 = mode_A \wedge mode_1 = manual \wedge mode_A = manual) \&$$
$$(Manual_2 \| ManualAreas)$$
$$\Box (mode_1 = mode_A \wedge mode_1 = automatic \wedge mode_A = automatic) \&$$
$$(Auto_2 \| AutoAreas)$$

Now, using a new law, we distribute the guards over the parallelism, slightly changing them.

$$= [B.5]$$
$$det?nz \rightarrow ActivateZone_1; lamp[ZoneId].nz!on \rightarrow alarm!firstStage \rightarrow$$
$$\left(\left(\begin{array}{c} mode_1 = mode_A \wedge \\ mode_1 = manual \end{array} \right) \& \atop Manual_2 \right) \| \left(\left(\begin{array}{c} mode_1 = mode_A \wedge \\ mode_A = manual \end{array} \right) \& \atop ManualAreas \right)$$
$$\Box \left(\left(\begin{array}{c} mode_1 = mode_A \wedge \\ mode_1 = automatic \end{array} \right) \& \atop Auto_2 \right) \| \left(\left(\begin{array}{c} mode_1 = mode_A \wedge \\ mode_A = automatic \end{array} \right) \& \atop AutoAreas \right)$$

Now, since the guards invalidate each other, we may apply an exchange law. Furthermore, we simplify the guards.

$$= [A.12, A.6]$$
$$det?nz \rightarrow ActivateZone_1; lamp[ZoneId].nz!on \rightarrow alarm!firstStage \rightarrow$$
$$\left(\begin{array}{c} (mode_1 = manual) \& Manual_2 \\ \Box (mode_1 = automatic) \& Auto_2 \end{array} \right) \| \left(\begin{array}{c} (mode_A = manual) \& ManualAreas \\ \Box (mode_A = automatic) \& AutoAreas \end{array} \right)$$

Next, we move the outputs channels to the left-hand side of the parallelism. This follows from the fact that the initial channels of both *ManualAreas* and *AutoAreas* are in Σ_2, and *alarm* and *lamp* are not.

$$= [B.1, A.11]$$
$$\{initials(ManualAreas) \cup initials(AutoAreas) \subseteq \Sigma_2\} \, \{\Sigma_2 \cap \{alarm, lamp\} = \emptyset\}$$
$$det?nz \rightarrow ActivateZone_1;$$

$$\left(\begin{array}{c} lamp[ZoneId].nz!on \rightarrow \\ alarm!firstStage \rightarrow \\ (mode_1 = manual) \, \& \\ Manual_2 \\ \Box \, (mode_1 = automatic) \, \& \\ Auto_2 \end{array}\right) \quad \| \quad \left(\begin{array}{c} (mode_A = manual) \, \& \\ ManualAreas \\ \Box \, (mode_A = automatic) \, \& \\ AutoAreas \end{array}\right)$$

The schema *ActivateZone₁* can easily be transformed to *ActivateZoneAS* using the schema calculus. The resulting schema can also be distributed over the parallelism. Finally, channel *det* can be distributed over the parallelism, since it is in Σ_2.

$$= [Schema \, Calculus, B.14, B.13, B.2] \, \{det \in \Sigma_2\}$$

$$\left(\begin{array}{c} det?nz \rightarrow lamp[ZoneId].nz!on \rightarrow \\ alarm!firstStage \rightarrow \\ (mode_1 = manual) \, \& \, Manual_2 \\ \Box \, (mode_1 = automatic) \, \& \, Auto_2 \end{array}\right) \quad \| \quad \left(\begin{array}{c} det?nz \rightarrow ActivateZoneAS; \\ (mode_A = manual) \, \& \\ ManualAreas \\ \Box \, (mode_A = automatic) \, \& \\ AutoAreas \end{array}\right)$$

Using similar strategies, we refine (5) and (6) to the following external choice.

$$(5, 6) = [\ldots]$$

$$\left(\begin{array}{c} actuatorsR \rightarrow \\ lamp[LampId].circFaultL!off \rightarrow \\ SwitchInternalFC2Auto; Reset_2 \end{array}\right) \quad \| \quad \left(\begin{array}{c} actuatorsR \rightarrow \\ SwitchAreas2Auto; \\ ResetAreas \end{array}\right)$$
$$\Box \, \left(\begin{array}{c} fault?faultId \rightarrow lamp[LampId].(getLampId \, faultId)!on \rightarrow \\ buzzer!on \rightarrow FireSys_2 \end{array}\right) \| AreasCycle$$

We are left with the external choice of parallel actions. Since the initial channels of the first three parallel actions are in the set Σ_2, we may apply the exchange law as follows.

$$= [A.12]$$
$$sysSt!fireSys_s \rightarrow$$

$$\left(\begin{array}{c} \left(\begin{array}{c} switchM?nm \rightarrow SwitchInternalFCMode; FireSys_2 \\ \Box \, det?nz \rightarrow lamp[ZoneId].nz!on \rightarrow alarm!firstStage \rightarrow \\ (mode_1 = manual) \, \& \, Manual_2 \\ \Box \, (mode_1 = automatic) \, \& \, Auto_2 \\ \Box \, actuatorsR \rightarrow lamp[LampId].circFaultL!off \rightarrow \\ SwitchInternalFC2Auto; Reset_2 \end{array}\right) \\ \| \\ \left(\begin{array}{c} switchM?nm \rightarrow SwitchAreasMode; AreasCycle \\ \Box \, det?nz \rightarrow ActivateZoneAS; \\ (mode_A = manual) \, \& \, ManualAreas \\ \Box \, (mode_A = automatic) \, \& \, AutoAreas \\ \Box \, actuatorsR \rightarrow SwitchAreas2Auto; ResetAreas \end{array}\right) \end{array}\right)$$
$$\Box \, \left(\begin{array}{c} fault?faultId \rightarrow lamp[LampId].(getLampId \, faultId)!on \rightarrow \\ buzzer!on \rightarrow FireSys_2 \end{array}\right) \| AreasCycle$$

With small rearrangements, we have that the right-hand side of the first parallelism corresponds to the definition of the action *AreasCycle*. So, we have that both branches of the external choice have this action as the right-hand side of the parallelism. Since all the initials of *AreasCycle* are in Σ_2, we may apply the distribution of parallelism over external choice.

$$= [A.13] \; \{initials(AreasCycle) \subseteq \Sigma_2\}$$
$$sysSt!fireSys_s \rightarrow$$

$$\left(
\begin{array}{l}
switchM?nm \rightarrow SwitchInternalFCMode; FireSys_2 \\
\square \; det?nz \rightarrow lamp[ZoneId].nz!on \rightarrow alarm!firstStage \rightarrow \\
\quad (mode_1 = manual) \; \& \; Manual_2 \\
\quad \square \; (mode_1 = automatic) \; \& \; Auto_2 \\
\square \; actuatorsR \rightarrow lamp[LampId].circFaultL!off \rightarrow \\
\quad SwitchInternalFC2Auto; Reset_2 \\
\square \; fault?faultId \rightarrow lamp[LampId].(getLampId\,faultId)!on \rightarrow \\
\quad buzzer!on \rightarrow FireSys_2
\end{array}
\right) \parallel AreasCycle$$

Finally, we can distribute *sysSt* and use the definition of $FireSys_2$ to conclude our proof. Again, this is valid because all the initials of *AreasCycle* are in Σ_2, and *sysSt* is not.

$$= [B.1, A.11] \; \{initials(AreasCycle) \subseteq \Sigma_2\} \; \{\Sigma_2 \cap \{sysSt\} = \emptyset\}$$

$$\left(
\begin{array}{l}
sysSt!fireSys_s \rightarrow \\
\quad switchM?nm \rightarrow SwitchInternalFCMode; FireSys_2 \\
\quad \square \; det?nz \rightarrow lamp[ZoneId].nz!on \rightarrow alarm!firstStage \rightarrow \\
\qquad (mode_1 = manual) \; \& \; Manual_2 \\
\qquad \square \; (mode_1 = automatic) \; \& \; Auto_2 \\
\quad \square \; actuatorsR \rightarrow lamp[LampId].circFaultL!off \rightarrow \\
\qquad SwitchInternalFC2Auto; Reset_2 \\
\quad \square \; fault?faultId \rightarrow lamp[LampId].(getLampId\,faultId)!on \rightarrow \\
\qquad buzzer!on \rightarrow FireSys_2
\end{array}
\right) \parallel AreasCycle$$

$$= [\text{Definition of } FireSys_2]$$
$$(FireSys_2 \parallel AreasCycle) \setminus GSync \qquad \qquad \square$$

Using these lemmas, and those related to the remaining actions, which are omitted here, we prove that FC_1 is refined by *ConcreteFC*.

Process Refinement We partitioned the state of the process FC_1 into *InternalFCSt* and *AreasSt*. Each partition has its own set of paragraphs, which are disjoint, since no action in one changes a state component in the other. Furthermore, the main action of the refined process is defined in terms of these two partitions. Therefore, we may apply Law A.18 in order to split process *ConcreteFC* into two independent processes as follows.

process *ConcreteFC* $\hat{=}$ (*InternalFC* $[\![\Sigma_2]\!]$ *Areas*) $\setminus$ *GSync*

The *ConcreteFC* is redefined as the parallel composition of *InternalFC* and *Areas*. Their definitions can be deduced from the definition of *ConcreteFC*.

3.2.3 Second Iteration: splitting InternalFC into two controllers

In this iteration, we split *InternalFC* into two separated partitions: the first one corresponds to the *FC* controller, and the other the *DisplayContoler* (see Figure 4).

Action Refinement We rewrite the actions so that the *FC* paragraphs no longer deal with the display events, which are dealt by *DisplayC*. The fire control state is left unchanged.

process *ConcreteInternalFC* $\hat{=}$ **begin**
$$FCSt \; \hat{=} \; [\, mode_1 : Mode \,]$$

Furthermore, the display controller has no state at all. The new state is defined as follows.

state $InternalFCSt_1 \mathrel{\hat{=}} FCSt$

The operations over the $InternalFCSt$ are slightly changed: they are renamed and affect the $FCSt$, which is the same as the $InternalFCSt$. Their definitions, and those of all actions over $FCSt$ have the same definition and description as those of FC. The display paragraphs are those of $DisplayC$, which can be found in Section 3.2.1.

The main action of the $ConcreteInternalFC$ is as follows.

- $(FireSysStart \parallel \alpha(FCSt) \mid \Sigma_2 \mid \alpha(DisplayCState) \parallel StartDisplay) \setminus DisplaySync$ **end**

We have the parallelism of action $FireSysStart$ and $StartDisplay$, with the channels used exclusively for their communication hidden. Again, since $FireSysStart_2$, $FireSysStart$, and $StartDisplay$ are defined using mutual recursion, we use Theorem 3.1 to prove that the process $InternalFC$ is refined by $ConcreteInternalFC$.

Process Refinement   Each partition in $ConcreteInternalFC$ has its own set of paragraphs, which are disjoint. Furthermore, we define the main action of the refined process in terms of these two partitions. Applying Law A.18, we get the following result.

process $ConcreteInternalFC \mathrel{\hat{=}} (FC \parallel \Sigma_1 \parallel DisplayC) \setminus DisplaySync$

The processes FC and the $DisplayC$ were already described in the specification of the concrete system in Section 3.2.1.

3.2.4   Third Iteration: splitting the Areas into individual Areas

This last iteration aims at splitting $Areas$ in individual processes $Area$ for each area.

Data Refinement   First, we must apply a data refinement to the original process $Areas$.

process $Areas_1 \mathrel{\hat{=}}$ **begin**

We introduce a local state $AreaState$ of an individual $Area$. Its definition is very similar to that of the concrete system, but includes an identifier $id : AreaId$. The global state $AreasSt$ is rewritten with a total function from $AreaId$ to local states. The invariant is slightly changed to handle the new data structure.

state

$$
\begin{array}{|l}
\hline
AreasSt_1 \underline{\qquad\qquad\qquad\qquad\qquad\qquad\qquad\qquad\qquad} \\
areas : AreaId \rightarrow AreaState \\
\hline
\forall a : AreaId \bullet (areas\,a).id = a \\
\qquad \wedge ((areas\,a).mode = automatic) \Rightarrow \\
\qquad\qquad (areas\,a).active = true \Leftrightarrow \#(areas\,a).actZns \geq 2 \\
\qquad \wedge ((areas\,a).mode = manual) \Rightarrow \\
\qquad\qquad (areas\,a).active = true \Leftrightarrow \#(areas\,a).actZns \geq 1 \\
\qquad \wedge (areas\,a).actZns \subseteq (areas\,a).controlZns \\
\qquad \wedge (areas\,a).controlZns = getZones\,a \\
\hline
\end{array}
$$

The retrieve relation is very simple and is defined below.

$$\begin{array}{|l}
\hline
\_RetrieveAreas _____ \\
AreasSt;\ AreasSt_1 \\
\hline
\forall a : AreaId \bullet (areas\ a).mode = mode_A \\
\qquad \land (areas\ a).controlZns = controlZns_1\ a \\
\qquad \land (areas\ a).actZns = actZns_1\ a \\
\qquad \land (areas\ a).discharge = true \Leftrightarrow a \in discharge_1 \\
\qquad \land (areas\ a).active = true \Leftrightarrow a \in active_1 \\
\hline
\end{array}$$

The mode in each of the local areas is that of *Areas*; the controlled and active zones of an area is defined as the corresponding image in the global state; a discharge has occurred in an area, if it is in $discharge_1$; and finally, the area is active if it is in $active_1$.

We introduce the paragraphs related to the local state *AreaState*. Basically, we have a corresponding local action for each global action. They are identical to those presented within the process *Area* in the concrete system, and are omitted at this point for conciseness.

Next, we redefine each of the global operations. Basically, all global operations have an effect in each of the individual local states. For instance, $InitAreas_1$ is refined below.

$$\begin{array}{|l}
\hline
\_InitAreas_1 _____ \\
AreasSt_1' \\
\hline
\forall a : AreaId \bullet (areas'\ a).actZns = \emptyset \land (areas'\ a).discharge = false \\
\qquad \land (areas'\ a).mode = automatic \\
\hline
\end{array}$$

The proof of the simulations are simple, but long. As before, for the main action, we rely on the fact that forwards simulation distributes through action constructors. The new actions have the same structure as the original ones, but use new schema actions.

$$StartAreas_1 \mathrel{\widehat{=}} switch \rightarrow InitAreas_1;\ AreasCycle_1$$
$$AreasCycle_1 \mathrel{\widehat{=}} actuatorsR \rightarrow SwitchAreas2Auto_1;ResetAreas_1$$
$$\qquad \Box\ switchM?nm \rightarrow SwitchAreasMode_1;\ AreasCycle_1$$
$$\qquad \Box\ det?nz \rightarrow ActivateZoneAS_1;$$
$$\qquad\qquad (\forall a : AreaId \bullet (areas\ a).mode = automatic)\ \&\ AutoAreas_1$$
$$\qquad\qquad \Box\ (\forall a : AreaId \bullet (areas\ a).mode = manual)\ \&\ ManualAreas_1$$

Since all the output and input values are not changed, in the application of Law A.2 we only rely on distribution. On the other hand, all the guards are changed. Both provisos raised by Law A.3 need to be proved. For instance, to prove the refinement of $AreasCycle_1$ we need the following lemma.

Lemma 3.4 *For any Mode m,*

$$\forall AreasSt;\ AreasSt_1 \bullet RetrieveAreas \Rightarrow$$
$$mode_A = M \Leftrightarrow \forall a : AreaId \bullet (areas\ a).mode = M$$

Proof. The proof of this lemma follows from predicate calculus, using the *RetrieveAreas* to relate $mode_A$ with each individual area's *mode*. $\qquad\qquad\Box$

The main action of the areas, $Areas_1$, is the simulation of the original action.

$\qquad \bullet\ StartAreas_1$ **end**

This concludes this data refinement step.

Action Refinement   In order to apply a process refinement that splits the *Areas* process into individual areas, we redefine each of the paragraphs within the processes areas as a promotion of the corresponding original one.

The local paragraphs and the global state remain unchanged. However, a promotion schema is introduced; it relates the local state to the global one.

$$
\begin{array}{l}
\underline{\textit{Promotion}} \\
\Delta AreasSt_1;\ \Delta AreaState;\ id? : AreaId \\
\hline
\theta AreaState = areas\ id?\ \wedge\ areas' = areas \oplus \{id? \mapsto \theta AreaState'\}
\end{array}
$$

The global operations are refined to a definition in terms of the corresponding local operations. For instance, the initialisation is refined as follows.

$$InitAreas_1 \cong \forall\, id? : AreaId \bullet InitArea \wedge Promotion$$

This can be proved using the action refinement laws presented in [12]. The redefinition of the remaining operations are trivially similar and omitted here.

The function **promote₂** promotes a given *Circus* action. The promotion of schemas is as in Z, and the promotion of *Skip*, *Stop*, *Chaos*, and channels do not change them.

$$\mathbf{promote_2}(c.e \rightarrow A) \cong c.\mathbf{promote_2}(e) \rightarrow \mathbf{promote_2}(A)$$

References to the local components have to become references to the corresponding component in the global state; all other references remain unchanged. An implicit parameter is a function f that maps indexes to instances of the local state. Another implicit parameter is the index i that identifies an instance of the local state in the global state.

$$\mathbf{promote_2}(x) \cong (f\,i).x \qquad\qquad \text{provided } x \text{ is a component of } L.st$$
$$\mathbf{promote_2}(x) \cong x \qquad\qquad\quad \text{provided } x \text{ is not a component of } L.st$$

This function is very similar to the function **promote** presented in [2]; however, it does not promote channels as the original one does.

Each action is defined as an iterated parallelism of the promotion of the corresponding local operation, but substituting the area *id* by the indexing variable *i*. Each branch of the parallelism may change its corresponding local state *areas i*; the remaining branches *j*, such that $j \neq i$, may change the remaining local states *areas j*. For instance, the actions *StartAreas₁* and *AreasCycle₁* can be rewritten as follows.

$$StartAreas_2 \cong\ \| i : AreaId \| \ \theta\,(areas\,i)\ |\ \Sigma_{areas}\ |\ \bigcup_{j:AreaId|j \neq i} \theta\,(areas\,j)\| \bullet$$
$$(\mathbf{promote_2}\ StartArea)\,[id, id? := i, i]$$

The remaining actions are rewritten in a very similar way. Finally, we replace the main action.

    • *StartAreas₂* **end**

Since *StartAreas₁* and *StartAreas₂* use mutual recursion, we use Theorem 3.1 again.

Process Refinement   This last process split needs a new process refinement law. Law 3.1 presented below applies to processes containing a local and a global state *LState* and *GState*, local paragraphs that do not affect the global state, a promotion schema, and global paragraphs expressed in terms of the promotion of local paragraphs to the global state using iterated parallelism. The operation *L.pps* ↑ *GState* conjoins each schema expression in the paragraphs *L.pps* with $\Xi GState$; this means that they do not change the components of *GState*. The results of this application are two processes: a local process *L* parametrised by an identifier *id* and a global process *G* defined as an iterated parallelism of local processes.

Law 3.1

> **process** $G \mathrel{\hat{=}}$ **begin**
> $\qquad LState \mathrel{\hat{=}} [\, id : Range;\ comps \mid pred_l\,]$
> $\qquad$ **state** $GState \mathrel{\hat{=}} [\, f : Range \to LState \mid \forall j : \mathrm{dom}\, f \bullet (f\, j).id = j \wedge pred_g\,]$
> $\qquad L.schema_j \uparrow GState$
> $\qquad L.action_k \uparrow GState$
> $\qquad L.act \uparrow GState$

> $\underline{\quad Promotion \underline{\hspace{8cm}}}$
> $\mid \quad \Delta LState;\ \Delta GState;\ id? : Range$
> $\mid \underline{\hspace{10cm}}$
> $\mid \quad \theta LState = f\, id? \wedge f' = f \oplus \{id? \mapsto \theta LState'\}$

> $\qquad G.schema_j \mathrel{\hat{=}} \forall id? : Range \bullet L.schema_j \wedge Promotion$
> $\qquad G.action_k \mathrel{\hat{=}} \ \| \, i : Range \, [\![\ \theta\,(f\, i) \mid cs \mid \bigcup_{j:Range \mid j \neq i} \theta\,(f\, j) \,]\!] \bullet$
> $\qquad\qquad\qquad\qquad (\textbf{promote}_2\ L.action_k)\,[id, id? := i, i]$
> $\qquad G.act \mathrel{\hat{=}} \ \| \, i : Range \, [\![\ \theta\,(f\, i) \mid cs \mid \bigcup_{j:Range \mid j \neq i} \theta\,(f\, j) \,]\!] \bullet$
> $\qquad\qquad\qquad\qquad (\textbf{promote}_2\ L.act)\,[id, id? := i, i]$
> $\qquad \bullet\ G.act$ **end**
> $= $ **process** $L \mathrel{\hat{=}} \ (id : Range \bullet$ **begin state** $LState \mathrel{\hat{=}} [\, comps \mid pred_l\,]$
> $\qquad\qquad\qquad\qquad\qquad\qquad\qquad\quad L.schema_j\ L.action_k \bullet L.act\ \textbf{end})$
> $\qquad$ **process** $G \mathrel{\hat{=}} \ \| \, id : Range \, [\![cs]\!] \bullet L(id)$

We can apply this law to $Areas_1$ in order to express the $Areas$ process as the following parallelism of individual $Area$ processes.

> **process** $ConcreteAreas \mathrel{\hat{=}} \ \| \, id : AreaId \, [\![\Sigma_{areas}]\!] \bullet Area(id)$

The $Area$ definition corresponds to that in the concrete system.

4 Conclusions

In this work, we present a development of a case study on the *Circus* refinement calculus. Using the refinement strategy presented in [2], we derive a distributed fire protection system from an abstract centralised specification. The result of the refinement presented here does not involve only executable constructs; additional simple schema refinements using [15] were omitted here. Our case study has motivated the proposal of new refinement laws; some of them can be found in Appendix B. There are more than fifty new laws, including process refinement laws. Their definitions can be found in [12]. Furthermore, some laws presented in [2] were found to be incorrect and corrected here. For instance, Law B.15 did not have any proviso in its original version in [2].

Refinement has been studied for combinations of Object-Z and CSP [16]; however, as far as we know, nothing has been proposed in a calculational style like ours. In [17], Olderog presents a stepwise refinement for action systems, in which most refinement steps involve sequential refinements; the decomposition of atomic actions introduces parallelism. The main difference of action systems formalism and *Circus* is that, using CSP operators, *Circus* has a much richer control flow than the flat structure of action systems, where auxiliary variables simulating program counters guarantee the proper sequencing of actions.

The development of programs is supported by a design calculus for occam-like [18] communicating programs in [19]; semantics of programs and specifications are presented in a uniform predicative style, which is close to that used in the unifying theories of programming. This work is another source of inspiration for *Circus* refinement laws.

In this paper, we show that, using *Circus*, we were able to specify elegantly both behavioural and data aspects of an industrial scale application. The refinement strategy presented in [2] was also proved to be applicable to large systems. In our case study, the development consists of three iterations: the first one splits the system into a system controller and the sensors. In the second iteration, the control is subdivided into two different controllers: one for the system and one for the display. Finally, the third iteration splits the sensors into individual processes, one for each area.

All the laws presented in [2] and [12] are currently being proved using the theorem prover ProofPower-Z. These proofs make the basis for a tool that supports our refinement strategy and the application of a considerable subset of the existing refinement laws of *Circus*. By providing this tool, we intend to transform the *Circus* refinement calculus into a largely used development method in industry.

References

[1] A. C. A. Sampaio, J. C. P. Woodcock, and A. L. C. Cavalcanti. Refinement in Circus. In L Eriksson and PA Lindsay, editors, *FME 2002: Formal Methods - Getting IT Right*, volume 2391 of *Lecture Notes in Computer Science*, pages 451–470. Springer-Verlag, unknown 2002.

[2] A. L. C. Cavalcanti, A. C. A. Sampaio, and J. C. P. Woodcock. A Refinement Strategy for Circus. *Formal Aspects of Computing*, 15(2-3):146–181, November 2003.

[3] J. C. P. Woodcock and J. Davies. *Using Z – Specification, Refinement, and Proof*. Prentice-Hall, 1996.

[4] J. M. Spivey. *The Z Notation: A Reference Manual*. Prentice-Hall, 2nd edition, 1992.

[5] A. W. Roscoe. *The Theory and Practice of Concurrency*. Prentice-Hall Series in Computer Science. Prentice-Hall, 1998.

[6] C. A. R. Hoare and J. He. *Unifying Theories of Programming*. Prentice-Hall, 1998.

[7] A. J. Galloway. *Integrated Formal Methods with Richer Methodological Profiles for the Development of Multi-perspective Systems*. PhD thesis, University of Teeside, School of Computing and Mathematics, 1996.

[8] K. Taguchi and K. Araki. The State-based CCS Semantics for Concurrent Z Specification. In M. Hinchey and Shaoying Liu, editors, *International Conference on Formal Engineering Methods*, pages 283 – 292. IEEE, 1997.

[9] A. W. Roscoe, J. C. P. Woodcock, and L. Wulf. Non-interference through Determinism. In D. Gollmann, editor, *ESORICS 94*, volume 1214 of *Lecture Notes in Computer Science*, pages 33 – 54. Springer-Verlag, 1994.

[10] C. Fischer. CSP-OZ: A combination of Object-Z and CSP. In H. Bowmann and J. Derrick, editors, *Formal Methods for Open Object-Based Distributed Systems (FMOODS'97)*, volume 2, pages 423 – 438. Chapman & Hall, 1997.

[11] Carroll Morgan. *Programming from Specifications*. Prentice-Hall, 2nd edition, 1994.

[12] M. V. M. Oliveira. The development of a fire control system in circus. Technical report, University of Kent, Computing Laboratory, University of Kent, Canterbury, Kent, CT2 7NF, UK, May 2004. At http://www.cs.kent.ac.uk/˜mvmo2/circus/fcs.pdf.

[13] Data Sheet MPE.130. At http://www.cs.kent.ac.uk/˜mvmo2/circus/mpe130.html.

[14] C. A. R. Hoare. *Communicating Sequential Processes*. Prentice-Hall International, 1985.

[15] A. L. C. Cavalcanti and J. C. P. Woodcock. ZRC - A Refinement Calculus for Z. *Formal Aspects of Computing*, 10(3):267 – 289, 1999.

[16] G. Smith and J. Derrick. Specification, refinement and verification of concurrent systems - an integration of Object-Z and CSP. *Formal Methods in Systems Design*, 18:249–284, May 2001.

[17] R. J. R. Back and K. Sere. Stepwise refinement of parallel algorithms. *Science of Computer Programming*, 13(2-3):133 – 180, 1990.

[18] G. Jones and M. Goldsmith. *Programming in occam 2*. Prentice-Hall, 1988.

[19] E. R. Olderog. Towards a design calculus for communicating programs. In J. C. M. Baeten and J. F. Groote, editors, *CONCUR'91: Proc. of the 2nd International Conference on Concurrency Theory*, pages 61–77. Springer, Berlin, Heidelberg, 1991.

A Existing Refinement Laws

Simulation Laws

Law A.1 $ASExp \preceq CSExp$
provided

- $\forall P_1.st;\ P_2.st;\ L \bullet R \wedge \text{pre } ASExp \Rightarrow \text{pre } CSExp$
- $\forall P_1.st;\ P_2.st;\ P_2.st';\ L \bullet R \wedge \text{pre } ASExp \wedge CSExp \Rightarrow (\exists P_1.st';\ L' \bullet R' \wedge ASExp)$

Law A.2 $c!ae \rightarrow A_1 \preceq c!ce \rightarrow A_2$
provided $\forall P_1.st;\ P_2.st;\ L \bullet R \Rightarrow ae = ce \text{ and } A_1 \preceq A_2.$

Law A.3 $ag\ \&\ A_1 \preceq cg\ \&\ A_2$
provided $\forall P_1.st;\ P_2.st;\ L \bullet R \Rightarrow (ag \Leftrightarrow cg) \text{ and } A_1 \preceq A_2.$

Action Refinement Laws

Law A.4 $\{g\};\ A = \{g\};\ g\ \&\ A$

Law A.5 $g_1\ \&\ (g_2\ \&\ A) = (g_1 \wedge g_2)\ \&\ A$

Law A.6 $g_2\ \&\ A \sqsubseteq_A g_3\ \&\ A$ **provided** $g_2 \Rightarrow g_3$

Law A.7 $\{p\};\ (A_1 \square A_2) = (\{p\};\ A_1) \square (\{p\};\ A_2)$

Law A.8 $\{g_1\};\ (g_2\ \&\ A) = \{g_1\};\ (g_3\ \&\ A)$ **provided** $g_1 \Rightarrow (g_2 \Leftrightarrow g_3)$

In the following law we refer to a predicate ass'. In general, for any predicate p, the predicate p' is formed by dashing all its free undecorated variables. We consider an arbitrary schema that specifies an action in *Circus*: it acts on a state St and, optionally, has input variables $i?$ of type T_i, and output variables $o!$ of type T_o.

Law A.9 $[\Delta St;\ i? : T_i;\ o! : T_o\ |\ p \wedge ass'] = [\Delta St;\ i? : T_i;\ o! : T_o\ |\ p \wedge ass'];\ \{ass\}$

Law A.10 $\{p\} \sqsubseteq_A Skip$

Law A.11 $(A_1;\ A_2) \| ns_1\ |\ cs\ |\ ns_2 \| A_3 = A_1;\ (A_2 \| ns_1\ |\ cs\ |\ ns_2 \| A_3)$
provided

- $initials(A_3) \subseteq cs;$
- $cs \cap usedC(A_1) = \emptyset;$
- $wrtV(A_1) \cap usedV(A_3) = \emptyset$

Law A.12 $(A_1 \| cs \| A_2) \square (B_1 \| cs \| B_2) = (A_1 \square B_1) \| cs \| (A_2 \square B_2)$
provided $A_1 \| cs \| B_2 = A_2 \| cs \| B_1 = Stop$

Law A.13 $A_1 \| cs \| (A_2 \square A_3) = (A_1 \| cs \| A_2) \square (A_1 \| cs \| A_3)$
provided $initials(A_1) \subseteq cs \text{ and } A_1 \text{ is deterministic}$

Law A.14 $c \to (A_1 \llbracket cs \rrbracket A_2) = (c \to A_1) \llbracket ns_1 \mid cs \cup \{\!\!\{c\}\!\!\} \mid ns_2 \rrbracket (c \to A_2)$
syntactic restriction $c \notin usedC(A_1) \cup usedC(A_2)$ or $c \in cs$

Law A.15 $F(A \setminus cs) = F(A) \setminus cs$ **provided** $cs \cap usedC(F(\_)) = \emptyset$

Law A.16 $Skip; A = A = A; Skip$

Law A.17

$$[\Delta S_1; \ \Delta S_2; \ i? : T \mid preS_1 \wedge preS_2 \wedge CS_1 \wedge CS_2]$$
$$=$$
$$[\Delta S_1; \ \Xi S_2; \ i? : T \mid preS_1 \wedge CS_1]; \ [\Xi S_1; \ \Delta S_2; \ i? : T \mid preS_2 \wedge CS_2]$$

syntactic restrictions

- $\alpha(S_1) \cap \alpha(S_2) = \emptyset$
- $FV(preS_1) \subseteq \alpha(S_1) \cup \{i?\}$ and $FV(preS_2) \subseteq \alpha(S_2) \cup \{i?\}$
- $DFV(CS_1) \subseteq \alpha(S_1')$ and $DFV(CS_2) \subseteq \alpha(S_2')$
- $UDFV(CS_2) \cap DFV(CS_1) = \emptyset$.

Process Refinement Laws

Law A.18 *Let qd and rd stand for the declarations of the processes Q and R, determined by Q.st, Q.pps, and Q.act, and R.st, R.pps, and R.act, respectively, and pd stand for the process declaration above. Then* $pd = (qd \ rd \ \textbf{process } P \mathrel{\hat=} F(Q, R))$ **provided** *Q.pps and R.pps are disjoint with respect to R.st and Q.st.*

B   New Refinement Laws.

Action Refinement Laws.

Law B.1 $c \to A = (c \to Skip); A$

Law B.2 $c?x \to (A_1 \llbracket ns_1 \mid cs \mid ns_2 \rrbracket A_2) = (c?x \to A_1) \llbracket ns_1 \mid cs \mid ns_2 \rrbracket (c?x \to A_2)$
provided $c \notin usedC(A_1) \cup usedC(A_2)$ or $c \in cs$

Law B.3 $[S_1'; \ S_2' \mid preS_1 \wedge preS_2 \wedge CS_1 \wedge CS_2] = [S_1' \mid preS_1 \wedge CS_1]; \ [S_2' \mid preS_2 \wedge CS_2]$
provided

- $\alpha(S_1) \cap \alpha(S_2) = \emptyset$
- $FV(preS_1) \subseteq \alpha(S_1)$ and $FV(preS_2) \subseteq \alpha(S_2)$
- $DFV(CS_1) \subseteq \alpha(S_1')$ and $DFV(CS_2) \subseteq \alpha(S_2')$
- $UDFV(CS_2) \cap DFV(CS_1) = \emptyset$

Law B.4 $\square_i \, g_i \, \& \, (A_i \llbracket ns_1 \mid cs \mid ns_2 \rrbracket A) = (\square_i \, g_i \, \& \, A_i) \llbracket ns_1 \mid cs \mid ns_2 \rrbracket A$
provided $initials(A) \subseteq cs$

Law B.5 $(g_1 \wedge g_2)$ & $(A_1 \llbracket ns_1 \mid cs \mid ns_2 \rrbracket A_2) = (g_1$ & $A_1) \llbracket ns_1 \mid cs \mid ns_2 \rrbracket (g_2$ & $A_2)$
provided $g_1 \Leftrightarrow g_2$ *or* $initials(A_1) \cup initials(A_2) \subseteq cs$

In the following law we refer to a predicate *assump'*.

Law B.6 $[State' \mid p \wedge assump'] = [State' \mid p \wedge assump']; \{assump\}$

Law B.7 $\{g_1\} \sqsubseteq_A \{g_2\}$ **provided** $g_1 \Rightarrow g_2$

Law B.8 $\mu P \bullet V(P) \sqsubseteq_A \mu P \bullet V(P)[\{g\}; F_i(P)/F_i(P)]$
provided $\{g\}; (F(P)$ before $X_i) \sqsubseteq_A (F(P)$ before $X_i); \{g\}$ for all $F(P)$ in $V(P)$
where $P = X_1, \ldots, X_n$, $V(P) = F_1(X_1, \ldots, X_n), \ldots, F_n(X_1, \ldots, X_n)$, *and* $V(P)[exp/F_i(P)]$
express the substitution of the i-th element of the vector $V(P)$ *by the expression exp.*

Law B.9 $\{g\}; c!x \to A = c!x \to \{g\}; A$

Law B.10 $\{g\}; c?x \to A = c?x \to \{g\}; A$ **provided** $x \notin FV(g)$

Law B.11 $\{g\}; c \to A = c \to \{g\}; A$

Law B.12 $\{g\}; [d \mid p] = [d \mid p]; \{g\}$ **provided** $g \wedge p \Rightarrow g'$

Law B.13

$(\square_i g_i$ & $SExp_i); (A_1 \llbracket ns_1 \mid cs \mid ns_2 \rrbracket A_2) \sqsubseteq_A ((\square_i g_i$ & $SExp_i); A_1) \llbracket ns_1 \mid cs \mid ns_2 \rrbracket \,$
provided

- $\bigcup_i wrtV(SExp_i) \subseteq ns_1 \cup ns_1'$
- $\bigcup_i wrtV(SExp_i) \cap usedV(A_2) = \emptyset$

Law B.14 $A_1 \llbracket ns_1 \mid cs \mid ns_2 \rrbracket A_2 = A_2 \llbracket ns_2 \mid cs \mid ns_1 \rrbracket A_1$

Law B.15 $A \llbracket cs \rrbracket Stop = Stop \llbracket cs \rrbracket A = Stop$ **provided** $initials(A) \subseteq cs$

Communicating Process Architectures 2004
Ian East, Jeremy Martin, Peter Welch, David Duce, and Mark Green (Eds.)
IOS Press, 2004

K-CSP: Component Based Development of Kernel Extensions

Bernhard SPUTH

DSP Centre, Ngee Ann Polytechnic, Block 8 #06-09,
Clementi Road 535, 599489 Singapore, Singapore
and
Department of Engineering, University of Aberdeen, Aberdeen, AB24 3UE, UK
bernhard@erg.abdn.ac.uk

Alastair R. ALLEN

Departments of Engineering and Bio-Medical Physics,
University of Aberdeen, Aberdeen, UK

Abstract. Kernel extension development suffers from two problems. Firstly, there is little to no code reuse. This is caused by the fact that most kernel extensions are coded in the C programming language. This language only allows code reuse either by using 'copy and paste' or by using libraries. Secondly, the poor separation of synchronisation and functionality code makes it difficult to change one without affecting the other. It is, therefore, difficult to use the synchronisation mechanisms correctly. The approach proposed in this paper tries to solve these problems by introducing a component based programming model for kernel extensions, and a system based on this proposal is implemented for the Linux kernel. The language used for the implementation is Objective-C, and as a synchronisation mechanism Communicating Sequential Processes is used. This model allows the functionality and synchronisation of a component to be developed separately. Furthermore, due to the use of Communicating Sequential Processes it is possible to verify the correctness of the synchronisation. An example given in this paper illustrates how easy it is to use the K-CSP environment for development.

1 Introduction

K-CSP is an extension to the Linux Kernel, which brings Component Based Programming into the domain of kernel extension development. K-CSP provides a proven synchronisation model in the form of Communicating Sequential Processes (CSP)[1]. Objective-C [2] is used as an object oriented environment to allow easy code reuse and therefore to increase code quality. The K-CSP architecture is generally applicable to any operating system based upon the C programming language.

Kernel extensions are runtime loadable modules which enhance the functionality of an operating system (OS) kernel. They are used to provide device drivers for new hardware or new file systems, without recompiling the kernel [3]. Once a module is loaded it becomes part of the kernel. A defective kernel extension may bring down the kernel and with it all other running programs, possibly resulting in data loss on the user's side. Therefore, it is necessary to develop kernel extensions in a defensive way. Defensive programming is characterised by performing consistency checks on variables before use. For instance, checking for null pointers in passed function parameters. This avoids errors caused by dereferencing such a pointer. A single null pointer dereference can cause mayhem in the running kernel.

Unfortunately, the kernel environment is not easy to work in. First of all, the kernel is a concurrent system with the ability to utilise multiple processors. This requires that kernel extensions have to be multiprocessor safe, by default. The kernel environment provides basic synchronisation mechanisms for this task, like spinlocks and semaphores. These synchronisation mechanisms must be used to guard critical code sequences in order to avoid concurrent access. Improper use of synchronisation mechanisms can cause deadlocks. Especially for an inexperienced developer, it is hard to judge whether a code sequence needs to be guarded or not. Another difficulty comes from the fact that an error in the synchronisation does not necessarily show up immediately. Even if it does, it may be hard to reproduce. Errors which cannot be reproduced are hard to fix, as there is no way to test whether the error is removed or not.

The next problem with classical synchronisation mechanisms is that functionality and synchronisation are mixed within the code. This makes it difficult to modify one without affecting the other. Especially if the code is modified at a later time, a previous working synchronisation might be broken. To avoid these problems, a synchronisation mechanism is required that allows the separation of synchronisation and functionality.

A first step towards this separation is access limitation. This is achieved by data hiding, a technique propagated by object oriented programming (OOP)[4]. In OOP, resources are contained within objects. Each resource has an access limiter assigned to it, allowing access from outside the object (unlimited) or not (limited). To access a resource with limited access, a method of the object needs to be called. This method performs all necessary synchronisation operations. Such methods can be used to synchronise access to resources. This soothes the synchronisation problems, but on the other hand it requires an object oriented environment in the kernel. An example of such an operating system is Apertos [5, 6, 7] which is object oriented from the ground up. This is great in terms of easy code reuse, which generally results in shorter development time and increasing the quality of the code. Unfortunately, the development of kernel extensions is limited in Apertos, because only a single thread of execution is allowed for each extension. While this is good for avoiding synchronisation problems, for some types of hardware it is necessary to have a second thread polling the device. This is, for instance, the case in kernel extensions using the isochronous stream of USB devices [8].

In order to support this type of hardware, an architecture is required that allows multiple threads of execution within a single kernel extension. Therefore, this approach needs to provide a means of abstraction for the packaging and synchronisation of threads. To encourage code reuse, it should be possible to create new kernel extensions out of pieces of already existing kernel extensions. These pieces of kernel extensions are so called *components* [9], and this is what Component Based Programming is about. The example given later in this document shows how easy it is with K-CSP to create components and use them. It also demonstrates the ease of developing multi-threaded kernel extensions with K-CSP.

2   Component Based Programming for Kernel Extensions

The K-CSP architecture attempts to bring component based programming into the domain of kernel extension development. This section gives an introduction to component based programming as well as traditional kernel extension development.

2.1   What is Component Based Programming?

Component Based Programming (CBP) is a programming methodology which focuses on easy and secure code reuse. It is the next logical step after Object Oriented Programming (OOP). The core idea is to build systems out of already existing components, instead of constantly *reinventing the wheel*. A component itself is a piece of self contained code providing a functionality, able to communicate with other components.

Component Based Programming is widely used in the field of User Interface development: examples are Desktop JavaBeans from Sun [10] or ActiveX Controls by Microsoft [11]. Components are also used in the field of distributed programming, for instance in Enterprise JavaBeans [12], or the CORBA Component Model [13].

Systems developed with CBP are more clearly structured and less error prone. CBP consists mainly of assembling components, rather than implementing functionality. This results in shifting the work of a developer from coding a hand tailored solution to designing a solution out of already available components. As each component only solves one problem, its size is most probably within the sweet spot of around 200 lines of code, where defect density is lowest according to Hatton [14]. Programs created with CBP are similar to block diagrams. This allows easier understanding of the programs, making them easy to debug, extend and modify.

2.2   Kernel Extension Development for the Linux Kernel

The Linux Kernel has been implemented using the C programming language [15]. Kernel extensions become part of the kernel once they are loaded. To be able to interface to the kernel, extensions need to comply with the kernel environment. This requires them to conform to the kernel calling conventions. Calling conventions are defined by the programming language. Therefore, kernel extensions are traditionally developed using the C programming language.

2.2.1   C Language Restrictions for CBP

The C programming language is a procedural programming language. Therefore, the highest layer of abstraction is a procedure or function. Data hiding above the function level is not supported by the C programming language. Free use of global variables is common and results, most of the time, in mayhem, when global variables are manipulated unexpectedly. This makes C unsuitable for a component based system. A component is self-contained and consists of code and data which must not be tampered with from outside the component.

Another point to consider is the lack of concurrency support by the C programming language. There are no language constructs for synchronisation. With no standardisation by the language, each OS provides its own synchronisation model. This makes it difficult to port kernel extensions, especially device drivers form one OS to another.

2.3   Comparison of Component Based Programming and Traditional Kernel Extension Programming

In the traditional way of developing kernel extensions, everything had to be implemented and tested from the ground up. This resulted in unstructured, error prone code. When using a component based approach, a programmer can rely on previously developed and tested components. The programmer's work changes from coding his own solution, to designing a solution out of already existing components. This hopefully increases the code quality of the solution. Therefore, a programmer becomes more an engineer than an artist. As components need to be created before they can be used, the component architecture needs to allow easy implementation and testing.

3   K-CSP Architecture

The aim of K-CSP is to bring component based programming into the Linux Kernel domain. Therefore, K-CSP has to become a part of the Linux Kernel, with all the previously mentioned limitations.

In order to develop an environment for component based programming the following requirements have to be met:

- Components need to be implementable in a self contained fashion. They should only allow interaction over fixed interfaces.

- Components must be able to be executed concurrently.

- There must be a safe way to connect components together.

In K-CSP, the function and the synchronisation have to be separated. This will avoid the chaos caused when changing one affects the other.

3.1   Components as Self-Contained Code

As component based programming is an evolutionary step from object oriented programming, it is sensible to base a component environment on an object oriented (OO) environment. Unfortunately, we cannot use C++ as a base, because the C++ namespace collides with the kernel headers. To use C++, the Linux Kernel would have to be reviewed and partly rewritten, according to the Linux Kernel FAQ [16]. In order to be able to use an OO-environment, we have two choices. We could develop our own OO-environment. The downside of this is that it will require a lot of work, and the solution is not reliable, because it is completely new. A new OO-environment would require the users to learn a new programming language. The second option we have is to take an already existing object oriented environment that conforms to the C conventions and port it into the kernel. Objective-C [2] is such an environment. Objective-C has the advantage that the code is translated into C before being compiled into a binary. This makes it possible to create kernel extensions which fully comply with the set of kernel requirements and at the same time have the data hiding capabilities of an object oriented environment.

3.2   Concurrent Execution of Components

Components need to react to requests from outside and inside. Outside requests, for a device driver, are for instance issued by the device. An example of such a request is an interrupt, which is handled by calling the interrupt service routine (ISR). This ISR is then executed concurrently with the remainder of the device driver. Requests coming from the user side are handled similarly. These components are implementable without using a thread: they are run using the thread of the caller. As they are used as an interface to the outside world of the kernel extension, they are called *Interfacing Components* (IC). These components do not execute in a recursive way.

Components that handle only internal requests are Control Components (CC). Control components perform monitoring or polling tasks. These components need to run recursively and therefore, they are executed in their own thread.

Both component types IC and CC can be modelled as CSP processes.

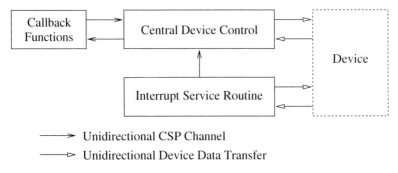

Figure 1: Example of a Device Driver implemented with K-CSP

3.3   Component Communication Infrastructure

With the components being executed concurrently, the communication between them has to be multi-thread safe, and for multiprocessor machines also multiprocessor safe. The channel construct introduced by CSP takes care of these problems and is intuitive to use. The component communication infrastructure is therefore implemented in the form of CSP Channels.

3.4   Resulting Model

The K-CSP architecture relies upon Objective-C to provide an object oriented environment, using a runtime library. In order to allow secure concurrency within K-CSP, a CSP subsystem will be created, which itself is based on the Objective-C runtime. With CSP as the synchronisation mechanism it is possible to prove the correct implementation of the synchronisation. The process and communication structure of a Device Driver implemented in K-CSP is shown in Figure 1. The figure gives a good abstraction of the different components and their interactions, like a block diagram.

4   Implementation Aspects of K-CSP

K-CSP is based upon Linux Kernel 2.6.3 [17]. GNU GCC version 3.3.x supplies the basis of the Objective-C runtime. The interface to the CSP subsystem is similar to that of JCSP [18].

4.1   Bringing Objective-C into the Kernel

The Linux Kernel is usually compiled using the C compiler of the GNU Compiler Collection (GCC) [19]. GCC also includes an Objective-C compiler. Therefore, the GNU *Objective-C Runtime Library* (runtime) can be used. But even with the runtime already available there are still a number of problems to solve:

- The runtime is meant to run in user mode. Therefore, it is necessary to port the code into kernel mode and resolve any incompatibilities.

- The Objective-C compiler utilises special segments in the ELF binary format [20], in order to register the classes of the program with the runtime. These segments are not supported by the module loader supplied by the Linux kernel.

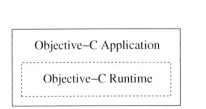

Figure 2: Tight coupling of Application and Objective-C Runtime

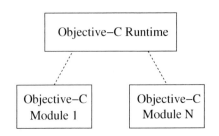

Figure 3: Loose coupling of Modules and Objective-C Runtime

- The Objective-C runtime is only meant to be used by one program, as shown in Figure 2. The runtime becomes part of the application and is terminated together with it. Therefore, the runtime does not support modules unregistering their classes when being unloaded. In the K-CSP implementation it is necessary to have multiple modules sharing the Objective-C runtime to enable usage of classes defined in other modules. This results in a loose coupling of Objective-C runtime and Modules, as illustrated in Figure 3. The kernel allows unloading of modules, if they are not in use. When unloaded, entries of these modules are still in the runtime registry and the next time a module tries to register entries of the same name the old entries are used. This is, for instance, the case when unloading and reloading a module. Loading and unloading of modules is not only a common practice during module development, but also in environments where hardware is connected to or disconnected from the system during runtime. The entries of the runtime registry contain pointers to the methods and members of the classes. The pointers must not stay valid when a module gets reloaded: if now an old entry is used it might refer the wrong location, resulting in a segmentation fault. To solve this problem entries of a module need to be purged from the runtime registry when a module gets unloaded.

4.1.1   Porting the Objective-C Runtime into the Linux Kernel

The availability of the GNU GCC Objective-C runtime in source code made the porting possible. The source code was developed in a modular way, encapsulating platform specific issues. All this made the porting a painless process. The most labour intensive task was to export the functions to the kernel, in order to make them accessible from outside the module.

4.1.2   Loading of Objective-C Kernel Extensions

The Linux Kernel is compiled in the ELF binary format [20], which is also used for kernel extensions. Objective-C programs are compiled in this file format. A binary complying with the ELF binary format consists also of multiple sections, each with a special purpose. The Objective-C compiler utilises the *.ctors* section (constructors) in order to register the classes contained in the binary with the runtime library. The routines specified in the *.ctors* segment are executed when loading the binary, before the main entry point is executed. For normal C binaries this is not necessary, therefore the module loader of the Linux Kernel, by default, ignores this segment. The kernel module loader had to be modified to execute available entries of the *.ctors* segment. With this modification it is possible to load kernel extensions developed with Objective-C with the Linux Kernel.

In order to execute a kernel extension it is necessary to supply a program entry point. For the Linux Kernel this entry point is defined to be a C function. Unfortunately, it is not possible to use a method of an object as entry point. This is due to the fact that an object first needs to be allocated and initialised, before a method of it can be called. Furthermore, methods in Objective-C get passed a hidden parameter, the *self* pointer. The *self* pointer is similar to the *this* pointer of C++ [21]. This automatically makes Objective-C methods unsuitable for callback functions of the Linux Kernel, because their fixed interface does not include the *self* pointer. This is the reason why it is necessary to provide wrapper functions, which get registered as callback functions and relay the parameters to the methods of an object.

4.1.3   Unloading of Modules

The original Objective-C runtime was designed to be used only by one program at a time. This is the reason why there was no concept of unloading. It is necessary to remove the previously registered entries from the Objective-C runtime, because the Linux Kernel requires the unloading functionality. So the runtime was extended with a function to remove the class definition for a specific class. This function needs to be parameterised, in order to unload the correct class definition. Therefore, each class of an Objective-C kernel extension has to come with its own call to the unload function. Removing a class definition while the objects of that class are still in use, results in the objects not working correctly. It is therefore of importance to only unload class definitions not in use. Assuming that no objects are in use after the execution of the module exit function by the kernel module loader, the module loader can safely execute the class definition unload functions provided by the module. To do so, these unload functions are registered as destructors in the *.dtors* section of the ELF binary format. This allows them to be found as long as the kernel extension is loaded.

After all these modifications to the Linux Kernel and the Objective-C runtime, we are now able to use Objective-C for development of Linux Kernel Extensions. This is the object oriented base upon which K-CSP is built.

4.2   CSP Subsystem Implementation

The CSP subsystem implementation is built on top of the Objective-C runtime. This allowed implementation of the CSP subsystem in an object oriented fashion and also aided as a test of the Objective-C runtime kernel port. Furthermore, this allows the porting of the CSP implementation to other OS where the Objective-C runtime is also available. At the moment the CSP subsystem supports the following CSP constructs:

- Process: In the K-CSP environment a Process is created by implementing the CSProcess protocol.

- Channel: The channel construct is only implemented in the form of a point to point channel (One2OneChannel). It supports alternation of channel inputs. Multi-point channels and call channels will follow soon.

- Alternative: The alternative construct only supports fair alternation selection methods. Extensions to priority selections are planned.

- Parallel: This is the normal parallel construct. It is used to implement a Process Network construct as available in JCSP.

5   Example of Utilising K-CSP

The ease of use of K-CSP is demonstrated in this section. The example is very simple, as it only shows one process sending messages to another process. Implementing something similar as a kernel extension without K-CSP would have required at least double the amount of code. The example given shows the power of Objective-C and CSP combined. This example demonstrates how the runtime type information system of the Objective-C environment can be used to terminate a process network, by sending poison messages. Before going into the example some background information on Objective-C and the K-CSP API is given.

5.1   Objective-C Background

In Objective-C all classes are derived from the class Object. As with Java, only single inheritance is allowed, but a class can implement multiple protocols. A protocol is the Objective-C version of an interface in Java. Objective-C separates the declaration of a class and its implementation. The declarations are stored in header files, just as in C/C++. The implementation is given in files with the extension 'm', called m-files. In the listing shown in this section, declaration and implementation are combined.

Every object in Objective-C provides methods for Runtime Type Information (RTTI)[22]. A few of these mechanisms are used in this example:

- `(const char *) name`
  This method returns the name of the class of this object.

- `(BOOL) isKindOf:` *class-object*
  Will return *YES* when the object is of type *class-object* or a descendant.

- `(BOOL) conformsTo:` *protocol*
  Returns *YES* if the object implements *protocol*.

5.2   K-CSP API

This example utilises the CSP subsystem of K-CSP. To be able to understand the code snippets, some information is given below on the API of the K-CSP elements used.

- `CSProcess`
  This protocol defines how processes have to be implemented.

- `One2OneChannel`
  This class provides a channel having one input and one output end. For interaction with processes two methods are provided.

    - `(BOOL) read:` `(id*)` *pMessage*
      This method is used by the receiver to read a message from the channel. This method returns a value of type BOOL, which can either be *YES* or *NO*. The method will return *NO* if an error has occurred. A reference to the message is passed to the *pMessage* parameter.

    - `(BOOL) write:` `(id)` *message*
      This method is used by the sender to pass a message to the receiving process. The boolean return value of the method indicates whether an error has occurred.

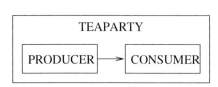

Figure 4: The TEAPARTY process network

Figure 5: Class tree for the different types of Tea

- Parallel
  The Parallel class provides a construct used to execute multiple processes in parallel.

  - (BOOL) add: (id) *object*
    The add method is used to add a process to an object of the Parallel class. The return value indicates whether the method completed successfully.

  - (BOOL) run
    The run method executes all processes added to the parallel object. It returns when all processes have finished execution. The return value of the run method is *YES* if no errors were encountered.

5.3 CSP Subsystem Internals

The CSP subsystem of K-CSP is designed in the form of a kernel extension. It is implemented in the Objective-C programming language. In K-CSP each created process is given its own thread using operating system functions. This allows the OS to distribute processes upon available CPUs. Operating system supplied synchronisation mechanisms are used for the implementation of Parallel, One2OneChannel and Alternative. The implementation of the CSP subsystem of K-CSP, shows that Objective-C indeed embeds nicely in a kernel environment designed for C.

5.4 Tea Party Example

This Tea Party example consists of two processes, PRODUCER and CONSUMER, which are connected using a One2OneChannel. They are combined to create a third process, called TEAPARTY. Figure 4 illustrates the resulting process network. The PRODUCER sends messages to the CONSUMER. The CONSUMER analyses the incoming messages. If they are objects implementing the Tea protocol, a text message is printed onto the standard output. If the message is of type Poison the CONSUMER terminates. The class tree for Tea is shown in Figure 5.

5.4.1 PRODUCER

The PRODUCER sends three messages, first EarlGrey, then Jasmine and finally Poison after which it terminates. Equation 1, shows the CSP version of the PRODUCER process. The implementation in K-CSP is shown in Listing 2. The translation of CSP into K-CSP has to be done manually for the time being.

$$PRODUCER = x!EarlGrey \rightarrow x!Jasmine \rightarrow x!Poison \rightarrow STOP \qquad (1)$$

Listing 2: K-CSP version of the PRODUCER process

```
 2  @interface PRODUCER: Object <CSProcess>
    {
 4      id<ChannelOutput> Out;
    }
 6  -(id) initWithChannelOutput: (id) ChannelOutput;
    @end

 8  @implementation PRODUCER
    -(id) initWithChannelOutput: (id) ChannelOutput;
10  {
        [super init];
12      Out = ChannelOutput;
        return self;
14  }
    -(BOOL) run
16  {
        // allocating, initializing and sending an EarlGrey
18      // object over the channel
        if(NO == [Out write: [[EarlGrey alloc] init]])
20      {
            dbgprint("Received Signal terminating\n");
22          return NO;
        }
24      if(NO == [Out write: [[Jasmine alloc] init]])
        {
26          dbgprint("Received Signal terminating\n");
            return NO;
28      }
        if(NO == [Out write: [[Poison alloc] init]])
30      {
            dbgprint("Received Signal terminating\n");
32          return NO;
        }
34      return YES;
    }
36  @end
    //This macro creates the required unload function to
38  //remove the entries of the class PRODUCER from the
    //runtime registry
40  KOBJC_CLASS(PRODUCER);
```

Listing 1: K-CSP version of the CONSUMER

```
 2  @interface CONSUMER: Object <CSProcess>
    {
 4      id<ChannelInput> In;
    }
 6  -(id) initWithChannelInput: (id) ChannelInput;
    @end

 8  @implementation CONSUMER
    -(id) initWithChannelInput: (id) ChannelInput;
10  {
        [super init];
12      In = ChannelInput;
        return self;
14  }
    -(BOOL) run
16  {
        id message;
18      while(1){
            if(NO == [In read: &message])
20          {
                dbgprint("Received Terminating Signal \n");
22              return NO;
            }
24          dbgprint("CONSUMER received a message of type: \
                %s\n",[message name]);
26          // checking whether this message is poisonous
            if([message isKindOf: [Poison class]] == YES){
28              dbgprint("CONSUMER received poison, now terminating\n");
                //releasing the message object.
30              [message free];
                return YES;
32          }
            // checking if the message implements the Tea protocol
34          if([message conformsTo:@protocol(Tea)] == YES){
                dbgprint("Received a cup of Tea, thank You\n");
36          }
            // releasing the message object
38          [message free];
        }
40  }
    @end
42  KOBJC_CLASS(CONSUMER);
```

5.4.2 CONSUMER

The CONSUMER process analyses every incoming message, to decide whether it is poisonous or not. If it is not poisonous, the message is further examined to determine if it is of type *Tea*, in which case a greeting will be printed. After printing the greeting the process will again wait for an incoming message. If the message received is poisonous, the process will immediately terminate. The CONSUMER CSP representation is given in Equation 2, with the K-CSP implementation in Listing 1.

$$CONSUMER = x?message : \{Tea, Poison\} \rightarrow P(message)$$
$$\text{where}$$
$$P(Tea) = printGreeting \rightarrow CONSUMER$$
$$P(Poison) = STOP \tag{2}$$
$$\text{with}$$
$$Tea = \{EarlGrey, Jasmine\}$$

5.4.3 TEAPARTY Process

The TEAPARTY process provides the environment for the ongoing tea party. Its main task is to interconnect the PRODUCER and CONSUMER processes, using a One2OneChannel and executing them in parallel. After the execution of the processes is completed the tea party is over and the TEAPARTY process terminates.

The CSP representation is given in Equation 3. The implementation using the K-CSP environment is shown in Listing 3. The console output of the TEAPARTY process is shown in Listing 4.

$$TEAPARTY = PRODUCER \parallel CONSUMER \tag{3}$$

Listing 3: K-CSP version of the TEAPARTY process network

```
   void TEAPARTY(void){
2      // Allocating and initialising a One2OneChannel object.
       One2OneChannel *chan = [[One2OneChannel alloc] init];
4      // Allocating and initialising the PRODUCER and CONSUMER process objects.
       PRODUCER *pro = [[PRODUCER alloc] initWithChannelOutput: chan];
6      CONSUMER *con = [[CONSUMER alloc] initWithChannelInput: chan];
       // Allocating and initialising an object of the class Parallel
8      Parallel *par = [[Parallel alloc] init];

10     // Adding the PRODUCER and CONSUMER objects to the parallel object.
       [par add: pro];
12     [par add: con];
       // Executing the processes using parallel.
14     if(NO == [par run]){
         dbgprint("TEAPARTY_run something is fishy\n");
16     }
       // cleaning up after the tea party, freeing all objects.
18     [par free];
       [con free];
20     [pro free];
       [chan free];
22     return;
   }
```

Listing 4: Output of the Tea Party onto the console

```
CONSUMER received a message of type: EarlGrey
Received a cup of Tea, thank You
CONSUMER received a message of type: Jasmine
Received a cup of Tea, thank You
CONSUMER received a message of type: Poison
CONSUMER received poison, now terminating
```

5.5   Comparing the K-CSP Implementation with a Traditional Implementation

The total time to implement the example was around two hours. The implementation of a kernel extension with similar functionality would have taken at least one day and resulted in a large amount of code. This is caused by the difficulty of creating and destroying threads in the kernel. Especially the secure stopping of a thread is not easy. But in K-CSP the programmer does not need to bother about it, which allows easier application of multithreading when necessary. Furthermore, due to the use of CSP channels it is possible to safely exchange data between the threads.

6   Conclusions

This paper gave an introduction to K-CSP, a component architecture for Linux kernel extensions. While K-CSP is still not fully developed, it is clear that the proposed model can make kernel extension development easier, faster and less error prone. The example given showed how simple it is with K-CSP to create components and use them. Due to the use of Objective-C as the object oriented environment and CSP as synchronisation mechanism, K-CSP can be easily ported to other Operating Systems which also use C as the development language. Such operating systems are: all linux flavors, FreeBSD, OpenBSD, Mac OS-X (based on BSD), Windows NT and its successors. This could lead to a simplification of kernel extension development, due to similar programming environments.

7   Further Work

With K-CSP still under development there are a lot of points still to be addressed. Of course an environment for component based programming must come with a set of components for the most common tasks. This enables programmers to benefit from CBP immediately. For programmers wanting to develop components for K-CSP, the components in this paper will act as examples. The CSP subsystem at the moment only comes with a limited set of CSP constructs: the number of supported constructs should be enlarged. An automatic translator from CSP to K-CSP, similar to that presented by G.S. Stiles in [23], could help to further increase code quality while decreasing development time. In order to avoid memory holes, the inclusion of a Garbage Collector (GC) would be appropriate. The Objective-C runtime comes with support for GC through an external library. The Linux Kernel build system at the moment does not support the use of the Objective-C compiler directly, which results in inserting calls to the Objective-C compiler in the makefiles. This could be avoided by enabling the build system to accept Objective-C files directly and using the Objective-C compiler. This is a point of enhancement for the convenience of the programmer.

References

[1] C.A.R. Hoare. Communicating sequential processes. *Communications of the ACM*, 21(8):666–677, August 1978.

[2] Brad J. Cox and Andrew J. Novobilski. *Object-Oriented Programming: An Evolutionary Approach.* Addison-Wesley Pub Co, 2nd edition, May 1991. ISBN: 0201548348.

[3] Alessandro Rubini and Jonathan Corbet. *Linux Device Drivers: Second Edition.* O'Reilly & Associates, Inc., 101 Morris Street, Sebastopol, CA 95472, 2nd edition, June 2001. 0-596-00008-1.

[4] Grady Booch. *Object Oriented analysis and design.* Addison Wesley Longman Inc., One Jacob Way, Reading, Massachusetts 01867 USA, 1993.

[5] Jun-ichiro Itoh and Yasuhiko Yokote. Concurrent object-oriented device driver programming in apertos operating system. Technical report, Sony Computer Science Laboratory, Keio University Department of Computer Science, August 1994.

[6] Jun-ichiro Itoh, Yasuhiko Yokote, and Mario Tokoro. SCONE: Using concurrent objects for low-level operating system programming. Technical report, Sony Computer Science Laboratory, Keio University Department of Computer Science, March 1995.

[7] Yasuhiko Yokote. The Apertos reflective operating system: The concept and its implementation. *ACM SIGPLAN Notices*, 27(10):414–434, 1992.

[8] Jan Axelson. *USB Complete: Everything you need to develop custom USB Peripherals.* Lakeview Research, 2209 Winnebago, St. Madison, WI 53704 USA, 2nd edition, 1999. ISBN: 0-9650819-3-1.

[9] Ju An Wang. Towards component-based software engineering. In *Proceedings of the eighth annual consortium on Computing in Small Colleges Rocky Mountain conference*, pages 177–189. The Consortium for Computing in Small Colleges, 2000.

[10] Desktop Java JavaBeans. Sun JavaBeans Website. http://java.sun.com/products/javabeans/.

[11] Microsoft COM technologies - information and resources for the component object model-based technologies. Website. http://www.microsoft.com/com/.

[12] Enterprise JavaBeans specification, version 2.1. Specification published by SUN Microsystems, November 2003. Version 2.1, Final Release. http://java.sun.com/products/ejb/docs.html.

[13] CORBA Component Model, v3.0. Specification of the Object Management Group, June 2002. http://www.omg.org/technology/documents/formal/components.htm.

[14] Les Hatton. Reexamining the fault density – component size connection. *IEEE Software*, 14(2):89–97, March/April 1997.

[15] Brian W. Kernighan and Dennis M. Ritchie. *The C Programming Language.* Prentice Hall PTR, Upper Saddle River, NJ 07458, USA, 2nd edition, March 1988. ISBN: 0131103628.

[16] The Linux kernel mailing list FAQ. Internet. http://www.tux.org/lkml/\#s15-3.

[17] The Linux kernel archives. Internet. http://www.kernel.org/.

[18] Communicating Sequential Processes for Java (JCSP). Internet. http://www.cs.kent.ac.uk/projects/ofa/jcsp/.

[19] GCC home page - GNU project - Free Software Foundation (FSF). Internet. http://gcc.gnu.org/.

[20] Hongjiu Lu. Elf: From the programmer's perspective. Technical report, NYNEX Science & Technology Inc., 500 Westchester Avenue, White Plains, NY 10604, USA, May 1995.

[21] Bjarne Stroustrup. *The C++ Programming Language.* Addison Wesley Longman Inc., One Jacob Way, Reading, Massachusetts 01867 USA, special edition, March 2000.

[22] Stephen G. Kochan. *Programming in Objective-C.* Sams Publishing, 800 East 96th Street, Indianapolis, Indiana 46240, USA, first edition, November 2003.

[23] G. S. Stiles, V. Raju, and L. Rong. Automatic Conversion of CSP to CTJ, JCSP, and CCSP. In Jan F. Broenink and Gerald H. Hilderink, editors, *Communicating Process Architectures 2003*, pages 63–81, 2003.

Communicating Process Architectures 2004
Ian East, Jeremy Martin, Peter Welch, David Duce, and Mark Green (Eds.)
IOS Press, 2004

Chaining Communications Algorithms with Process Networks

Oliver FAUST, Bernhard SPUTH and David ENDLER

DSP Centre, Ngee Ann Polytechnic, Block 8 #06-09,
Clementi Road 535, 599489 Singapore, Singapore
faust_o@web.de, bernhard@erg.abdn.ac.uk, david.endler@t-online.de

Alastair R. ALLEN

Departments of Engineering and Bio-Medical Physics,
University of Aberdeen, Aberdeen, UK

Abstract. *Software Defined Radio* (SDR) requires a reliable, fast and flexible method to chain parametrisable algorithms. *Communicating Sequential Processes* (CSP) is a design methodology, which offers exactly these properties. This paper explores the idea of using a Java implementation of CSP (JCSP) to model a flexible algorithm chain for Software Defined Radio. JCSP offers the opportunity to distribute algorithms on different processors in a multiprocessor environment, which gives a speed up and keeps the system flexible. If more processing power is required another processor can be added. In order to cope with the high data rate requirement of SDR, optimized data transfer schemes were developed. The goal was to increase the overall system efficiency by reducing the synchronisation overhead of a data transfer between two algorithms. To justify the use of CSP in SDR, a system incorporating CSP was compared with a conventional system, in single and multiprocessor environments.

1 Introduction

A Software Defined Radio (SDR) is a single device which is capable of performing different wireless communications functions at different times [1, 2]. Such devices avoid communication breakdowns by adjusting to new environments. Such a breakdown happened during the first gulf war (1991): the U.S. military observed that their operations were hindered by incompatible radio equipment. This was the reason why the SPEAKeasy project [3] was launched by different branches of the U.S. military as one of the first attempts to create a Software Defined Radio.

Algorithms are used to model the functionality of an SDR device at a specific time. It is not efficient to state a specific functionality in the form of a single sequential algorithm, because this does not allow for reusing parts of the algorithm to model other functionality. Therefore, it is desirable to have general parametrisable algorithms, generic enough to be employed in different models. This requires the ability to execute multiple algorithms and to move data freely between them. The execution of the individual algorithm should only depend on the data, such that only data processing, and not waiting for data, requires processing resources. This reduces the processing time, because one processor, or a processor network, can be shared among multiple algorithms. The design of such systems is one of the goals of Communicating Sequential Processes (CSP) [4]. The sharing of processing resources is achieved by executing multiple processes concurrently. A process incorporates a rule defining the relationship between data input and output. For Software Defined Radio the rules are stated as algorithms. Data can be exchanged between processes by means of channels connecting the individual processes. Part of the power of CSP is the way the data exchange is synchronised between individual processes. The formal correctness of a given CSP system can be proved mathematically. This allows the separation of the functionality from the synchronisation, leading to data driven systems. The SDR concept is an extension of a data driven system, such that not only the data exchange between algorithms is data dependent, but even the algorithms themselves depend on the data, i.e. the algorithms change depending on the data to be processed.

The price for having parallelism in an SDR system is the increased synchronisation overhead, which decreases the data throughput. But data throughput is one of the factors which limits the capability of a particular SDR system. The practical part of this paper (Section 4) details buffer reuse as one of the methods to increase the data throughput. For a particular channel, the total time spent on synchronisation depends on the synchronisation overhead and on how often the channel is used. If a fixed data-rate is assumed for a particular channel, then the data frame size will determine how frequently a channel is used. The effect of different frame sizes on the data throughput is shown in the measurements detailed in Section 6.

2   Discussion: Sequential versus Concurrent Data Processing

Data processing is a repeating three-step process: fetching a data block, processing it and storing the result. Based on this definition it is possible to state the optimal condition for data processing: A data processing system is called optimal if it can meet the processing requirements while utilising as little resources as possible. Under these constraints a data processing design which utilises a single processor to 100% is optimal, due to the fact that the processor is the limiting resource. In a sequential design the three steps for data processing are performed in a single loop. Under practical considerations a sequential design has several problems.

In a real-time environment, the data fetching, processing, and result storage steps run with a constant data rate. This means that data fetching and storing steps require time. The processor does not perform these steps, these are done by external entities. The processor waits for these entities to signal completion. If the data processing is performed sequentially, the wait time cannot be utilised for data processing. To achieve the desired output rate, the processing has to be done in the remaining time, which requires a faster processor. Therefore, a sequential design is not an optimal solution for real-time signal processing. The situation worsens when executing a sequential design in a multiprocessor environment, because only one processor is utilized. The only way to speed up a given sequential design is to use a faster processor! There is a linear relationship between the execution speed of a sequential design and the processor speed.

To utilise wait times as well as multiple processors, the fetching, processing and storing steps should be performed concurrently. Each of the steps forms a small-scale sequential algorithm. These concurrently executing steps need to exchange the results of their labour. These exchanges must be safe, i.e. the concurrent operating steps must perform synchronised data exchange. The synchronisation of the interconnects requires processing power, but this is a small price to pay for a nearly full utilisation of multiple processors.

3   Some SDR Algorithms

An algorithm produces specific output from specific input, and the input-output relationship is normally expressed in mathematical terms. The discussion here is restricted to the algorithms used in the system implementation (see Section 4). These algorithms come from the area of digital communications, which is a field where Software Defined Radios are widely employed.

Most of the transmission signals used for digital communications are defined in the baseband domain. This allows the description of the signal independently from the actual transmission frequency. In a transmitter a Digital Up Converter (DUC) is used to shift the base band signal to a transmission band. A receiver incorporates a Digital Down Converter (DDC) for the inverse operation. To state a distributed model for both the DUC and DDC functionality, the following five different algorithms are required:

- Up-Sampler, **L ↑**;
- Finite Impulse Response Filter, **FIR**;
- I/Q Combiner, **IQ/IF**;
- I/Q Splitter, **IF/IQ**;
- Down-Sampler, **L ↓**;

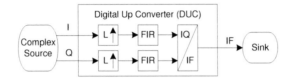

Figure 1: Digital Up Converter algorithm chain

A detailed description of these algorithms can be found in various Digital Signal Processing text books [5, 6]. Figure 1 shows how these algorithms are connected in order to represent the DUC functionality. The output of the source is an arbitrary complex baseband signal, the real part of this signal is represented by an I (Inphase) signal and the imaginary part is represented by a Q (Quadrature) signal. Representing the base band signal via I and Q has the advantage that the subsequent algorithms process real instead of complex numbers: this simplifies the algorithm implementation. The upsampling and filtering combination is used to increase the sample frequency of the baseband signal. This operation allows the I/Q Combiner to shift the baseband signal into an intermediate frequency (IF). The IF signal is a real valued transmission signal. The value of the IF (intermediate frequency) must be stated as a rational number (numerator and denominator) to ensure that the signal can be created with a digital system. In other words, it must be possible to represent one or multiple periods with a finite (integer) number of samples.

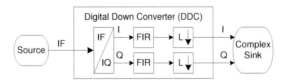

Figure 2: Digital Down Converter algorithm chain

Figure 2 details the block diagram for the DDC. The I/Q splitter shifts the received IF signal down into the baseband domain. This baseband signal has an unnecessarily high sample frequency, i.e. the highest possible signal frequency is much lower than half of the sample frequency [7]. The filtering and down sampler combination reduces the sample frequency. This operation is necessary because the sample frequency determines the processing speed for the subsequent baseband processing algorithms. For simplicity these algorithms are represented by the complex sink block in Figure 2.

If the FIR algorithm is parametrisable, the same implementation can be used for DUC and DDC. This reduces the implementation time and improves the quality of the result, because well known standard implementations can be used. Due to the fact that a receiver merely performs the inverse operations of a transmitter, such synergy effects are quite frequent in digital communication systems. For SDR, the synergy effects are not limited to transmitter and receiver symmetries, they extend to similarities between different standards [8]. The DUC and DDC functionalities are perfect examples of synergies across different standards. If the individual algorithms can be parametrised, there is only one implementation required to accommodate a multitude of different standards.

4   Implementation Aspects

SDR systems can be used in various types of environments, such as client PCs, broadcasting or embedded systems. As the algorithms stay the same, they should be executable in the different environments without any changes. In the Java environment, the compiler translates the source code into Java Byte code, which is executable by a Java Virtual Machine (JVM). JVMs are available for nearly all types of environments, making the Java environment ideal for implementing SDR systems.

The system under discussion here consists of the algorithm chains shown in Figures 1 and 2. To be able to verify the correct functioning of the algorithm chain, it was decided to process files compatible with the FhG Software Radio [9]. This is software that decodes signals according to the Digital Radio Mondiale (DRM) standard [10]. The FhG Software Radio is able to decode files containing DRM signals in either IF or IQ format. The files contain samples of 16 bit resolution, which corresponds to the short data type in Java. As all the algorithm implementations operate with integer values, a data conversion has to be performed.

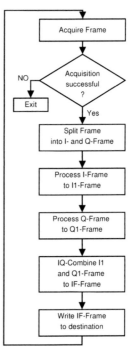

Figure 3: Finite State Machine of the DUC chain.

For the Digital Up Converter (DUC) of Figure 1 a complex source, providing the I and Q components, is required. As the file format stores these two signal components in a multiplexed form, a de-multiplexing step is required. This de-multiplexing step will also perform the data type conversion from short to integer. For the Digital Down Converter (DDC) of Figure 2, an IQ-Multiplexer is required in order to write files compatible with the Fraunhofer Software.

Processing single samples introduces a high number of function calls, which in turn decreases the performance of the system. To avoid this, groups of samples, so-called frames, are constructed and processed together. Increasing the frame-size results in a greater delay, as the system has to wait longer for the frames to become available. The frame-size depends on the processing system and the particular application. In SDR the applications are not fixed, some applications allow more delay than others. For example, a broadcast standard allows more delay than a communication standard, because a human is able to detect communication delays that are larger than 20ms. This is the reason why in the SDR system under discussion the frame size must be flexible. This is relatively unusual for CSP systems; normally all parameters are optimised for fastest processing without latency constraints.

4.1   Sequential Implementation

For implementing the sequential approach, each algorithm of the DUC and DDC chains is implemented as a Java class. The DUC and DDC chains require the signal data to be processed by the algorithms in a fixed way. Therefore, each chain is represented by a function, which instantiates the algorithms and calls each of them according to the schedule. This is equivalent to a finite state machine, as shown in Figure 3 for the DUC chain.

4.1.1   Optimisation of the Sequential Implementation

In the sequential implementation each algorithm allocates a new output buffer and disposes of the input buffer. Both allocation and disposing of buffers takes time, which could be spared if the output buffer could be recycled. Since only one algorithm is executing at a time, and the frame-size does not change during runtime, recycling of the buffer is possible.

4.2   Concurrent Implementation using CSP

CSP is not included in the standard Java distribution, so a Java implementation of CSP had to be found. *Communicating Threads for Java* (CTJ) [11, 12, 13, 14] and *Communicating Sequential Processes for Java* (JCSP) [15, 16, 13, 14] seemed to be what we were looking for. JCSP and CTJ have a similar goal and therefore provide a similar functionality, and to choose between them was not easy. In the end, the exhaustive documentation, with lots of examples plus lots of other support material, made JCSP the implementation of choice.

In CSP, each process executes independently from other processes: this makes it possible to execute multiple processes concurrently. Data exchange between processes is only possible by using unidirectional channels which act as a synchronisation mechanism. Every process has channel-inputs and channel-outputs, depending on its communication requirements. The combination of processes and their interconnection channels is called a process network.

To convert the sequential implementation into a concurrent implementation, we have to transfer the sequential algorithm chain into a process network. To create this process network it is necessary to identify the independent components of the sequential algorithm chain, and convert each into a process. Taking a look at block diagrams, Figures 1 and 2, identifies that each block performs its operation independently from other blocks. Therefore, each block is converted into a process. This is done by implementing a wrapper class. This wrapper class has an instance of the algorithm class as member, whilst providing a CSP conforming interface. To create the corresponding process network is now only a matter of interconnecting the processes according to the block diagrams.

As the concurrent approach can only utilise as many processors as it has processes, a large number of processes is desirable. For the developer, on the other hand, a large number of processes becomes difficult to handle. It is difficult for the programmer to maintain an overview of the complete method/function: this leads to insecurity. Fortunately, CSP allows the creation of components and their use in a hierarchical fashion [17]. This is enabled by the fact that a process network in CSP is nothing else than a process. Therefore, it is possible to use predefined process networks, as components, to build a larger process network. This process network's interface will simply consist of externally connected channel inputs and outputs. This technique of component building was used to create the DUC and DDC processes of Figures 1 and 2. The process-networks for the IQ-Combiner and IQ-Splitter are shown in Figure 4.

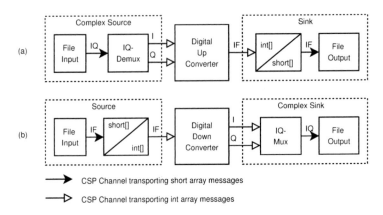

Figure 4: Process Networks for IQ-Combiner and IQ-Splitter.

4.2.1 Improving the Data Throughput

As previously stated, it is desirable to avoid unnecessary buffer allocation and disposal. In the sequential implementation this was achieved by allocating a single output buffer, which was then used as input by the following algorithm. Using the same scheme in the concurrent implementation, where the algorithms are executed in parallel, could result in one algorithm writing to the buffer while another reads from the same buffer. The result would be wrong, rendering this implementation useless.

If we assume that each algorithm / process only operates on a single buffer per channel at one time, it is sufficient to use two buffers which are exchanged between two processes. This approach has two drawbacks. First, the size of the output buffers is fixed over the complete runtime of the network. Second, each passing of output frames requires two channel communications: one to send the new output buffer and one to receive the now empty output buffer. The two communications increase the synchronisation overheads, increasing the runtime.

In order to avoid the second channel operation, the sending process needs to keep a reference to both output buffers. One buffer is marked as *output-buffer*, to store processing results, while the other buffer is marked as *away-buffer*. The *away-buffer* is used by the next process as its input. Once the process has completed processing its input, it sends the *output-buffer* to the next process and swaps *output-buffer* and *away-buffer*. The switching of the buffers is handled by a so-called BufferKeeper object. Figure 5 illustrates the working of the scheme.

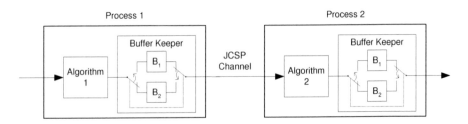

Figure 5: Buffer Reuse Scheme in the Algorithm Chain

For this scheme to work it is important to know when the receiver has processed the previous buffer. This is solved by constraining the receiver to request a new buffer only after the previous buffer is processed. With this method it is safe to perform the output buffer switch after the sending operation has succeeded.

5 Comparison between Sequential and Concurrent Implementation

The concurrent implementation has multiple advantages over the sequential implementation.

5.1 Easy to Apply, Easy to Debug

It is easy to convert sequential algorithms into CSP processes. This is done by creating a process which performs the channel operations, and uses the algorithm implementation to create the desired output from the input. This approach provides a clean division between functionality and synchronisation. This scheme allows the development and verification of functionality and synchronisation separately. This results in simpler test setups and therefore faster development.

5.2 CSP Enables Compact Designs

In CSP everything is a process, resulting in process networks also being processes. This enables the abstraction of recurring process networks in the form of processes. For the user of the resulting process it does not matter if there is a single process or a process network inside. These processes allow us to build components [17], which can be tested individually (unit testing) [18]. This component based approach accelerates and simplifies the development of algorithm chains, due to the use of previously developed and tested components. The ability to layer CSP based systems produces compact designs: these can be easier to understand and are therefore desirable [19]. The DUC chain, for instance, has two layers:

1. Top Layer: Complex Source, Digital Up Converter, Sink.

2. Bottom Layer:

   - Complex Source: File Input, IQ-Demux
   - Digital Up Converter: I-UpSampler, I-FIR, Q-UpSampler, Q-FIR, IQ-Combiner
   - Sink: Int2Short, File Output.

5.3 Taking Advantage of Multiple CPUs

A concurrent implementation can provide a speedup S on multiple CPUs. The speedup is defined as [20]:

$$S = \frac{T_S}{T_N} \tag{1}$$

with

- T_S = optimal sequential processing time; the best time that can be achieved on a single processor using the best sequential algorithm

- T_N = concurrent processing time; the actual time achieved on an N-processor system with the concurrent algorithm and a specific scheduling method being considered.

In our case, the time of the sequential implementation is considered as T_S. The scheduling is fixed by the fact that the sequence of the algorithms is fixed by the task itself. The runtime of the sequential implementation is nearly independent of the frame-size. For the concurrent approach, larger frame-sizes result in fewer channel operations and therefore in less synchronisation overhead. That means its runtime decreases with increasing frame-sizes. A graph

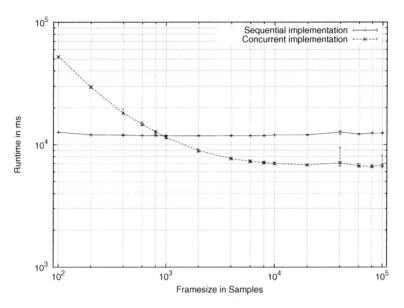

Figure 6: Comparing the runtime of concurrent and sequential implementation, on a dual CPU machine.

showing the dependency of the runtime of sequential and concurrent implementations on the frame-size is given in Figure 6.

More interesting than the raw speedup, which depends on the number of CPUs, is whether the efficiency of the concurrent implementation scales on multiple CPUs. The efficiency E, of a concurrent implementation is defined as:

$$E = \frac{S}{N} = \frac{T_S}{T_N \cdot N} \tag{2}$$

with N as the number of CPUs in the system. A plot of the efficiency versus the frame-size is given in Figure 7.

5.4   Wait Cycles Introduced by the IO Subsystem can be used for Signal Processing

The runtime of the sequential approach is defined as the summation of all steps of processing:

$$T_S = \sum_{i=1}^{m} t_i \tag{3}$$

with:

- t_i = execution time for one step of a sequential implementation
- m = number of steps in a sequential implementations.

Assuming that the sequential algorithm chain is connected to a slow source or sink, the time spent waiting for the IO subsystem is reflected in the processing time. The concurrent implementation can utilise this wait time to perform processing. The processing time is determined solely by the IO subsystem if the processing is faster than the acquiring or storing of the data. Due to this fact a concurrent implementation, on a single CPU system, can be faster than a sequential implementation.

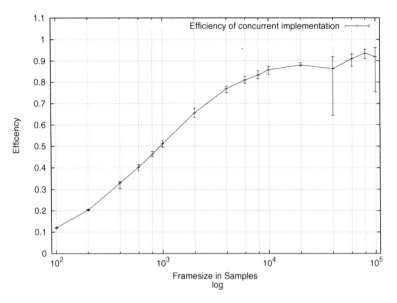

Figure 7: Efficiency of the JCSP implementation, on a dual CPU machine over the frame size.

6 Measurements

All measurements were performed using an HP workstation x4000, equipped with two Intel P4 Xeon 1.5GHz CPUs with 256kB cache and 512MB Rambus RAM. J2SDK build 1.4.2_01-b06 for Linux, available from Sun, was used as the Java environment. The Java environment was installed on Slackware Linux 9.1 running Linux Kernel 2.6.3, from kernel.org.

For all measurements, the Digital Up and Down Converter chains were parametrised:

DUC chain:

- Up-sampling factor: 4

- Numerator: 1

- Denominator: 4

DDC chain:

- Down-sampling factor: 4

- Numerator: 1

- Denominator: 4

All measurements represent the combined runtime of the DUC and the DDC chain.

6.1 Efficiency

Measurement Setup: In order to avoid undue influence by the IO sub-system, a source and sink which operate with virtually no latency were developed. The source supplies a specific number of samples before signalling end of data. To show that the runtime depends on the frame-size, the source is able to supply frames of any size. The implementation of the sink is an empty function, which gets called, but does not perform any processing. This setup allows us to measure the runtime of the algorithm chains without disturbance from the IO sub-system.

The runtime of the implementations were measured assuming a round trip, first digital up converting the data, then digital down converting it. The DUC chain is sourced with $6 \cdot 10^6$ IQ-samples producing $24 \cdot 10^6$ IF-samples – due to the performed up-sampling. The DUC chain is sourced with these $24 \cdot 10^6$ samples.

For measuring the optimal sequential processing time (T_S), the machine was loaded with a single CPU kernel. For each frame-size, ten runtime measurements were taken and the lowest result was taken as T_S for this frame-size.

To determine the concurrent processing time (T_N), also ten measurements per frame-size were performed.

Measurement Results: The efficiency graph in Figure 7, shows the dependency of the concurrent implementation on the frame-size. Generally speaking, the larger the frames get, the less synchronisation overhead is introduced. In our case the efficiency is over 80% with frame-sizes of 6000 samples upwards.

6.2   Slow IO Sub-system

The aim of this measurement was to show that a concurrent implementation has advantages even on a single CPU system. This is for instance the case when a single CPU system acquires the data to process from a slow IO sub-system without caching.

Measurement Setup: In order to create reproducible measurement results, a data rate controlled source was developed. The data rate was specified as samples per second sps. The source holds a variable containing the number of available samples, the *as-counter*. The as-counter gets incremented, with a samples per tick value spt, by a periodic timer thread. In Java (on Linux) a periodic timer thread can have a minimum period length of 1ms (1000 ticks per second tps). The particular kernel version used, provided the necessary timer resolution. This results in $spt = \frac{sps}{tps}$. Once the periodic timer thread has performed the increment, it wakes up a possibly waiting receiver. If the as-counter value is larger or equal to the frame-size, the receiver decrements the frame-size from the counter and processes the data. This scheme provides a stable source for data rates that are integer multiples of 1000. This source represents a data rate controlled source with cache, since the periodic timer thread always increments the as-counter. The flowchart of the source is shown in Figure 8. For reasons of simplicity, the synchronisation is not included.

To remove the caching feature from this source, it is necessary to stop incrementing the as-counter while there is no reader waiting. This was done by introducing a reader waiting flag, which is only set when a reader is waiting. The periodic timer thread checks this flag and only when it is set increments the as-counter. The only problem is, that in the case that the processing of a frame takes less than 1ms, the runtime is only determined by the source. This is due to the fact that for the timer thread the receiver-waiting flag is constantly set. This results in a measurement where the sequential approach would have always requested the next frame, before it processed the current frame. In short, the source would behave as if it would perform caching. Therefore, the measurements were done only with large frame-sizes, which in any case took longer to process than 1ms. The source was parametrised to provide a total of $72 \cdot 10^6$ samples with a sample rate of $1 \cdot 10^6$ samples/s. This results in the source requiring $72s$ to provide the data.

For this test run a frame-size of $100,000$ samples was chosen. For each test case, 10 runs were performed and the mean value used to produce Figure 9.

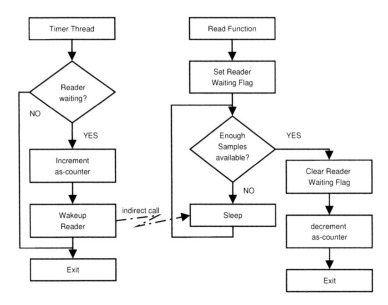

Figure 8: Flowchart of the rate controlled cache less source

Measurement Results: The bar graph in Figure 9 compares the runtime of sequential and concurrent implementations, using different sources. The sequential implementation requires $96s$ to process data from a slow source. The slow source alone requires $72s$ to provide the data, leaving $96s - 72s = 24s$, which is the processing time of the sequential implementation. The sequential implementation sourced by the low latency (fast) source requires $24.6s$ to process the same amount of data. This supports the validity of the statement made in Equation 3 that the runtime of the sequential approach is the summation of all steps of processing.

The concurrent implementation, on the other hand, requires $72.1s$, which is very close to the $72s$ the source requires to provide the data. This shows that a concurrent implementation can utilise wait times introduced by external entities to perform processing. A concurrent implementation can have runtime advantages even on a single processor system.

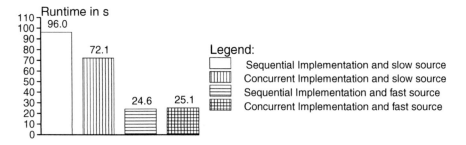

Figure 9: Impact of a slow source on the runtime of the different implementations on a single CPU machine

7   Conclusions

The use of CSP technology in SDR systems is beneficial, because of increased flexibility and reliability. Compared with other, monolithic, implementations the CSP approach offers a speedup in multiprocessor systems, because the algorithms can be executed in parallel. Multiprocessor systems require some sort of synchronization in order to keep track of which algorithm is used to process what data. For Software Defined Radio systems these synchronization methods are not the core problem, therefore it is advisable to use a standard method. CSP represents such a standard method, which offers the opportunity to prove the absence of deadlocks. Other implementations which cater for parallel processing require sophisticated synchronization methods. In the best case these other synchronization methods are reinventions, but most of the time they fall short in reliability and flexibility compared with the CSP approach.

A flexible way of distributing the processor load is required in order to make full use of a multiprocessor environment. CSP offers the opportunity to utilize additional processing resources. The question is: how good are the algorithms when distributed over the available processors. SDR requires mainly an algorithm chain where the processing speed is determined by the time requirement of the slowest process in the chain. The goal for a load balancer is to find an optimal processing load distribution in a multiprocessor system. This task is left for a future undertaking.

References

[1] Joseph Mitola. *The software radio architecture*. IEEE Commun. Mag., no.5, pp.26-38, May 1995.

[2] Joseph Mitola. *Software radio architecture: A mathematical perspective*. IEEE J. Sel. Areas Commun., vol.17, no.4, pp.514-538, April 1999.

[3] R. J. Lackey and D. W. Upmal. *Speakeasy: The Military Software Radio*. IEEE Communications Magazine, vol. 33, no. 5, pp. 56-61, May 1995.

[4] C.A.R. Hoare. *Communicating Sequential Processes*. Prentice Hall, 2003.

[5] Sanjit K. Mitra. *Digital Signal Processing – A Computer-Based Approach*. Mc Graw Hill, Avenue of the Americans, New York, NY 10020 United States of America, second edition, 2001.

[6] John G. Proakis and Dimitris G. Manolakis. *Digital Signal Processing Principles, Algorithms, And Applications*. Prentice Hall, Upper Saddle River, New Jersey 07485 United States of America, 1996.

[7] C.E. Shannon.   A mathematical theory of communication.   *The Bell System Technical Journal*, July/October 1948.

[8] Jeffrey H. Reed. *Software Radio: A Modern Approach to Radio Engineering*. Prentice Hall, Upper Saddle River, New Jersey 07485 United States of America, 2002.

[9] Fraunhofer.   *Homepage FhG Software Radio*.   http://www.iis.fraunhofer.de/dab/products/drmreceiver/.

[10] *DRM standard IEC 62272-1 Ed. 1: Digital Radio Mondiale (DRM) - Part 1: System Specification*. International Electrotechnical Commission, IEC Central Office 3, rue de Varemb? P.O. Box 131 CH - 1211 GENEVA 20 Switzerland, 2003-03.

[11] André W. P. Bakkers, Jan F. Broenink, Gerald H. Hilderink, and Wiek Vervoort. Communicating Java Threads. In André W. P. Bakkers, editor, *Proceedings of WoTUG-20: Parallel Programming and Java*, pages 48–76. IOS Press, the Netherlands, 1997.

[12] Gerald H. Hilderink. CTJ (Communicating Threads for Java) Home Page. Available at: http://www.ce.utwente.nl/javapp/ Retrieved July, 2004.

[13] Peter H. Welch, André W. P. Bakkers, G. S. Stiles, and Gerald H. Hilderink. CSP for Java: Multithreading for All. In Barry M. Cook, editor, *Proceedings of WoTUG-22: Architectures, Languages and Techniques for Concurrent Systems*, pages 277–278. IOS Press, the Netherlands, 1999.

[14] Peter H. Welch, Gerald H. Hilderink, and Nan C. Schaller. Using Java for Parallel Computing - JCSP versus CTJ. In Peter H. Welch and Andr W. P. Bakkers, editors, *Communicating Process Architectures 2000*, pages 205–226. IOS Press, the Netherlands, 2000.

[15] Peter H. Welch. Process Oriented Design for Java: Concurrency for All. In H.R.Arabnia, editor, *Proceedings of the International Conference on Parallel and Distributed Processing Techniques and Applications (PDPTA'2000)*, volume 1, pages 51–57. CSREA, CSREA Press, June 2000.

[16] Peter H. Welch. Java Communicating Sequential Processes Home Page. Available at: http://www.cs.ukc.ac.uk/projects/ofa/jcsp/ Retrieved July, 2004.

[17] Peter H. Welch. Communicating Processes, Components and Scalable Systems. Homepage, May 2001. http://www.cs.ukc.ac.uk/projects/ofa/jcsp/components.pdf.

[18] Steven C. McConnell. *Code Complete: A Practical Handbook of Software Construction*. Microsoft Press, One Microsoft Way, Redmond, Washington, 1993.

[19] Eric Steven Raymond. *The Art of Unix Programming*. Pearson Education, Inc., Pearson Education Inc, Rights and Contracts Department, 75 Arlington Street, Suite 300, Boston, MA 02116, first edition, 2004.

[20] Randy Chow and Theodore Johnson. *Distributed Operating Systems & Algorithms*. Addison Wesley, 2725 Sand Hill Road, Menlo Park, CA 94025, 1997.

Communicating Process Architectures 2004
Ian East, Jeremy Martin, Peter Welch, David Duce, and Mark Green (Eds.)
IOS Press, 2004

339

Using CSP to Verify Aspects of an
occam-to-FPGA Compiler

Roger M.A. PEEL and WONG Han Feng

Department of Computing, University of Surrey, Guildford, Surrey GU2 7XH, United Kingdom

Abstract. This paper reports on the progress made in developing techniques for the verification of an **occam** to FPGA compiler. The compiler converts **occam** [1] programs into logic circuits that are suitable for loading into field-programmable gate arrays (FPGAs). Several levels of abstraction of these circuits provide links to conventional hardware implementations. Communicating Sequential Processes (CSP) has then been used to model these circuits. This CSP has been subjected to tests for deadlock and livelock freedom using the Failures-Divergence Refinement tool (FDR). In addition, FDR has been used to prove that the circuits emitted have behaviours equivalent to CSP specifications of the original **occam** source codes.

1 Introduction

occam is a language that permits parallel processes and blocking inter-process communications to be specified in a fine-grained structure which is particularly suitable for the implementation of embedded systems [1]. It forms the basis for languages such as Handel-C [2] which can be compiled directly to a form that may be run on field-programmable gate arrays. Since **occam**'s process and communication structure is derived from Hoare's Communicating Sequential Processes (CSP) [3], many **occam** programs are therefore easily specified in CSP.

Currently, a new version of the authors' **occam** to FPGA compiler [4] is being built to incorporate better circuit optimisation and further language features. During this re-implementation, it has become clear that design or coding faults in the logic generated by the compiler are very difficult to find. This is because all of the logic gates operate in every clock cycle, and values are latched into the flip-flops of the FPGA in parallel when required. In contrast to sequential programs, much more can go wrong in parallel logic – and then trigger other faults – in each clock cycle. Thus, techniques have been developed that allow for the circuits to be checked for accuracy, such as building a dedicated simulator and circuit visualiser within the compiler, and developing the formal verification technique presented in this paper. By checking a number of such circuits, it should be possible to gain confidence in the code generation of each section of the compiler.

The immediate application of the work reported in this paper, therefore, is to provide an automatic mechanism for reference tests of elementary compiler functions. This could also be performed by simulating the logic circuits that are generated, using suitable test vectors, and then pattern-matching for particular results. On the other hand, running FDR [5] trace refinements should be easier to automate, because small changes to the compiler would probably affect the test vectors required by the alternative approach. A second application is for the verification of building-block processes that are then combined to build larger systems.

---

[1] **occam** is a trademark of ST Microelectronics

Later on, it should be possible to reason about the behaviour of complete embedded systems, either by modelling them in their entireties, or by composing these sectional results.

Section 2 of this paper provides further details of the background to this work, and lists some of the alternative approaches that are employed. In Section 3, we explain how we used CSP to model logic circuits. In Section 4, we show how a small occam counter program was represented in CSP, and how we refinement-checked it against a CSP specification of the task. Section 5 discusses occam channel communications, and Section 6 provides some concluding remarks.

2 Background

Field-programmable gate array (FPGA) devices are components which contain configurable blocks of low-level logic, typically comprising flip-flop storage elements, combinatorial logic, and maybe special data processing units, memory blocks and even complete processors such as the PowerPC [6]. There are many ways to program FPGAs. Each manufacturer usually provides basic schematic capture tools that allow low-level circuits to be drawn on a computer screen, possibly incorporating macro elements that describe common sub-circuits such as adders and multipliers. These diagrammatic representations are then optimised and converted to the format that is sent to the FPGA at power-up, at which time it is configured to perform the desired task. Some FPGAs may be entirely, or partially, re-configured later on, too. The problem with designing at such a low level is that it is difficult to reason about the circuits that have been constructed, leaving complicated simulations or hardware probing and debugging as the main development techniques. As FPGAs become larger, this mechanism scales poorly.

The VHDL design language provides a very low-level way to specify either the physical or the behavioural characteristics of FPGA logic, in a way that allows a hierarchy of modules to be built. Many library components are available for tasks such as arithmetic, and blocks of logic (IP, or intellectual property) may be purchased for incorporation into larger designs. Each of these blocks, as well as all of the more basic logic, operates in parallel, which can lead to high performance, but which can also introduce concurrency issues that are not supported well by the design method. As in the schematic capture approach, VHDL designs are usually tested through simulation. In order to evaluate the interaction of two asynchronous components, the simulation test vectors must exercise all possible situations in which critical interactions might occur – a very demanding requirement.

JHDL [7] represents logic elements as specially-developed Java classes, and provides methods to allow the designer to specify their interconnections. The technique also provides methods that can be used in the simulation phase, as well as back-end support for configuring several popular FPGA device families.

At a higher-level of abstraction, it is possible to use conventional programming languages to program FPGAs. Various authors and organisations have written compilers that convert programs written in sequential languages such as C into logic for FPGAs. This approach is limited by the amount of parallelism that can be discovered automatically in the C source code. Better, non-standard parallel constructs can be added to a sequential language to represent various forms of parallelism. SystemC [8] does this in a thread-like manner; it also implements event methods that provide a basis for synchronised communications. Handel-C [2, 9] does the same, but was developed from an occam prototype and more closely follows that model. Handel-C uses a synchronous message-passing, CSP-based, framework that was originally modelled on occam. Unfortunately, it is possible to use the flexibility of its C-like capabilities to defeat the security of the message-passing framework.

The authors therefore have chosen to retain an occam-like structure in their new compiler. The aim of the work is to develop a compilation environment that allows embedded-system designers to incorporate a high degree of message-passing parallelism in their designs, to provide good timing properties and optimisations, and to be able to take advantage of proof and verification techniques developed by the CSP community.

The compiler currently generates one-hot logic [10], in which a series of flip-flops are set active when the program statements that they relate to are being executed. Further flip-flops store each bit of each declared variable. In this way, program control is passed from one statement to the next by activating the next flip-flop in a chain and clearing the previous one. In sequential code, therefore, one flip-flop is in its active state (or hot) at any time – hence *one-hot*. When a parallel program forks, the one-hot predecessor stage activates all of the initial stages of the parallel processes; upon completion, the par-end must collect together all of the parallel one-hot termination signals and only activate the following process when all of its predecessors have terminated. Notice that each parallel process runs truly in parallel – there is no concept of time-sharing as is seen in an implementation of a parallel (or threaded) language on a uniprocessor. The flip-flops that hold the values of variables are triggered to store a new value by the one-hot flip-flop that represents a particular assignment statement or channel receive event.

In the future, other forms of logic, such as asynchronous, might be used by the compiler as alternatives to clocked synchronous logic. This could well still use a one-hot structure, but all of the logic elements would run at their own pace and synchronise with their neighbours independently of a common clock. This scheme is more complicated to design, but typically has a lower power consumption and generates lower levels of radio-frequency emissions.

The authors are aware that there are issues of metastability in all clocked digital logic circuits. Metastability arises because a flip-flop (or single-bit storage cell) normally samples its input on an incoming clock edge and reflects that value shortly thereafter. Unfortunately, if the value of the input signal changes at the time of the clock edge, or shortly before it, or shortly afterwards, then the value of the input is indeterminate and thus the value of the output is unpredictable. Worse still, in this circumstance, the signal level on the flip-flop logic output may not settle to the high or the low digital logic voltage level for a substantial period, which upsets the logic that it feeds, too. Provided that the input signal does not change for a specified *set-up time* before the clock is asserted, and provided that the input signal does not change for a specified *hold time* afterwards, then the vendors of the implementation logic are prepared to guarantee the metastable behaviour of their devices. In the circuits generated by our compiler, the inputs to all of the flip-flops are generated from combinations of the outputs of other flip-flops (see Figure 1), so the round-trip times can easily be determined and the configuration software can determine the maximum clock rate within which metastability should not occur. The work presented in this paper does not address these issues further. Provided that the vendors of the implementation logic are prepared to guarantee the metastable behaviour of their devices, then our techniques – and those of every other digital designer - are considered to be sound in this respect.

Another technique that is being used to generate fault-free logic for FPGAs is to start with a formal algebra such as CSP and then to compile this directly to FPGAs, or alternatively to target an intermediate stage such as Handel-C [11], or the various Java-based CSP implementations [12]. CSP currently provides most of the facilities required for embedded systems, but issues such as timing, data structures and arithmetic capabilities still need good solutions.

3   Method

3.1   Process Algebra and Model Checking

The scheme that has been employed in our research utilises the Communicating Sequential Processes algebra to model both the behaviour of source occam programs and also of the target logic circuits generated by the occam-to-FPGA compiler. The Failures-Divergence Refinement (FDR) tool [5], produced by Formal Systems Europe Ltd, may then be used to prove various properties of both the initial source and of the compiled logic circuits. These properties can include deadlock freedom, livelock freedom, the behavioural equivalence of two circuits, and the equivalence of a circuit with its formal (CSP) specification.

Although CSP has been used in our research, many forms of temporal logic would also be appropriate to this task. SPIN and PROMELA have been used in [13]. Denis Nicole has had success with SMV in [14]. However, he also concludes that state-space explosion can easily occur as the systems under test increase in size. We chose CSP primarily so that we could use the FDR model checker, which has proved to be very suitable.

3.2   Compiled Circuits

At present, our occam-to-FPGA compiler generates circuits using a relatively limited number of components – edge-triggered D-type and T-Type flip-flops, AND gates, OR gates, inverters and input/output buffers. Each of these components has been modelled in CSP, and thus a complete model of a circuit can be described using a number of these components, connected by CSP channels, all running in parallel.

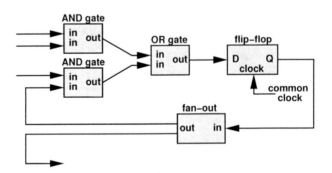

Figure 1: an example of part of a clocked FPGA circuit

Figure 1 shows just one flip-flop in a typical FPGA configuration, together with an OR-gate and a layer of AND-gates. It also shows a fan-out (or delta) stage, which is not needed in real hardware but is needed in a channel-based implementation when the channel output of a process is copied to a number of process inputs. Although FPGAs are capable of containing logic that is more complicated than this sum-of-products form, and although our occam compiler generates such logic, this simple figure could be generalised to illustrate any valid circuit. This example corresponds to the contents of a simple configurable logic block (or CLB) of a typical Xilinx FPGA [6]. Notice that there is a cycle in this figure, and that the flip-flop component is part of this cycle.

3.3 Modelling the Circuits with occam

In order to gain confidence with our strategy of modelling logic circuits in CSP, we started by using occam to simulate some small circuits. Initially, we built an occam program that models a 3-input NAND gate. This program was run successfully using the Kent Retargettable occam compiler (KRoC) [15]. The combinatorial 3-input NAND circuit has three inputs and one output and each combination of its binary inputs can be exercised in turn to prove that it operates as expected. This was done by supplying all eight possible combinations of the three input signals and verifying the eight outputs in a simple occam test harness.

```
WHILE running          -- I/O-PAR process
  SEQ
    ...   parallel I/O (once on each channel)
    ...   compute

WHILE running          -- I/O-SEQ process
  SEQ
    ...   parallel inputs (once on each input channel)
    ...   compute
    ...   parallel outputs (once on each output channel)
    ...   compute
```

Figure 2: I/O-PAR and I/O-SEQ processes

Welch [16] introduces the concepts of I/O-PAR and I/O-SEQ processes, whose structures are illustrated in Figure 2. In the former, all inputs and outputs operate in parallel and, thus, each channel is used on every 'heartbeat' of the whole circuit, with each process locked into step with its neighbours. Note that this is not a *global* lockstep – although that would be a valid, but inefficient, refinement of these *nearest-neighbour* locksteps. In I/O-SEQ processes, all of their inputs operate in parallel, but sequentially with the parallel combination of all of their outputs.

Programs which contain just I/O-PAR processes, or those with mixtures of I/O-PAR and I/O-SEQ processes, in which there are no cycles of just I/O-SEQ processes, are proven deadlock-free [16, 17, 18, 19, 20]. This is a restrictive condition, of course; many programs that do not follow these rules also turn out to be deadlock-free, especially if sufficient buffer processes are provided.

Our NAND gate process was initially written as an I/O-PAR component. In this configuration, each of its inputs and outputs is communicated in parallel precisely once, then the new state is determined. and then the parallel inputs and output are performed again, and so on. In this way, arbitrary collections of NAND gates may be composed into a larger circuit with no danger of deadlock. Furthermore, each combination will also be I/O-PAR and may itself be composed with other components to make an even larger I/O-PAR program.

Six such NAND gates were then connected together in an occam program to form a D-type flip-flop, using techniques similar to those also found in [16]. The circuit used, shown in Figure 3, is one that is provided in dozens of digital logic text books and TTL data books (e.g. [21]). This program was also executed using KRoC.

Welch notes in [16] that the I/O-PAR NAND gates each have a propagation delay of one I/O-PAR cycle, and thus the set-up and hold times for the input signals had to be controlled to ensure that the flip-flop's data inputs were not changed within three cycles of the clock edges. Variations of this constraint account for different numbers of delay cycles throughout the work reported in this paper, and are seen in the set-up and hold times of all hardware flip-flops, too.

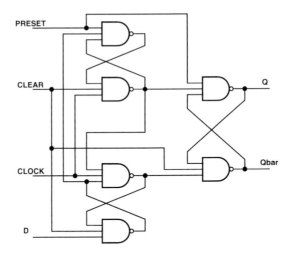

Figure 3: the edge-triggered D-type flip-flop initially implemented

3.4   Modelling the Circuits with CSP

Having experimented with occam models of these logic elements, we encoded the 3-input NAND gate in CSP, composed six of them into a D-type flip-flop, and were then able to experiment using FDR. Initially, we built an I/O-PAR version of the NAND gate in CSP, but later we also built a version of the D-type flip-flop with I/O-SEQ NAND gates, together with I/O-PAR output buffers (which render the whole ensemble I/O-PAR when the six NAND processes are combined) to ensure deadlock freedom. Again, the programs worked as expected, and FDR was able to prove their deadlock properties and equivalence-check each of them against the original version. By providing a filter process to translate a common stream of input signals to that required to satisfy the set-up and hold time requirements of the different clock regimes, and by hiding all of the signals internal to that process, the effects of the circuits could be proved to be equivalent.

The snag with these versions of our D-type flip-flop was that they generated very large state spaces in FDR, although FDR was able to compact their initial requirements considerably. Despite this, however, it became clear that this 6-NAND mechanism for building clocked logic elements was far too expensive to be built into large circuits.

Rather than building our flip-flops from first principles (e.g. 6 NAND gates), a more practical approach turned out to be to build direct behavioural models and use them as base components for the modelling of larger circuits. The equivalence between these behavioural models and those structured out of NAND gates can easily be separately verified.

3.5   Problems with Modelling in CSP

We use the behavioural modelling in CSP of these flip-flops to illustrate one of the difficulties CSP has in expressing certain simple patterns of behaviour – one of these being I/O-PAR!

Figure 4 shows the occam expression of these flip-flops. They are clearly I/O-PAR with respect to their in and out channels. The clock represents a (general multiway) event that other design rules (for the circuits constructed with this flip-flop) guarantee will not block indefinitely – and, hence, may be safely considered part of the *compute* body of the I/O-PAR cycle [20].

```
PROC dff (CHAN OF BOOL in, out,      PROC tff (CHAN OF BOOL in, out,
          CHAN OF BOOL clock)                  CHAN OF BOOL clock)
  INITIAL BOOL state IS FALSE:         INITIAL BOOL state IS FALSE:
  WHILE TRUE                           WHILE TRUE
    BOOL next:                           BOOL flip:
    SEQ                                  SEQ
      PAR                                  PAR
        in ? next                            in ? flip
        out ! state                          out ! state
      BOOL any:                            BOOL any:
      clock ? any                          clock ? any
      state := next                        IF
  :                                          flip
                                               state := ~state
                                             TRUE
                                               SKIP
                                     :
```

Figure 4: The occam D-type and T-type flip-flops

There are no direct expressions in CSP of the patterns in Figure 4. However, there are in Circus [22, 23] – an extension of CSP that includes state variables and assignment (and formal Z specifications of state transformation).

Circus expressions for these flip-flops are shown in Figure 5. The loops are turned into tail recursion with the state, whose value is preserved between loop cycles, becoming a parameter. This is a standard CSP mechanism.

The strange Circus idiom, *dff_in?tmp* → *(next := tmp)*, precisely captures the semantics of the occam process, in ? next. There is no equivalent in CSP.

The CSP process, *c?x* → *P (x)*, introduces a variable, *x*, whose scope extends only to the process to the right of the arrow. Circus, which incorporates CSP, maintains this semantics and is why we cannot simply write: *dff_in?next* → *Skip*.

Unfortunately, we cannot use the Circus equations of Figure 5 in our work since, currently, model checkers do not exist for this algebra. We must translate into classical CSP to be able to use FDR. There are two ways to do this, although neither is particularly elegant.

The first is to *add* more concurrency, as shown in Figure 6. The explicit Circus variable is modelled by a separate CSP process, running in parallel with the flip-flop. Assignment and reading of the variable are accomplished by channel communications (hidden from the view of users of the flip-flop). The external I/O-PAR structure is explicitly preserved, although it is seriously confused by the internal concurrency.

$$DFF \ (state \in \{0, 1\}) = \mathbf{var} \ next \in \{0, 1\} \ \bullet$$
$$(dff\_out!state \rightarrow Skip \ ||| \ dff\_in?tmp \rightarrow (next := tmp));$$
$$clock \rightarrow DFF \ (next)$$
$$DFLIPFLOP = DFF \ (0)$$

$$TFF \ (state \in \{0, 1\}) = \mathbf{var} \ flip \in \{0, 1\} \ \bullet$$
$$(tff\_out!state \rightarrow Skip \ ||| \ tff\_in?tmp \rightarrow (flip := tmp));$$
$$clock \rightarrow if \ (flip = 0) \ then \ TFF \ (state) \ else \ TFF \ (1 - state)$$
$$TFLIPFLOP = TFF \ (0)$$

Figure 5: The Circus D-type and T-type flip-flops

$VARIABLE\ (value)\ =\ (put?x \rightarrow VARIABLE\ (x)\ \square\ get!value \rightarrow VARIABLE\ (value))$

$DFF\ (state)\ =\ (dff\_out!state \rightarrow Skip\ |||\ dff\_in?tmp \rightarrow put!tmp \rightarrow Skip);$
$\qquad\qquad\qquad clock \rightarrow get?next \rightarrow DFF\ (next)$
$DFLIPFLOP\ =\ (DFF\ (0)\quad ||\quad VARIABLE\ (0))\ \backslash\ \{put, get\}$
$\qquad\qquad\qquad\qquad _{\{put,\ get\}}$

$TFF\ (state)\ =\ (tff\_out!state \rightarrow Skip\ |||\ tff\_in?tmp \rightarrow put!tmp \rightarrow Skip);$
$\qquad\qquad\qquad clock \rightarrow get?flip \rightarrow if\ (flip = 0)\ then\ TFF\ (state)\ else\ TFF\ (1 - state)$
$TFLIPFLOP\ =\ (TFF\ (0)\quad ||\quad VARIABLE\ (0))\ \backslash\ \{put, get\}$
$\qquad\qquad\qquad\qquad _{\{put,\ get\}}$

Figure 6: The CSP D-type and T-type flip-flops – version 1

In fact, we prefer a solution that *removes* the explicit I/O-PAR concurrency, leaving sets of external choices whose input variables retain sufficient scope to complete the recursion – Figure 7. It's not pretty but it yields relatively small state spaces for FDR to search.

$DFF\ (state)\ =\ dff\_out!state \rightarrow dff\_in?next \rightarrow clock \rightarrow DFF\ (next)$
$\qquad\qquad\qquad\quad \square$
$\qquad\qquad\qquad dff\_in?next \rightarrow dff\_out!state \rightarrow clock \rightarrow DFF\ (next)$
$DFLIPFLOP\ =\ DFF\ (0)$

$TFF\ (state)\ =\ tff\_in?1 \rightarrow tff\_out!state \rightarrow clock \rightarrow TFF\ (1 - state)$
$\qquad\qquad\qquad\quad \square$
$\qquad\qquad\qquad tff\_in?0 \rightarrow tff\_out!state \rightarrow clock \rightarrow TFF\ state)$
$\qquad\qquad\qquad\quad \square$
$\qquad\qquad\qquad tff\_out!state \rightarrow (tff\_in?1 \rightarrow clock \rightarrow TFF\ (1 - state)$
$\qquad\qquad\qquad\quad \square$
$\qquad\qquad\qquad\qquad tff\_in?0 \rightarrow clock \rightarrow TFF\ (state))$
$TFLIPFLOP\ =\ TFF\ (0)$

Figure 7: The CSP D-type and T-type flip-flops – version 2

3.6   Modelling Higher-Level Circuits with CSP

The flip-flops in Section 3.5 were written according to the I/O-PAR rules in order to fit into the higher-level circuit models of the form shown in Figure 9. We took advantage of the characteristics of the FPGA target architecture of our occam compiler to produce a flip-flop model that only requires a single CSP synchronisation event to signal the transition from one circuit state to the next. We would need to use two clocks in an equivalent occam program, to allow for the distributed nature of the individual clock channels in this environment. Our new model uses considerably fewer states than the original flip-flop built from NAND gates.

The new, behavioural, CSP flip-flop model of Figure 7 replicates the start-up state of real Xilinx FPGAs – all flip-flop values are initialised to zero when they are powered up.

Although true for the 6-NAND flip-flop as well, the new flip-flop follows the *event-based time* model discussed in [24] and [25]. Rather than using specific timed CSP primitives, event-based time relies on the distribution of a global *tock* signal which causes all of the recipients to synchronise, thereby stepping simulated time forward by one cycle.

It was possible to use the trace refinement mechanisms in FDR to prove that the new flip-flop – as well as all of the intermediate versions – behaved identically to the original one, again allowing for their different clocking and setup / hold time regimes. When an implementation process refines a CSP specification, it will not undertake any activities that the specification is not prepared to perform. Trace refinement is the special case where the activities referred to are CSP traces – lists of events. In order to verify that two processes behave identically, one tests that one process refines the second, and that the second refines the first. It is this result that we primarily used to compare our flip-flop designs, after taking account of their different clocking requirements.

Whilst looking to minimise the state that FDR needs to analyse each component, it was also discovered that it would be more economical to compose larger AND and OR gates from combinations of 2-input devices. The CSP combinatorial AND and OR processes were made I/O-SEQ in nature, rather than the I/O-PAR of the NAND gates used in the original experiments. This is valid because they only appear as part of the input logic to the I/O-PAR flip-flop components in our circuits, and thus cannot appear in cycles of solely I/O-SEQ components. This is the condition required in [16] to ensure deadlock freedom – the original NAND circuit had cycles around the NAND gates and thus required them to be I/O-PAR to satisfy this rule.

4 Verifying Compiler Output

Having gained experience with small CSP processes modelling FPGA circuit elements, we went on to examine the output of our occam-to-FPGA compiler in a similar manner. Initially we tested the small occam program that is shown in Figure 8.

```
UINT2 x :                -- a 2-bit unsigned integer, explained below.
WHILE TRUE
  SEQ
    x := x PLUS 1
    DELAY ()             -- a one-cycle delay, explained below.
```

Figure 8: the counter program source code

This program simply loops, incrementing the variable x each time. It separates each addition from the next with a DELAY() process. This is a compiler *built-in* PROC that translates into a guaranteed one-cycle delay. It is introduced here to prevent an optimisation in our compiler from scheduling successive assignments to be executed in consecutive clock cycles – which would have been confusing to debug and analyse at the circuit level.

The program in Figure 8 uses a two-bit, unsigned, value for x – but this could be extended to any number of bits with no impact on the results in this paper. It compiles to produce three edge-triggered D-type flip-flops, which provide the sequencing logic, two T-Type flip-flops which store the two bits of variable x, and a block of combinatorial logic that implements the adder logic for the PLUS operator, together with the gating logic that stores the incremented value when the assignment statement is active. These are shown in Figure 9.

This configuration can be implemented on a CPLD or on an FPGA directly, using its single, common clock. The device manufacturers specify the maximum clock rate for which such a configuration is guaranteed to operate properly. As mentioned in Section 3.6, a single clock process in occam, outputting tock events on a single channel, would need to use a fan-out process to clock each individual flip-flop, and would need to send two clock ticks in each flip-flop cycle to ensure that all of the data values presented to the flip-flops were set-up and held properly.

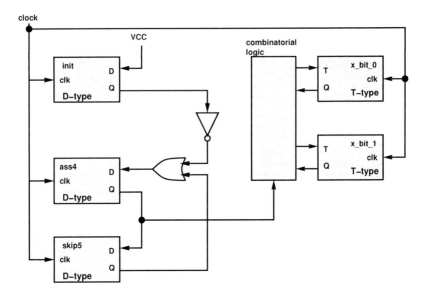

Figure 9: the counter circuit

This circuit was converted into CSP by hand, utilising the flip-flop and combinatorial components described above. Once the technique becomes routine, we intend to produce a CSP output route from our compiler, to generate CSP in FDR's required textual notation automatically.

Using FDR, it was then possible to prove that this circuit was deadlock and livelock free, and to show that the trace of output values of the variable x counted 0, 1, 2, 3, 0, 1, 2, 3, ... , and so on.

Furthermore, it was possible to build a small CSP specification of this counting cycle and to verify, using FDR trace-refinement, that the compiled occam program generates the same sequence of outputs as its specification. This CSP specification is shown in Figure 10.

$$COUNTER = out!0 \rightarrow out!0 \rightarrow out!1 \rightarrow out!1 \rightarrow out!2 \rightarrow out!2 \rightarrow out!3 \rightarrow out!3 \rightarrow COUNTER$$

Figure 10: the CSP specification of the counter process

The CSP *COUNTER* generates output values along a channel, out, whilst the occam program shown in Figure 8 simply stores updated values into the bits of variable x. In order to reconcile these two representations of the counter output, a CSP process has been written to convert the values of the T-type flip-flops into a single channel that carries integer values. This CSP is not illustrated in this paper. The reason that the CSP processes that represent representing flip-flops store *integer* values (i.e. 0 and 1) rather than *Booleans* is due to the complexity of this conversion process. Other ways of converting, outputting and comparing integer values will be explored in the future.

The repetition of the outputs in Figure 10 is required because the simulations are cycle-realistic – and one CSP event takes place on each simulated clock cycle. The repeated operations are caused by the DELAY() process in the original program shown in Figure 8. In occam programs with more complicated timing properties, such as the evaluation of expressions which might take a variable number of cycles, we intend just to compare selected events rather than all of them. This could be done by hiding more of the internal state of the CSP processes before conducting the refinement checks. Of course, cycle-realistic timing might be an important circuit property, for instance in the video output buffer in [4], in which case this behaviour could be examined directly.

There were some initialisation issues in the CSP simulation of the circuit, which showed up as extra values emitted on the outputs of the flip-flops at start-up. These were caused by the internal I/O-PAR nature of the combinatorial components and had to be replicated in the CSP program specification, or avoided by comparing traces of just assignments or just occam channel communications. We have now eliminated them from the generated circuit by using I/O-SEQ processes for the combinatorial components throughout. The flip-flop processes remain I/O-PAR, of course, and thus appear in every cycle of the programs and keep them deadlock-free. Consequently, circuits modelled using CSP specifications generate exactly the same traces in FDR as in the FPGA logic simulator.

Having obtained the CSP results described above, we also implemented this counter circuit in occam, making a high-level simulation of our FPGA circuit. In this case, the flip-flops were still made I/O-PAR, and the combinatorial logic components were I/O-SEQ. Because the FPGA clock signal was represented as a fanned-out group of clock channels, it was theoretically necessary to introduce a double-clock arrangement to ensure that all of the combinatorial elements had completed their actions before the flip-flops triggered to start the next clock cycle. This particular counter circuit is sufficiently regular in operation that the round-robin scheduling of KRoC causes the processes to execute in the right order even without the double-edged clock, but this cannot be guaranteed to happen – future schedulers and multi-processor implementations may be different. The actual occam codes used for the flip-flops in this simulation, therefore, were the same as those in Figure 4 *except* that the `clock ? any` lines are duplicated – i.e. they pause in each cycle for two clock channel communications, corresponding to falling and rising edges in an electronic implementation.

Our counter circuit, manually translated to 240 lines of occam and interfaced to input and output conversion processes, ran perfectly and generated the expected incrementing counter values.

5 Further Work – Channel Communications

While the example in the previous section is very small and simple, it it does demonstrate an endless loop, a simple ripple carry adder, read and write access to a variable, a delay process and sequential composition. Much more important – to the implementation of the compiler – will be correctness proofs of occam channel communication, a circuit's behaviour at the beginning and end of parallel constructs, channel alternation (ALT), and the handling of input and output ports on the periphery of the circuit.

Figure 11 shows the occam source code of a program that explores the relationships between channel communications whose transmitter and receiver become ready in the same cycle, or when the transmitter becomes ready first or when the receiver becomes ready first. The logic circuits generated by our compiler implement the blocking behaviour of the channel communications in these cases. The delays provide additional cycles to ensure that, following the previous synchronising channel communication, the intended process becomes ready first for the next communication. More delays are provided than strictly needed to provide the necessary timing relationships, but the extras allow the operation of the successive channel communications to be completely separated in time – this assists manual inspection of the FPGA simulator and CSP traces. This circuit compiles down to 29 flip-flops with several rather large sum-of-products (AND/OR/NOT) equations.

```
CHAN OF UINT2 a:
PAR
                          UINT2 w, x, y:
      SEQ                 SEQ
         DELAY ()            DELAY ()          -- sender and receiver
         a ! 2               a ? w             -- become ready simultaneously
         DELAY ()            DELAY ()
         a ! 3               DELAY ()          -- sender ready
                             DELAY ()          -- before
                             a ? x             -- receiver
         DELAY ()            DELAY ()
         DELAY ()            a ? y             -- receiver ready
         DELAY ()                              -- before
         a ! 1                                 -- sender
```

Figure 11: A channel communication test *(where the parallel processes have been laid out side-by-side to reflect their timing behaviour)*

It has not yet been possible to generate its CSP equivalent manually. Instead, we have worked on the three separate timing circumstances individually, and these are shown in Figure 12.

```
-- sender first        -- receiver first      -- simultaneous

CHAN OF UINT2 ch:      CHAN OF UINT2 ch:      CHAN OF UINT2 ch:
PAR                    PAR                    PAR

   UINT2 rx:             UINT2 rx:              UINT2 rx:
   SEQ                   SEQ                    SEQ
      DELAY ()              ch ? rx                DELAY ()
      ch ? rx                                      ch ? rx
                          SEQ
   SEQ                      DELAY ()            SEQ
      ch ! 3                ch ! 1                 DELAY ()
                                                   ch ! 2
```

Figure 12: Three channel communication sub-tests

The correct re-use of channel a three times in the original program cannot be tested in the three separate sub-programs, so the verification of the combined program in Figure 11, possibly with some of the DELAY()s removed, will still be required to provide complete confidence of the compiler's generation of the channel communication logic. Verifying the re-use of variables and channels is just the sort of proof for which this CSP technique will be most useful. In practice, using separate channels in Figure 11 would reduce the gating logic considerably and would be the preferred choice. Similarly, if a variable is used to store two independent values at different times in the execution of a program, it is usually beneficial to use two variables when the program is compiled to FPGA. Indeed, a source-code-level optimiser could identify where separate channels or variables would be more economical than re-used ones and spawn the separate instances appropriately.

The three occam programs in Figure 12 compile to 8, 8 and 10 flip-flops, respectively. The re-use of channel a, as well as the replicated start-up logic, explains why the number of flip-flops does not sum to 29.

These three programs were laboriously hand-converted to CSP – yielding files of approximately 1100, 1100 and 1200 lines of machine-readable CSP in the three cases. The three programs are very similar – essentially the simultaneous one has two delays before communication starts on the channels, and the other two have one of these delays removed. Careful use of the FDR `sbisim()` compression routine is able to keep the state space manageable in these cases, and the trace refinements take around five to ten seconds each (on a modestly-powerful PC). In each case, the value transmitted is seen to arrive in the bits of the destination variable.

Since enlargement of the circuits being verified very quickly leads to a huge number of circuit states being explored in FDR, we have developed informal strategies for combining the CSP representations of circuit components, using `sbisim()`, in an efficient manner. Basically, pairs of gates that share relatively few inputs, and that are directly connected by signals that do not propagate anywhere else, are good candidates for compression. However, it does not yet appear to be straightforward to automate this activity in our compiler.

6   Conclusions

So far, it has been possible to demonstrate that small occam programs, compiled into digital logic circuits suitable for running on FPGAs, have the same behaviours as their CSP specifications. The stages used to construct these assertions may be traced back to the most basic fundamentals of digital logic, and these building blocks are very small and thus also easy to justify as correct on pragmatic grounds. Our experience is that logic circuits that have undergone analysis using these techniques behave predictably and correctly on real hardware.

The scheme introduced above shows considerable promise in allowing circuits generated from occam programs to be validated. This is currently being exploited to automate the reference-testing of successive iterations of the compiler. In addition, it is possible to verify complete parallel processes, together with their simple test harnesses, before building them into embedded systems. Provided that the compiler's composition logic has also been verified, this should provide considerable confidence that the embedded programs are accurate.

Jonathan Phillips and Dyke Stiles at Utah State University are working on the automated translation of an occam-like subset of CSP to Handel-C [11], for onward translation to FPGA logic. The work reported in this paper could provide an interesting verification route for their developments, too.

Acknowledgements

We would like to thank Peter Welch, Dyke Stiles, Jim Woodcock and Alistair McEwan for their discussions and the suggestions that they have made – directly and indirectly – during the production of this paper.

References

[1] INMOS Limited. Occam2 Reference Manual. Prentice-Hall, 1988. ISBN 0-13-629312-3.

[2] I. Page & W. Luk. Compiling occam into FPGAs. In W. Moore & W. Luk, eds, *FPGAs* , pages 271-283, Abingdon EE&CS books, 1991.

[3] C.A.R. Hoare. Communicating Sequential Processes. Prentice-Hall, 1985, ISBN 0-13-153289-8.

[4] R.M.A. Peel & B.M. Cook. Occam on Field Programmable Gate Arrays - Fast Prototyping of Parallel Embedded Systems In H.R. Arabnia, ed, *the Proceedings of the International Conference on Parallel and*

Distributed Processing Techniques and Applications (PDPTA'2000), pages 2523-2529, CSREA Press, June 2000. ISBN 1-892512-51-3.

[5]   Formal Systems (Europe) Ltd., Oxford. Failures-Divergence Refinement – the FDR User Manual, version 2.80. 2003.

[6]   Refer to www.xilinx.com for datasheets and product overviews on the Xilinx Virtex-II Pro.

[7]   Peter Bellows and Brad Hutchings. JHDL – An HDL for Reconfigurable Systems. in *Proceedings of the IEEE Symposium on Field-Programmable Custom Computing Machines*, April 1998.

[8]   Stuart Swan. An Introduction to System Level Modeling in SystemC 2.0. available at http://www.systemc.org/projects/sitedocs/document/v201_White_Paper/en/1, 2001, referenced July 2004.

[9]   Ian Page et al. Advanced Silicon Prototyping in a Reconfigurable Environment. in P.H. Welch et al., eds, *Proceedings of WoTUG-21*, pages 81 - 92, IOS Press, Amsterdam, 1998, ISBN 90-5199-391-9.

[10] S. Knapp. Accelerate FPGA Macros with One-Hot Approach. in *Electronic Design*, 13th Sept. 1990.

[11] J.D. Phillips. An Automatic Translation of CSP to Handel-C. M.Sc. Thesis, Utah State University, 2004.

[12] V. Raju, L. Rong and G.S. Stiles. Automatic Conversion of CSP to CTJ, JCSP, and CCSP. in Jan F. Broenink and Gerald H. Hilderink, eds, *Communicating Process Architectures 2003*, pages 63-81, IOS Press, Amsterdam, 2003, ISBN 1-58603-381-6.

[13] J. Pascoe and R. Loader. Consolidating The Agreement Problem Protocol Verification Environment. in *Communicating Process Architectures 2002*. IOS Press, Amsterdam, 2002, ISBN 1-58603-268-2.

[14] D.A. Nicole, S. Ellis and S.Hancock. occam for reliable embedded systems: lightweight runtime and model checking. in *Communicating Process Architectures 2003*, pages 167-172, IOS Press, Amsterdam, 2003, ISBN 1-58603-381-6.

[15] D.C. Wood and P.H. Welch. The Kent Retargettable occam Compiler. in *Proceedings of WoTUG-19*, pages 143-166, IOS Press, Amsterdam, April 1996, ISBN 90-5199-261-0.

[16] P.H. Welch. Emulating Digital Logic using Transputer Networks (very high parallelism = simplicity = performance). in *Proc. PARLE'87 – Parallel Architectures and Languages Europe*, pages 357-373, Springer-Verlag, 1987.

[17] P.H. Welch and G.R. Justo. On the serialisation of parallel programs. in J. Edwards, ed, *Proceedings of WoTUG-14*, pages 159-180, IOS Press, Amsterdam, 1991, ISBN 90-5199-063-4.

[18] P.H. Welch, G.R. Justo, and C.J. Willcock. Higher-Level Paradigms for Deadlock-Free High-Performance Systems. In *Transputer Applications and Systems '93*, pages 981–1004, Aachen, Germany, September 1993. IOS Press, Netherlands. ISBN 90-5199-140-1.

[19] J.M.R. Martin, I. East, and S. Jassim. Design Rules for Deadlock Freedom. *Transputer Communications*, 3(2):121–133, September 1994. John Wiley and Sons. 1070-454X.

[20] J.M.R. Martin and P.H. Welch. A Design Strategy for Deadlock-Free Concurrent Systems. *Transputer Communications*, 3(4):215–232, October 1996. John Wiley and Sons. 1070-454X.

[21] Texas Instruments. The TTL Data Book. 3rd edition, 1979 (ISBN 0-904047-27-X).

[22] A.L.C. Cavalcanti, A.C.A. Sampaio, and J.C.P. Woodcock. A Refinement Strategy for Circus. *Formal Aspects of Computing*, 15(2-3):146–181, November 2003.

[23] M. Oliveira, A.L.C. Cavalcanti, and J. Woodcock. Refining Industrial Scale Systems in Circus. In *Communicating Process Architectures 2004*, WoTUG-27, ISSN 1383-7575, pages 281–309, IOS Press, Amsterdam, The Netherlands, September 2004.

[24] A.W. Roscoe. The Theory and Practice of Concurrency. Prentice Hall, 1998.

[25] Steve Schneider. *Concurrent and Real-Time Systems: the CSP approach*, John Wiley & Sons Ltd., 2000

Communicating Process Architectures 2004
Ian East, Jeremy Martin, Peter Welch, David Duce, and Mark Green (Eds.)
IOS Press, 2004

Focusing on Traces to Link $\mathcal{VCR}$ and CSP

Marc L. SMITH

Department of Computer Science, Colby College, Waterville, Maine 04901-8858, USA

Abstract. View-Centric Reasoning ($\mathcal{VCR}$) replaces CSP's [1] *perfect observer* with multiple, possibly imperfect observers. To employ view-centric reasoning within existing CSP models [2] requires a bookkeeping change. Specifically, $\mathcal{VCR}$ [3] introduces parallel events as a new primitive for constructing traces, and distinguishes two types of traces: histories and views. Previously, we gave the operational semantics of $\mathcal{VCR}$ [4], and demonstrated the utility of parallel traces to reason for the first time unambiguously about the meaning of the Linda predicate operations rdp() and inp(). The choice of using an operational semantics to describe $\mathcal{VCR}$ makes direct comparison with CSP difficult; therefore, work is ongoing to recast $\mathcal{VCR}$ denotationally, then link $\mathcal{VCR}$ with the other CSP models within Hoare and He's *Unifying Theories of Programming* [5]. Initial efforts in this direction [6] led to a comparison of $\mathcal{VCR}$ with Lawrence's $\mathcal{HCSP}$ [7]. In this paper, we present some recent insights and abstractions – inspired by modern quantum physics – that have emerged whilst contemplating parallel traces in light of the unifying theories. These insights lead to a more natural expression of $\mathcal{VCR}$ traces, in the sense that they more closely resemble CSP traces, thus forming a basis for linking $\mathcal{VCR}$ and CSP.

1 Introduction

According to Hoare and He [5], a programming theory consists of elements from three orthogonal dimensions. First, there is a set of primitive concepts, or *alphabet*, at some desired level of abstraction. Elements of an alphabet are those variables and constants that may be used in the specification of, or observed during the execution of, a program. Second, the *signature* of a programming theory is the set of primitive statements, and rules for statement composition, that may be used to specify programs. Third, a theory has a mathematical foundation, with a corresponding set of provable equations, or *laws*, that aid in the design of programs with desired properties. To compare two or more programming theories, one compares elements of their respective alphabets, signatures, and laws. Programming theories are unified by their shared elements and differentiated by their unique (relative to each other) elements. To link one theory of programming to another is to relate the two somehow, e.g., a subset or refinement relationship.

The main thrust of Hoare and He's Unifying Theories of Programming (UToP) [5] is to develop links between different theories of programming, within the discipline of computing science. Establishing these links between all theories of programming is the basis for Hoare and He's grand challenge of unification (in much the same way that Physics seeks to discover a Grand Unified Theory that accounts for all four known fundamental forces in the universe). UToP is thus not a completed body of work, but rather, a thorough and important starting point for ongoing research. View-centric reasoning ($\mathcal{VCR}$) [3] wasn't initially developed with UToP in mind; instead, $\mathcal{VCR}$ was based on CSP [1]. $\mathcal{VCR}$ replaced CSP's interleaved trace of a single observer with the *views* (traces of non-interleaved, parallel events) of multiple, possibly imperfect observers. In support of this grand challenge of unification, the current goal is to both define $\mathcal{VCR}$ as its own programming theory and link it to existing CSP models within UToP. Indeed, CSP is one of the theories of programming illuminated in UToP, and it is linked as a subtheory of other theories of programming.

The approach of this paper departs from Smith et al. [6], where the authors began to establish links between $\mathcal{VCR}$ and Lawrence's $\mathcal{HCSP}$ [7]. $\mathcal{HCSP}$ has merged events and bags, similar in spirit to $\mathcal{VCR}$'s parallel events. Our justification for this former approach was that it made sense to link to a CSP model that has $\mathcal{VCR}$'s abstraction of parallel events. However, linking to $\mathcal{HCSP}$ represented more work than linking to the Traces model of CSP, $\mathcal{T}$, and $\mathcal{VCR}$'s abstractions were originally meant to extend $\mathcal{T}$. The work to link $\mathcal{VCR}$ to $\mathcal{T}$ is ongoing, and not presented in this paper, but new insights into traces have emerged, consistent with the approach of UToP and the theories of modern quantum physics UToP embraces, as cited in UToP [5]. Ultimately, linking $\mathcal{VCR}$ to $\mathcal{T}$ will satisfy the desire to characterize $\mathcal{VCR}$ in a way that is most accessible to the CSP community, thus permitting a more direct basis for comparison.

The remainder of this paper is organized as follows. Section 2 gives background information concerning UToP's perspectives on observation of computation within an environment, as well as the history and major tenets of $\mathcal{VCR}$. Section 3 contains the heart of this paper, describing a new characterization of traces. We conclude and discuss future work in Section 5.

2   Background

Before we present a new characterization of recording traces, some background information is in order. Beyond the information presented in this section, the reader is encouraged to consult the complete treatments of Hoare and He's Unifying Theories of Programming (UToP) [5] and Smith et al.'s View-Centric Reasoning ($\mathcal{VCR}$) [8, 4]. Section 2.1 emphasizes those aspects of UToP impacted by the inclusion of View-Centric Reasoning ($\mathcal{VCR}$) into the unifying theories. Pertinent aspects of $\mathcal{VCR}$ are introduced in Section 2.2.

2.1   *UToP Perspectives on Environment and Observation*

Hoare and He present theories of reactive processes in their Unifying Theories of Programming [5]. In terms of linking theories of programming, the theory of reactive processes is a subtheory of the imperative theory of designs; CSP is a further subtheory of the theory of reactive processes. The notion of environment is elucidated early in this presentation, as environment is essential to theories of reactive processes, examples of which include CSP and its derivative models. Essentially, the environment is the medium within which processes compute. Equivalently, the environment is the medium within which processes may be observed. The behavior of a sequential process may be sufficiently described by making observations only of its inputs and corresponding outputs. In contrast, the behavior of a reactive process may require additional intermediate observations.

Regarding these observations, Hoare and He borrow insight from modern quantum physics. Namely, they view the act of observation to be an interaction between a process and one or more observers in the environment. Furthermore, the roles of observers in the environment may be (and often are) played by the processes themselves! As one would expect, an interaction between such processes often affects the behavior of the processes involved.

A process, in its role as observer, may sequentially record the interactions in which it participates. Recall participation includes the act of observation. Naturally, in an environment of multiple reactive processes, simultaneous interactions may be observed. Hoare and He define a *trace* as "the sequence of interactions recorded up to some given moment in time." Thus a trace represents an ongoing chronological record of observable events that occur within the environment of a program's execution. Traditionally, simultaneous events are recorded in some arbitrary order, since traces are considered partially, not totally, ordered. An event that represents the synchronization of multiple processes is recorded once. It is sometimes useful to consider the occurrence of an individual event to be synchronization with the environment. Likewise, an observer could be the environment, or a process within the environment.

2.2   Origins and Evolution of VCR

View-Centric Reasoning was inspired by Hoare's CSP [1]. In particular, the central role traces play in reasoning about the behavior of processes, and the metaphor of a computation's history being recorded by an idealized observer were the basis for VCR, before learning of Hoare and He's UToP. In its original form, view-centric reasoning was a parameterized operational semantics for reasoning about properties of concurrency. That is, VCR was a meta model, capable of individual instantiation via parameter specification: by passing in different sets of parameter values to VCR's operational semantics, the VCR semantics could assume the characteristics of other existing models of concurrency. The idea of developing a meta model was inspired by the author's desire to discover abstractions common to all models of parallel and distributed computation. The author does not claim to have discovered all common abstractions for concurrency, but indeed, many abstractions and parameters emerged, and VCR was successfully instantiated for two very different models of concurrency: Agha's Actors [9] and Gelernter's Linda [10]. For more information about early work on VCR, see Smith [3] and more recently Smith et al. [4, 8].

From the beginning, the inspiration for VCR has been Hoare's CSP [1], and the elegance of using traces to reason about properties of computation. Still, VCR departed from CSP in several noticeable ways: the operational semantics; multiple, possibly imperfect observers (in contrast to CSP's perfect observer, an imperfect observer is capable of occasionally "blinking," and thus nondeterministically miss recording zero or more events); parallel events to obviate the need for arbitrary interleaving; and the distinction of a computation's history and views. In VCR's operational semantics, CSP's rich process algebra was abstracted away; processes were represented at a higher level of abstraction by their continuations. These process continuations were interpreted by meaning functions, as part of VCR's transition relation; that is, upon invocation, given a process's continuation, a meaning function simulates computational progress, returning the process's new continuation and any resulting observable events of interprocess communication. VCR, not surprisingly, focused solely on constructing a computation's history and views to support view-centric reasoning. Using an operational semantics for VCR was an excellent choice for reasoning at this level of abstraction.

Since the environment as well as the processes within the environment could all be observers of a program's computation, VCR permits these multiple observers to each record their own trace. Furthermore, to account for the multiple, possibly imperfect perspectives, VCR introduces some bookkeeping changes. Recognizing the possibility of event simultaneity in the absence of synchronization, and the possibility for different perspectives among observers, unordered and ordered parallel events become the new primitives for recording traces in VCR. A parallel event is represented as a multiset of events. Furthermore, two types of traces are distinguished: histories and views. A computation's history is a trace that consists of a sequence of unordered parallel events. Multiple views may be constructed from a given history, in the form of traces that consist of sequences of correspondingly ordered parallel events.

Around the time of Smith et al. [4] several points became clear. First, Hoare and He's Unifying Theories of Programming (UToP) [5] shared the goals of VCR, but encompassed a far broader range of concerns. Next, UToP was more mature than $\mathcal{VCR}$, and already well established. Finally, there were important benefits to linking $\mathcal{VCR}$ with the other CSP theories of programming within UToP, and UToP explicitly addresses linking together theories of programming. This last point revealed a notable disadvantage to continuing to develop $\mathcal{VCR}$ solely as an operational semantics. To draw $\mathcal{VCR}$ within the unifying theories, it would have to be expressed in the alphabetized relational calculus, and so began the authors' efforts to do so in Smith et al. [6].

3   Revisiting the CSP Trace

The original CSP metaphor concerning traces involves an infallible observer who watches a process performing a computation. Each time an observable event occurs, the observer faithfully records the event's name in a notebook. The events are recorded in the order they occur; thus the trace is chronologically ordered... almost. We are instructed to disregard the possibility that two or more events may occur simultaneously, since the observer will merely record all such events in some arbitrary sequence. Thus, to be more precise, CSP traces are partially ordered, chronologically. Consider the following example of a CSP trace:

$$tr = \langle a, b, c, d, e, f, g \rangle$$

The interpretation of trace tr is pronounced, "a then b then c...". But when reasoning about tr it is not clear which consecutive events occurred sequentially, and which consecutive events (if any) appeared to occur simultaneously from the olympian observer's frame of reference (true simultaneity, not just the perception of simultaneity by a single observer, is problematic in light of relativity, and the inspiration for views in $\mathcal{VCR}$). Since tr is partially ordered, rather than delimit the events of tr with commas, it might be clearer to delimit tr's events with the partial order relation, $\leq$, thus representing both possibilities. For further clarity, we could decorate this relation with a subscripted c, $\leq_c$, to reflect the chronological nature of the partial order. Once again, the same CSP trace, newly delimited:

$$tr' = \langle a \leq_c b \leq_c c \leq_c d \leq_c e \leq_c f \leq_c g \rangle$$

The interpretation of trace tr' is pronounced, "a before-or-with b before-or-with c...". It is reasonable to wonder what is accomplished by substituting the event delimiters of the trace. It would seem nothing, beyond the acknowledgment of two chronological possibilities between consecutive events in the original tr. If only we could look more closely at each individual $\leq_c$ relation in tr', and discern which of the two possibilities holds. Indeed, there is a way. Recall the CSP observer: as each event occurs, the observer *knows* in that instant whether it occurred in sequence or simultaneously with other events. In other words, total order knowledge existed even though it isn't preserved in CSP's partial order traces.

To overcome this obstacle, we borrow an abstraction from modern quantum physics: superposition. Consider $\leq_c$ to be a *quantum relation*, and instances of $\leq_c$ in tr' to be in a state of superposition. That is, for each $\leq_c$ in tr', *both* "$<_c$" and "$=_c$" remain possible states, until one relation or the other is observed upon reasoning about tr'. The observed underlying state for each $\leq_c$ relation would correspond to the CSP observer's knowledge at the time its related events were recorded. Once each $\leq_c$ relation has been observed in tr', the partially ordered trace becomes a total ordering (a "strict" interleaving) and might for example look like this:

$$tr'' = \langle a <_c b =_c c <_c d =_c e =_c f <_c g \rangle$$

The interpretation of trace tr'' is pronounced, "a before b-with-c before d-with-e-with-f before g." It is straightforward to see that trace tr'' would be equivalently expressed in a $\mathcal{VCR}$ history trace like this:

$$tr'' = \langle \{a\}, \{b,c\}, \{d,e,f\}, \{g\} \rangle$$

where event multisets represent parallel events. From either of the above two forms of tr'', $\mathcal{VCR}$ views of the other, possibly imperfect, observers (represented as lists of lists, or lists of traces) could be generated. The inner traces in $\mathcal{VCR}$ are called ROPEs (Randomly Ordered Parallel Events). Here are some of the many possible views of tr'':

$$\langle \langle a \rangle, \langle b,c \rangle, \langle d,e,f \rangle, \langle g \rangle \rangle$$

$$\langle \langle a \rangle, \langle b,c \rangle, \langle d,f,e \rangle, \langle g \rangle \rangle$$

$$\langle \langle a \rangle, \langle b,c \rangle, \langle f,e,d \rangle, \langle g \rangle \rangle$$

$$\langle \langle a \rangle, \langle b,c \rangle, \langle e,d,f \rangle, \langle g \rangle \rangle$$

$$\langle \langle a \rangle, \langle c,b \rangle, \langle d,e,f \rangle, \langle g \rangle \rangle$$

$$\langle \langle a \rangle, \langle c,b \rangle, \langle d,f \rangle, \langle \rangle \rangle$$

Furthermore, the views of tr'' could also be expressed in the strict interleaving form of tr'', thus avoiding the additional syntax required by a list of ROPEs:

$$\langle a <_c b =_c c <_c d =_c e =_c f <_c g \rangle$$

$$\langle a <_c b =_c c <_c d =_c f =_c e <_c g \rangle$$

$$\langle a <_c b =_c c <_c f =_c e =_c d <_c g \rangle$$

$$\langle a <_c b =_c c <_c e =_c d =_c f <_c g \rangle$$

$$\langle a <_c c =_c b <_c d =_c e =_c f <_c g \rangle$$

$$\langle a <_c c =_c b <_c d =_c f \rangle$$

There is at least one disadvantage to this new form of views, namely, the ability to reason about imperfect observation is limited in the case of empty ROPEs (compare the corresponding last views, where event g is missing).

Before we leave this new approach to recording traces, some overall characterization is desirable. There is more than one way to proceed from here. Briefly, we describe two.

For the first characterization, let the Olympian CSP observer record the trace of a computation, introducing no changes to existing CSP models. Thus, for some computing process P, let

$$tr \in traces(P)$$

where tr's partially ordered elements are as before. Since tr is partially ordered, chronologically, we can immediately represent the trace of events, tr', delimited by $\leq_c$ relations rather than as a comma-separated list:

$$tr' = \langle a \leq_c b \leq_c c \leq_c d \leq_c e \leq_c f \leq_c g \rangle$$

Next, we could consider a focus oracle, $focus()$, whose domain is the set of partially ordered CSP traces, and whose range is the set of totally ordered (strictly interleaved) traces, as before. The focus oracle magically reveals the state of each $\leq_c$ relation that corresponds to what the CSP observer witnessed when recording tr. Thus,

$$focus(tr') = \langle a <_c b =_c c <_c d =_c e =_c f <_c g \rangle$$

If the thought of utilizing the quantum physics abstraction of superposition seems troublesome, we offer one additional interpretation, from Computer Science: There is a sense in which the tr' trace is a lazy data structure, whose $\leq$'s are not yet elaborated. Under this premise, the focus oracle merely elaborates those parts of the trace not yet elaborated. The oracle is still magic, and correctly focuses on the total ordering known to the CSP observer.

For the second characterization, let the *environment* of P be a distinguished observer who records traces directly as a total order with "<" and "=" to delimit recorded events, rather than the comma-separated trace of the CSP observer. That is, the environment is implicitly able to observe each quantum "$\leq$" and record the observed operator.

Conveniently, both approaches characterized are equally backward-compatible with CSP simply by replacing "$<_c$"s and "$=_c$"s with commas in the totally ordered trace. Thus any trace analyzed using view-centric reasoning is also analyzable with the other existing CSP models.

4   Motivating Parallel Events

Given the unqualified success of CSP's approach to representing concurrency via sequentially interleaved traces, it is reasonable to ask, why introduce parallel events at all? One reason is that it is not always possible to determine from an interleaved trace, or even the set of all such possible traces, of a computation, whether two or more events occurred simultaneously (that is, simultaneously from the CSP observer's frame of reference). The best way to illustrate this point is with a degenerate example. Consider the interleaved trace:

$$\langle a, a, a, a, a \rangle$$

This is a degenerate example because the set of all possible traces of this computation would be a singleton containing just the above trace. Now suppose what we wished to reason about is the degree of parallelism that occurred during this computation. Using our new approach to focusing on this trace, we quickly realize many actual possibilities exist. For example:

$$\langle a <_c a <_c a <_c a <_c a \rangle$$

$$\langle a =_c a <_c a <_c a <_c a \rangle$$

$$\langle a =_c a =_c a <_c a <_c a \rangle$$

$$\langle a <_c a =_c a =_c a <_c a \rangle$$

$$\langle a =_c a <_c a =_c a <_c a \rangle$$

Clearly, these are not all the possibilities. Yet not one of these possibilities could be identified – with certainty – from the given comma-delimited, interleaved trace as the actual corresponding computation recorded by the CSP observer.

Perhaps a more practical example deserves the attention of $\mathcal{VCR}$'s parallel event semantics. I/O-PAR (and I/O-SEQ) are design patterns described by Welch, Martin and others in [11, 12, 13, 14]. The reason these design patterns are appealing is because *arbitrary topology* networks of I/O-PAR processes are guaranteed to be deadlock/livelock free, and thus they are desirable components for building systems (or parts of systems).

Informally, a process P is considered I/O-PAR if it operates deterministically and cyclically, such that, once per cycle, it synchronizes in parallel on all the events in its alphabet. For example, processes P and Q, given by the following CSP equations, are I/O-PAR:

$$P = (a \rightarrow SKIP \ ||| \ b \rightarrow SKIP); \ P$$

$$Q = (b \rightarrow SKIP \ ||| \ c \rightarrow SKIP); \ Q$$

Using the focused trace notation presented in this paper, the traces of P and Q are, respectively, all prefixes of tr_P and tr_Q:

$$tr_P = \langle a =_c b <_c a =_c b <_c a =_c b <_c \ \ldots \rangle$$

$$tr_Q = \langle b =_c c <_c b =_c c <_c b =_c c <_c \ \ldots \rangle$$

Notice how elegantly these focused traces capture the essence of the behavior of processes P and Q. If one were to attempt to represent the behavior of P and Q using traditional comma-separated traces, the effort would be more tedious and cumbersome.

5   Conclusions and Future Work

This paper presented recent insights into the nature of CSP's traces that emerged while studying Hoare and He's Unified Theories of Programming. The goal of expressing $\mathcal{VCR}$ in the alphabetized relational calculus and linking a $\mathcal{VCR}$ theory of programming to existing CSP models in the unifying theories remains. However, we are much closer to our goal now that we've identified ways to map from classic CSP traces to the parallel traces of $\mathcal{VCR}$, via the $focus()$ oracle. Furthermore, we can map back to CSP traces from $\mathcal{VCR}$ traces and views. Finally, we are encouraged by the relationship and resemblance of CSP's traces to those of $\mathcal{VCR}$, and remain optimistic that $\mathcal{VCR}$ will soon be linked within the unifying theories.

While the basis for linking $\mathcal{VCR}$ to CSP is established, work remains to define $\mathcal{VCR}$ as a theory of programming given in the alphabetized relational calculus. Along this path, a new goal has emerged, to extend parallel events from traces alone to the specification of processes that engage directly in parallel events. For example, in Section 4, how would one express process P in terms of parallel events? Furthermore, how would one represent the process that results from pipelining P into Q, and so on? In general, the semantic description of I/O-PAR should benefit from such a desired algebra, one that is capable of manipulating parallel events. Such an abstraction could ultimately help enhance our insights into the design and verification of concurrent systems.

Acknowledgments

Professor Charles E. Hughes and Dr. Rebecca J. Parsons were original collaborators during the development of the $\mathcal{VCR}$ model as a parameterized operational semantics. Professor Jim Woodcock provided valuable feedback for an earlier CPA conference paper [4], as well as the current roadmap toward linking $\mathcal{VCR}$ within the Unifying Theories of Programming. In particular, Professor Peter Welch suggested the I/O-PAR design pattern to motivate and illustrate the value of parallel event semantics, which helped to focus this paper's presentation and point the way toward future work. Finally, the author wishes to thank the anonymous referees, whose remarks and insights helped improve the *focus* and content of this paper.

References

[1] C.A.R. Hoare. *Communicating Sequential Processes*. Prentice Hall International Series in Computer Science. Prentice-Hall International, UK, Ltd., UK, 1985.

[2] A. W. Roscoe. *The Theory and Practice of Concurrency*. Prentice Hall International Series in Computer Science. Prentice Hall Europe, 1998.

[3] Marc L. Smith. *View-centric Reasoning about Parallel and Distributed Computation*. PhD thesis, University of Central Florida, Orlando, Florida 32816-2362, December 2000.

[4] Marc L. Smith, Rebecca J. Parsons, and Charles E. Hughes. View-centric reasoning for linda and tuple space computation. In J. S. Pascoe, P. H. Welch, R. J. Loader, and V. S. Sunderam, editors, *Communicating Process Architectures 2002*, volume 60 of *Concurrent Systems Engineering Series*, pages 223–254, Amsterdam, 2002. IOS Press.

[5] C.A.R. Hoare and Jifeng He. *Unifying Theories of Programming*. Prentice Hall Series in Computer Science. Prentice Hall Europe, 1998.

[6] Marc L. Smith, Charles E. Hughes, and Kyle W. Burke. The denotational semantics of view-centric reasoning. In J.F. Broenink and G.H. Hilderink, editors, *Communicating Process Architectures 2003*, volume 61 of *Concurrent Systems Engineering Series*, pages 91–96, Amsterdam, 2003. IOS Press.

[7] Adrian E. Lawrence. Hcsp: Imperative state and true concurrency. In J. S. Pascoe, P. H. Welch, R. J. Loader, and V. S. Sunderam, editors, *Communicating Process Architectures – 2002*, Concurrent Systems Engineering, pages 39–55, Amsterdam, 2002. IOS Press.

[8] Marc L. Smith, Rebecca J. Parsons, and Charles E. Hughes. View-centric reasoning for linda and tuple space computation. *IEE Proceedings–Software*, 150(2):71–84, apr 2003.

[9] Gul A. Agha. *ACTORS: A Model of Concurrent Computation in Distributed Systems*. The MIT Press Series in Artificial Intelligence. The MIT Press, Cambridge, Massachusetts, 1986.

[10] David Gelernter. Generative communication in linda. *ACM Transactions on Programming Languages and Systems*, 7(1), January 1985.

[11] P.H. Welch. Emulating Digital Logic using Transputer Networks (Very High Parallelism = Simplicity = Performance). *International Journal of Parallel Computing*, 9, January 1989. North-Holland.

[12] P.H. Welch, G.R.R. Justo, and C.J. Willcock. Higher-Level Paradigms for Deadlock-Free High-Performance Systems. In R. Grebe, J. Hektor, S.C. Hilton, M.R. Jane, and P.H. Welch, editors, *Transputer Applications and Systems '93, Proceedings of the 1993 World Transputer Congress*, volume 2, pages 981–1004, Aachen, Germany, September 1993. IOS Press, Netherlands. ISBN 90-5199-140-1.

[13] J.M.R. Martin, I. East, and S. Jassim. Design Rules for Deadlock Freedom. *Transputer Communications*, 3(2):121–133, September 1994. John Wiley and Sons. 1070-454X.

[14] J.M.R. Martin and P.H. Welch. A Design Strategy for Deadlock-Free Concurrent Systems. *Transputer Communications*, 3(4):215–232, October 1996. John Wiley and Sons. 1070-454X.

Communicating Process Architectures 2004
Ian East, Jeremy Martin, Peter Welch, David Duce, and Mark Green (Eds.)
IOS Press, 2004

Design of a Transputer Core and its Implementation in an FPGA

Makoto TANAKA, Naoya FUKUCHI, Yutaka OOKI and Chikara FUKUNAGA

Tokyo Metropolitan University 1-1 Minami-Osawa, Hachoiji, Tokyo, 192-0397, Japan

Abstract. We have made an IP (Intellectual Property) core for the T425 transputer. The same machine instructions as the transputer are executable in this IP core (which we call the TPCORE). To create an IP core for the transputer has two aspects. On one hand, if we could succeed in building our own one and putting it in an FPGA (or VLSI chip), we could apply it as a core processor in a distributed system. On the other hand, if we can extend our transputer development from a very conventional one to more sophisticated ones, as Inmos proceeded to the T9000, we hope to find technological breakthroughs for the bottlenecks that the original transputer had – such as the restriction of the number of communication channels. It is important to have an IP core for the transputer. Although the TPCORE uses the same register set with the same functionality as the transputer and follows the same mechanisms for the link communication between two processes and interrupt handling, the implementation must be very different from original transputer. We have extensively used micro-code ROM to describe any states that the TPCORE must take. Using this micro-code ROM for the state transition description, we could implement the TPCORE economically on FPGA space and achieve efficient performance.

1 Introduction

The transputer was once widely used as a core processor in parallel or distributed systems extensively all over the world in the 1980s. However as Inmos Ltd. of the day could not supply a new generation transputer in the early 1990s in timely manner, many users gave up using the transputer as a core processor of their parallel systems or were forced to look for architectures other than a parallel one for their applications.

There may be still many people like the authors themselves who hope to run occam codes developed for transputers or to design a parallel system with occam. Although the occam compiler has been evolved and facilitated to execute on a Linux machine (KRoC , the Kent Retargettable occam Compiler project [1]), we could not find easily a hardware object, which is optimized for occam execution like the transputer – even though the technology of hardware implementation on silicon has significantly developed.

We have two motivations to have an IP core of transputer: one is an intention still to apply the transputer in our home-made distributed systems; and the other one is an intention to make a start point to find a solution for new transputer architecture rather than T9000. If we have the IP core, we may be able to try to find our way to overcome, for example, the case of an excess of the number of communication channels over the number of physical links between processes running in different transputers; we may propose new schemes for load distribution and scheduling algorithms; and we may find an idea for a fast cross-bar switching algorithm by implementing multiple cores into one chip.

In order to develop such a processor like an occam machine, we have firstly analyzed the instruction set of transputer T425 and tried to resolve every instruction in detail, which has been not described explicitly in the data sheet [2]. We then made an IP core (TPCORE), using Verilog/VHDL, to be able to process all the instruction set of T425. We have aimed to construct an IP core which can run an occam program compiled, linked, loaded and downloaded with the transputer toolset developed by Inmos [3]. We then made a realization of TPCORE using FPGA, and carried out some performance tests. We report in this article TPCORE development, logical structures we have chosen, hardware implementation for the CPU, link, interrupt and process control blocks. Finally, we present some results of performance for the execution of occam programs, which were compiled with occ.

2   Fundamental Architecture of TPCORE

The overall block diagram of TPCORE is shown in Figure 1. TPCORE comprises a CPU, a Link block, Memory Controller and Memory. The memory consists of four 4Kbyte blocks. The Link block has four interfaces (link) to communicate (exchange data) with other TP-COREs.

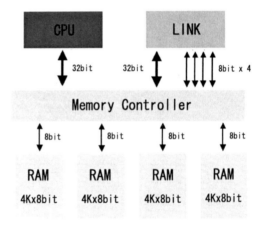

Figure 1: TPCORE block diagram

2.1   Memory Controller

The memory controller accepts either the memory access requests from the CPU or from the link interfaces, and adjusts the requests according to the specification of the the memory (device) actually embedded in an FPGA. In this way we can simply modify the verilog code for the memory controller and keep the CPU and link block untouched even if we implement TPCORE in another FPGA which has a different memory device of the size or data transfer technology.

The memory controller manages one address and one data bus. Although the address space can be extended over about 4GB, which is expressed with 32 bits, presently we use only 15 bits for the address specification (32kB space). In the original transputer, there was a special address space, which we could access it with faster cycle than the other address space. TPCORE handles, however, all the address space uniformly.

We have not made a dedicated communication bus between the CPU and the link. The data exchange between them is performed using the common data bus managed by the memory controller. If the link block occupies the memory block for communication with external modules, execution in the CPU is blocked.

2.2 CPU

The block diagram of the CPU is shown in Figure 2. The address and data buses shown in the figure are controlled by the memory block. In order to follow the instruction set of the transputer as much as possible, we implement six almost identical registers in TPCORE. These registers are the instruction pointer (Iptr), the operand (Oreg), the work space pointer (Wptr), and three stack registers (Areg, Breg and Creg). We have given these registers identical roles to the ones of transputer. The value stored in Wptr is recognized as Process ID for a process. The CPU block uses this value to make a local address for the process. The local address for the process is set using Oreg and the lower 4bit of Iptr in addition to Wptr. The least significant bit is used to distinguish the process priority.

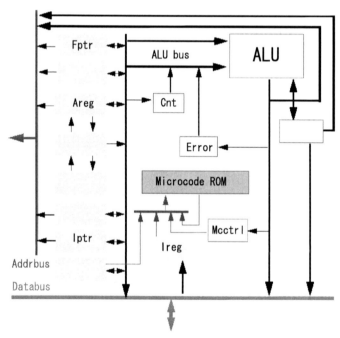

Figure 2: CPU block diagram

Beside these six registers, we have prepared (private) registers for the error handling (Error), loop counting (Cnt), and temporal data storage (Temp). Although the existence of these registers has not been described explicitly in various transputer data books, it is naturally required to be installed in a CPU object. We have implemented them in order not to influence other logic structures reconstructed though the references. Especially we have carefully designed the arithmetic logical unit (ALU) concerning these private registers. ALU has two input and two output streams. As shown in Figure 2, the register Cnt will be an input, and Temp will be an output while Error will be either input or output source of ALU.

Table 1: Micro-code ROM 64bit specification

bit number	Contents
63–61	Not used
60,55,36-33	Condition branch for the micro-code ROM
59–57	memory access privilege
56,54	Behavior of the Link interfaces
53-50	Output destination for the data bus
49-37,23	Behavior of various registers
32-24	Input source selection for ALU
22,21	Input selection for the address bus
20-17	Input selection for the data bus
16-14	Process priority
13-9	Instruction code for ALU
8-0	Next address of the micro-code ROM

2.3   State Transition Table in Micro-code ROM

All possible states described with items listed in Table 1 in all the components of TPCORE (the memory controller, the link block, and the CPU) are stored in the micro-code ROM. The micro-code ROM has the depth of 512 and the width of 64bit.

We have found two advantages to use the micro-code ROM for description of states and their transitions; one is that we can modify and adjust performance of an instruction by changing appropriate bits of the appropriate address of the micro-code ROM without modifying the verilog code of TPCORE, and the another one is that we can reduce the FPGA space since we pack all the state transitions into an internally embedded memory, and we do not need to install state transition machines into the FPGA wired-space.

Several examples of the contents of the micro-code ROM are given below.

Instruction Fetch State
In order to fetch the instruction to be executed next:

1. Iptr must be selected to Input for the address bus in which Iptr contains the address for the next instruction,

2. memory must be selected to the source for the data bus since the address to be executed next which is kept in Iptr must loaded on the address bus,

3. Ireg must be set to the output destination for the data bus, and

4. the next address of the micro-code ROM must be set to 0x001 to go to the instruction decode state.

The specification is given in this state and is described in the micro-code ROM at address 0x000..

Instruction Decode State
The contents of four higher bits of Ireg or Oreg 32bit are used to specify the next instruction to be done. The next address of the micro-code ROM is then determined conditionally according to the instruction decoded.

Instruction Execution State

If the instruction to be executed is finished in one state transition, then the next state will be back to the Instruction Fetch. Instead if the instruction needs other states to complete, then the next address for the micro-code ROM is an appropriate one for the next state.

3 Hardware for Parallel Processing

3.1 Process Control

The mechanism of the process control in TPCORE follows basically the one used for transputer as faithfully as possible. The value in Wptr is regarded as the process ID. The first address to be executed in the process is stored in Wptr-4, and the ID of the next process to be executed is stored in Wptr-8. Thus the process itself has the information for the next process. This chain structure for the process queue is prepared separately for the high and low priorities, and the structures are retained in the registers of fptr0, fptr1, bptr0 and bptr1. Since a change of one of these registers in the process scheduling is regarded as the state transition, the process control is also managed by the micro-code ROM.

3.2 Interrupt Process

The mechanism for the interrupt handling is also derived from the one used in transputer. The save or reload of the relevant registers at the beginning and end of an interrupt is described in state changes. The handling of the interrupt is described with the micro-code ROM. Once an interrupt is occurred, the address for the next micro-code ROM is changed to point the addresses to initiate or terminate the interrupt handling (18 and 22 states for the interrupt and return from interrupt respectively). Afterwards normal state transition cycle is resumed.

3.3 Link Communication

The communication between two processes in TPCORE is done through channels as is done in the transputer. The communication is one to one and synchronous. The channel facilitates no buffer for data to be transferred. A 32bit word in the memory is used for a channel between two processes running in the same TPCORE while one of a total of four link interfaces (also implemented in a special address space in memory) is used for a channel to communicate with a process running in a different TPCORE. The assembly instructions for communication like in and out distinguish internal and external communication from the address used for the channel. The stack register Creg is used for a pointer to specify the address of the data, Breg is the channel address, and Areg is used to specify the number of bytes to be transferred.

If, for example, out is executed with Breg=0x80000000, the link interface0 will be used to output the message externally, and the CPU asks to the link block to do the external communication by giving contents of the stack registers and the current process ID. Suspending the execution of the process currently executed, the CPU starts the next process taken from the scheduling queue. Once the link communication is over, then the CPU restores the stack registers and the process ID, and resumes the suspended process. The link protocol for the external communication is the same one as defined as Inmos protocol. The TPCORE has a link interface to accept the data over RS232C line. The protocol for data transfer over RS232C is the same one as the Inmos link protocol.

3.4   ALT Procedure

TPCORE implements ALT construction in the following way.

1. Address (Wptr-12) is prepared for ALT processing to keep the status of the ALT process. There are three statuses; Enabling, Waiting and Ready.

2. The status becomes Enabling when alt instruction is executed at the beginning of ALT construction.

3. Then enbc is executed to check whether a guard channel already received data. If so, then the status is set Ready, and altwt is over. If not, altwt sets the status to Waiting, and yields other process to proceed.

4. An out instruction of an another process, which is linked with an input guard channel of the ALT recognizes that altwt is being executed, and set remotely Ready to the status, and altwt is terminated.

5. If a guard channel receives data, an interrupt is generated to resume the ALT process, disc instruction is executed to sweep out altwt remnant, and it determines an appropriate address for execute of instructions for the established guard, then altend is executed to jump the address that disc specified.

4   Implementation and Verification

The design of the TPCORE Hardware has been done with the following steps,

1. **Analysis of the transputer instruction set**
   In order to investigate what changes are occurred in the internal registers or memory for execution of an instruction, we have extensively used a program "isim", which is an application involved in Inmos transputer toolset [3]. As we could observe changes of the registers and relevant memories with transputer instructions one by one, isim was very useful tool to look into the internal state transitions caused by some complicated instructions such as ones associated with PAR or ALT constructions.

2. **Description of the micro-code ROM**
   Once the changes in the registers or memories by the instructions were understood, we have summarized it in the framework of the state transition model. The model is implemented into the micro-code ROM. We also include state transitions caused by the interrupt, external link communication etc. into the micro-code ROM.

3. **Hardware design**
   Once the format of the micro-code ROM has been established and the contents of it have been filled, we have begun to design the hardware parts (the CPU block, memory controller, and the link block) using verilog. The verilog code was verified with the simulation. The verification of the hardware design also contains the validity check of the description in the micro-code ROM. An example of the simulation is shown in Figure 3. We have used ModelSimXEII5.6e [4] for the verilog simulation of both the register transfer and gate levels, and used ISE6.1i [5] for the logic synthesis.

Figure 3 shows following steps of the simulation:

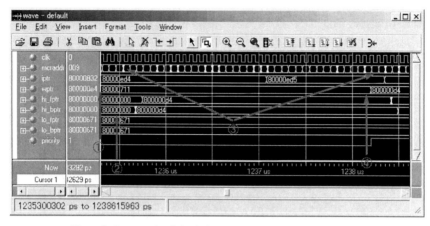

Figure 3: An example of simulation output: generation of an interrupt.

1. the lowest bit of Wptr is set to one as TPCORE executes a lower priority process in the beginning,

2. a higher priority process is generated, and its Wptr (0x80000711) is put in hi_fptr at about 1235.5us,

3. the address of the micro-code ROM (mcraddr) must be changed simply from 0x16e to 0x000 unless an interrupt is generated, but is changed to 0x000 through 0x1d3, 0x1d4,...,0x1e4, these 18 extra addresses of the micro-code ROM contains the states during the interrupt handling, and

4. after the state transition by the interrupt is over at around 1238.5us, a higher priority process is going to be executed.

Table 2: Implementation detail

Working frequency	24MHz (max. estimated 31.5MHz)
Number of gates	1371928 (1.4M) gates (64% used)
Memory size	32kByte
Memory access rate	24MByte/s
Number of instructions	96

We have implemented TPCORE developed in this way on an FPGA of Xilinx Virtex II. The result of this implementation is summarized in Table 2. Note that TPCORE has implemented only 96 instructions while the T425 has 103. We have implemented no timer instructions as yet.

TPCORE must do the following steps (some routes are indicated in Figure 2) within one cycle of the clock in order to do (a part of) an instruction;

1. input sources for ALU are assigned to ALU buses by micro-code ROM controller (Mc-ctrl) according to the micro-code ROM description,

2. ALU put an output as a result on the ALU output bus and sets various condition codes, and

3. Mcctrl decodes the data on the ALU output bus and calculates the next micro-code ROM address to refer.

TPCORE will do one 64bit subtraction, one 32bit addition and three steps of 32 to 64bit multiplexing operations for the above process in one clock. This complication limits the working frequency to 24MHz in the FPGA implementation.

Figure 4 shows a signal sequence actually observed in TPCORE implemented in Virtex II. This sequence expresses an interrupt generation. In Figure 4 HIQEMP and LOQEMP

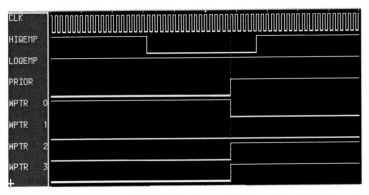

Figure 4: A signal sequence observed in TPCORE implemented in Xilinx Virtex II for interrupt generation.

mean empty flags of high and low priority queues respectively, PRIOR indicates the priority of the process currently being executed. The WPTR0 to WPTR4 are the four least significant bits of Wptr. The sequence of the signals in the figure is interpreted as follows,

1. a low priority process is being executed since Wptr0 is set to high at the beginning,

2. HIQEMP is transited to low at some time, namely a high priority process is entered in a waiting queue, and

3. after some clocks, the lowest significant bit of Wptr is changed from high to low, this indicates the high priority process was entered in an execution state from the waiting queue.

In Table 3 we listed comparison of TPCORE with T425 for the number of cycles needed for typical instructions. PS and B used in Table 3 denote the number of cycles needed to change processes and the highest bit number in which 1 is set in Areg, respectively. In TPCORE the number of cycles needed to change an active process depends on the conditions (priorities and number of queues). An interrupt is occurred when a process is put in a high priority queue during execution of a low priority process. In this case we need 18 cycles to exchange processes. It takes only four cycles to exchange two low priority processes. The column for the number of cycles for altwt (alt wait) in T425 in this table has been left blank. Accroding to [6], number of cycles for this instruction in T425 can not be explicitly defined since timer instructions will be used for the guard. Timer instructions have not been implemented in TPCORE, the number for TPCORE for altwt is one in case of not using timer instructions.

Finally we demonstrate two examples of the occam program execution; one is a prime number search with the algorithm of the so-called 'Sieve of Eratosthenes' (Figure 5), and the other one is 'Knight's Tour' on a chess board (Figure 7). The programs were loaded

Table 3: Comparison of the number of cycles needed for typical instructions for TPCORE with T425.

Instruction	Description	T425	TPCORE
j	jump	3	1
ldc	load constant	1	1
ldl	load local	2	2
ldnl	load non local	2	2
eqc	equal constant	2	1
pfix	prefix	1	1
call	call	7	7
wcnt	word count	5	6
in (internal)	input mssg	16	16+7B+PS
out (internal)	output mssg	16	16+7B+PS
altwt	alt wait		7+PS
enbc	Enable Channel	7	8
add	add	1	1
rem	remainder	37	45

by iserver into TPCORE and the output messages were printed on the host PC screen with various subroutines in hostio.lib of the occam2 toolset library.

Figure 6(a) shows the elapsed time of the prime number search program (the Sieve of Eratosthenes) versus the integer upper limit for the search range. Since we have not installed any instructions related to timer, we have measured the time with a logic analyzer. An occam code fragment for testing the primeness of an integer (denoted as max in the code below) is shown below.

```
SEQ
  j, check, going := 2, TRUE, TRUE
  WHILE going
    SEQ
      pcheck := max REM j
      IF
        max = j
          check, going := TRUE, FALSE
        pcheck = 0
          check, going := FALSE, FALSE
        TRUE
          j := j+1
```

The elapsed time is not linear with the search region. If we count, however, the number of repeat times for this loop in a search and plot the execution time versus this count, we could find a linear relation between two quantities as shown in Figure 6(b). One can calculate 4.8 microseconds/loop from the slope of the line in this figure. The number of cycles needed to execute this loop once is expected as 74 after we analyze the assembler code for this part. We find, therefore, that one cycle needs about 66ns, which corresponds to 16MHz working frequency. We are still analyzing reasons that this frequency is far below 24MHz; the norminal working frequency of TPCORE.

```
D:¥Work¥BOOTCH~1¥Linkboot>iserver prime
Please Type Number :1000
1000:
    2    3    5    7   11   13   17   19   23   29
   31   37   41   43   47   53   59   61   67   71
   73   79   83   89   97  101  103  107  109  113
  127  131  137  139  149  151  157  163  167  173
  179  181  191  193  197  199  211  223  227  229
  233  239  241  251  257  263  269  271  277  281
  283  293  307  311  313  317  331  337  347  349
  353  359  367  373  379  383  389  397  401  409
  419  421  431  433  439  443  449  457  461  463
  467  479  487  491  499  503  509  521  523  541
  547  557  563  569  571  577  587  593  599  601
  607  613  617  619  631  641  643  647  653  659
  661  673  677  683  691  701  709  719  727  733
  739  743  751  757  761  769  773  787  797  809
  811  821  823  827  829  839  853  857  859  863
  877  881  883  887  907  911  919  929  937  941
  947  953  967  971  977  983  991  997
D:¥Work¥Bootcheck¥Linkboot>
```

Figure 5: 'Sieve of Eratosthenes' executed in TPCORE for prime number search.

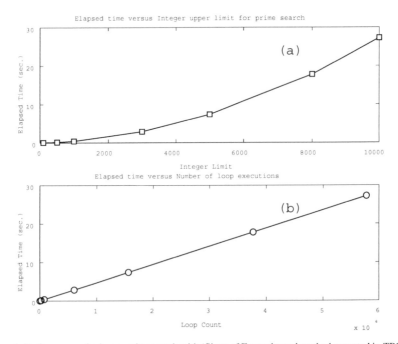

Figure 6: Performance of prime number search with 'Sieve of Eratosthenes' method executed in TPCORE.

```
D:\Work\Bootcheck\Linkboot>iserver knight
Input Boardsize : 8
Initialize knight point
 X : 1
 Y : 1
Path searching start. Please wait.
Knight`s Tour path is
  1 60 39 34 31 18  9 64
 38 35 32 61 10 63 30 17
 59  2 37 40 33 28 19  8
 36 49 42 27 62 11 16 29
 43 58  3 50 41 24  7 20
 48 51 46 55 26 21 12 15
 57 44 53  4 23 14 25  6
 52 47 56 45 54  5 22 13

D:\Work\Bootcheck\Linkboot>_
```

Figure 7: 'Knight's Tour' on a 8 by 8 chess board.

5   Summary and Outlook

We have made an IP core of the transputer T425, called TPCORE. TPCORE can execute a program written in occam, which is compiled with occ and linked with ilink. We can use iserver to download the executable program from a host PC to TPCORE. We expressed all the state transitions caused by execution of the CPU instructions, link and interrupt processing as well as process scheduling, and put them into the micro-code ROM. This implementation allows easier modification and extension of TPCORE performance and saves resource in an FPGA.

Almost all the instructions prepared for transputer T425 have been successfully implemented into TPCORE. Instructions concerning time sharing have not yet been implemented in TPCORE. These instructions are inserted by the occam compiler automatically, for example, when a long loop instruction is used in an occam program. The detailed behaviour of these instructions are neither given in [6] or obtained through isim running. To implement these time sharing instructions, we must execute them in an actual transputer and debug the relevant registers. This is an issue to be done in the next step.

Although the occam programs demonstrated in the previous section use the constructors PAR or ALT, the parallelization or multiplexing of processes are done within a single TPCORE. We have not yet checked the validity of the link block logic particularly carefully and, hence, communications with a process running in another TPCORE. By upgrading the FPGA or increasing the number of FPGAs, we will soon start the validity check of external link communications with this block.

Acknowledgement

We acknowledge Dr. M. Imori of the University of Tokyo for his advice and comments during the study. We are grateful to Mr. K. Matsui of Prominent Network Inc. for giving us the information about the CPA conference and suggesting us to submit a paper based on this study to this conference.

References

[1] Kent University KRoC Web cite: http://www.cs.kent.ac.uk/projects/ofa/kroc/

[2] SGS-THOMSON Micorelectronics, Transputer IMS T425 data sheet 1996

[3] SGS-THOMSON Micorelectronics, IMS D0305 "Occam 2 Transputer toolset Reference Manual" 1983

[4] Mentor Graphics Corporation, http://www.mentor.com

[5] Xilinx, Inc., http://www.xilinx.com

[6] Inmos Ltd., "Transputer Instruction set – A Compiler Writer's Guide", Prentice Hall 1988,

Communicating Process Architectures 2004
Ian East, Jeremy Martin, Peter Welch, David Duce, and Mark Green (Eds.)
IOS Press, 2004

Derivation of Scalable Message-Passing Algorithms Using Parallel Combinatorial List Generator Functions

Ali E. ABDALLAH and John HAWKINS

Research Institute for Computing,
London South Bank University,
103 Borough Road,
London SE1 0AA,
United Kingdom.

A.Abdallah@lsbu.ac.uk, John.Hawkins@reading.ac.uk

Abstract. We present the transformational derivations of several efficient, scalable, message-passing parallel algorithms from clear functional specifications. The starting algorithms rely on some commonly used combinatorial list generator functions such as *tails*, *inits*, *splits* and *cp* (Cartesian product) for generating useful intermediate results. This paper provides generic parallel algorithms for efficiently implementing a small library of useful combinatorial list generator functions. It also provides a framework for relating key higher order functions such as *map*, *reduce*, and *scan* with communicating processes with different configurations. The parallelisation of many interesting functional algorithms can then be systematically synthesized by taking an "off the shelf" parallel implementation of the list generator and composing it with appropriate parallel implementations of instances of higher order functions. Efficiency in the final message-passing algorithms is achieved by exploiting data parallelism, for generating the intermediate results in parallel; and functional parallelism, for processing intermediate results in stages such that the output of one stage is simultaneously input to the next one. This approach is then illustrated with a number of case studies which include: testing whether all the elements of a given list are distinct, the maximum segment sum problem, the minimum distance of two sets of points, and rank sort. In each case we progress from a quadratic time initial functional specification of the problem to a linear time parallel message-passing implementation which uses a linear number of communicating sequential processes. Bird-Meertens Formalism is used to concisely carry out the transformations.

1 Introduction

The design of efficient algorithms for many interesting programming problems often relies on the generation of combinatorial rearrangements of their input lists. A generic description of such an algorithm can then be seen as taking a list of values, generating useful rearrangements of the input list and processing those intermediate lists, possibly in parallel, in order to construct the final result. Examples of combinatorial list generator functions include: *inits*, *tails* and *segs* which generate, from a given list, the list of all its prefixes, suffixes, and segments (contiguous sublists) respectively. An algorithm which operates on a combinatorial list generator function, say *gen*, usually has the following form:

$$alg\ s = (phase_n \circ phase_{n-1} \circ \cdots \circ phase_1)\ (gen\ s)$$

where $phase_i$ is usually an instance of a higher order library function. The sequential implementation of such an algorithm normally exhibits, at least, a quadratic time behaviour. This is mainly because the size of the intermediate data generated by $(gen\ s)$ is, at least, quadratic. In [1, 2] it was shown that the above form can be correctly refined to a pipe of $(n+1)$ communicating processes, as shown in Fig 1. Here the first process $GEN(s)$ generates sequentially the result of $(gen\ s)$ and passes it to the process PH_1; and in turn to each of the processes PH_i (where $1 \le i \le n$), which implements the corresponding function $phase_i$.

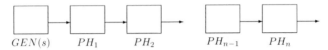

$GEN(s)$ $\qquad$ PH_1 $\qquad$ PH_2 $\qquad\qquad$ PH_{n-1} $\qquad$ PH_n

Figure 1: A pipelined implementation of $ALG(s)$

The above refinement obtained solely by exploiting pipelined parallelism is still quadratic, at best, on account of the size of the output of $GEN(s)$. Therefore, for this kind of algorithm pipelining alone may not lead to significant improvement in terms of speed. Hence, the only way to make a substantial improvement is to remove the bottleneck imposed by the sequential generation of $(gen\ s)$ and proceed by generating all the elements of $(gen\ s)$ in parallel, in a data-parallel fashion, each element on a separate channel. This ensures that all the sublists are generated in parallel in linear time. The structure of the pipelining solution stays unchanged but this time each phase in the pipe has internal parallelism; it takes inputs and produces outputs on a *vector* of channels as opposed to a single channel.

This paper provides a number of scalable and efficient message-passing algorithms for implementing a small library of list generator functions. It exploits both data parallelism, for generating all the elements of the resulting list in parallel; and pipelining parallelism, for processing intermediate results in stages such that the output of one stage is simultaneously input to the next one. To ensure scalability, global communications are eliminated and replaced by efficient local communications for routing shared data to all the relevant processing elements.

We also associate each of several key higher order functions such as *map*, *reduce*, and *scan* with two communicating processes which have different layouts: one, operating on a vector of values, which is suitable for data parallelism; and the other, operating on a stream of values, which is suitable for functional (or pipelined) parallelism. We show how the composition of higher order functions can be correctly implemented as (generalized) piping of the processes which implement each of these functions.

Since implementations of these library functions are readily available from a repertoire of parallel designs, the design of many message passing algorithms can then be systematically derived by simple program transformations and refinements. The parallelisation of many interesting functional algorithms is directly obtained from "off the shelf" parallel implementations of list generators and composition with appropriate parallel implementations of instances of higher order functions. This approach is then illustrated with a number of case studies which include: testing whether all the elements of a given list are distinct, the maximum segment sum problem, the minimum distance of two sets of points, and rank sort. In each case we progress from a quadratic time initial functional specification of the problem to a linear time parallel message-passing implementation which uses a linear number of communicating sequential processes. Bird-Meertens Formalism is used to concisely carry out the transformations.

The rest of this paper is organized as follows. Section 2 introduces some notation based on BMF and briefly explains some concepts for associating key higher order functions with communicating processes. Section 3 introduces several combinatorial list generator functions and provides efficient scalable parallel message-passing algorithms for implementing them. Section 4 illustrates how the concepts and techniques of the previous two sections can be used to systematically derive efficient parallel solutions to a number of small case studies. Section 5 briefly describes related work and, finally, Section 6 concludes this paper.

2   Notation and Basic Concepts

Throughout this paper, we will use the functional notation and calculus developed by Bird and Meertens [3, 4, 5] for specifying algorithmics and reasoning about them and will use a CSP style environment (as developed by Hoare [8]) for specifying processes and reasoning about them. We give a brief summary of the notation and conventions used in this paper. The reader is advised to consult the above references for further details.

2.1   Lists, Streams and Vectors

Lists are finite sequences of values of the same type. The list concatenation operator is denoted by ++ and the list construction operator is denoted by :. The elements of a list are displayed between square brackets and separated by commas.

Conventionally we have modelled lists in our parallel implementation as a *stream*, a serial sequence of messages on a channel. So for a list $[x_1, x_2, ..., x_n]$, we first send x_1 along our channel, then x_2 and so on up to x_n which is then followed by the special message *eot* to denote the end of the transmission. However, as has been explained, this can, in certain cases, introduce unacceptable bottlenecks into a network. Thus we have the alternative to streams which we call *vectors*. Here a separate channel is used for each item in the list and as such the whole list can then be communicated in parallel. This not only alleviates this bottleneck for many algorithms but also introduces scope for some data parallelism in our networks.

2.2   The Map Operator

The operator ∗ (pronounced "map") takes a function on the left, a list on the right, and applies the function to each element of the list. Informally, we have:

$$f * [a_1, a_2, \cdots, a_n] \;=\; [f(a_1), f(a_2), \cdots, f(a_n)]$$

We can associate with this function two different processes, the first, MAP, corresponds to functional or task parallelism. It takes a stream of inputs on one channel, say *in*, and produces a stream of output on a channel, say *out*. This can be pictured as seen in Figure 2.

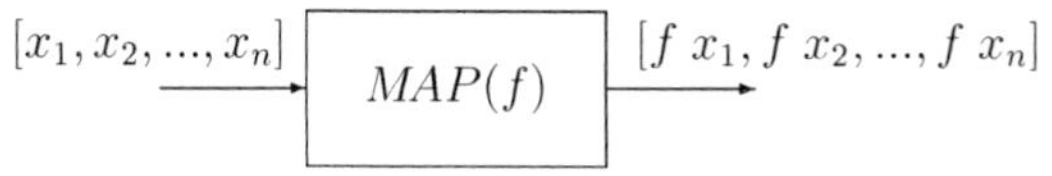

Figure 2: The Process MAP.

The second implementation, $VMAP$, corresponds to data or vector parallelism. It takes the list of values as inputs on a list of channels (one channel per value) and produces the resulting list on a list of channels one value per channel. This can be pictured as seen in Figure 3.

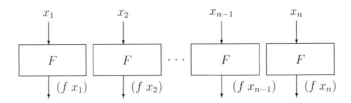

Figure 3: The Process $VMAP$.

2.3 Reduction Operators

The operator $/$ (pronounced "reduce") takes an associative binary operator on the left, a list of values on the right and returns the "summation" of all the elements of the list. This can be informally described as follows

$$(\oplus)/[a_1, a_2, \cdots, a_n] \quad = \quad a_1 \oplus a_2 \oplus \cdots \oplus a_n$$

The left reduction operator $(\oplus \not\rightarrow e)$ (also known as $foldl$) corresponds to a specific interpretation of reduction in which the computation of a list starts with e, as an initial value, and the result is gradually accumulated by successively applying the operator $\oplus$ while traversing the list from left to right. Informally, we have:

$$(\oplus \not\rightarrow e)\,[a_1, a_2, \cdots, a_n] \quad = \quad (\cdots((e \oplus a_1) \oplus a_2) \oplus \cdots) \oplus a_n$$

The right reduction operator $(\oplus \not\leftarrow e)$ (also known as $foldr$) is similar to $(\oplus \not\rightarrow e)$ except that the computation proceeds by traversing the list in the opposite direction, that is, from right to left.

$$(\oplus \not\leftarrow e)\,[a_1, a_2, \cdots, a_n] \quad = \quad a_1 \oplus (a_2 \oplus (\cdots \oplus (a_n \oplus e) \cdots))$$

Note that the operator used with directed reductions (both left and right) may not be associative.

As regards implementation of the fold operators, again we have two choices. The first two processes, $FOLDL$ and $FOLDR$, again, correspond to functional parallelism. $FOLDL$ is depicted in Figure 4, and $FOLDR$ would have a similar appearance. Here the process takes in a stream and returns either a stream or a single result, depending on the nature of the function used.

$$[x_1, x_2, .., x_n] \longrightarrow \boxed{FOLDL(\oplus, e)} \longrightarrow (...((e \oplus x_1) \oplus x_2)...) \oplus x_n$$

Figure 4: The Process $FOLDL$.

As before, the introduction of vectors requires that we also have a second view of the operators when the issue of implementation arises. Here we need to envisage a process that takes in a vector and produces the same result as the previous processes. Thus we have the process VFOLDL (as seen in Figure 5). Again, VFOLDR has a similar layout.

We may also require fold operators that do not take a base value, often termed as the functions $foldl1$ and $foldr1$, named as such due to only being defined on lists of length 1 or greater. This can be achieved in the implementation simply by removing the input of e, and,

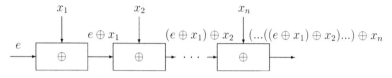

Figure 5: The process $VFOLDL$

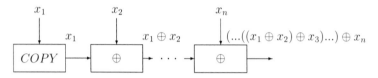

Figure 6: The process $VFOLDL1$

to compensate, replacing the first instance of the folding function with $COPY$, which simply mimics its input as its output. This can be seen in Figure 6 for a refinement of $foldl1$ applied to a vector. A similar implementation can be achieved for $foldr1$ via the same techniques.

2.4 Sections and Function Composition

Binary operators can be *sectioned*. This means that $(a\oplus)$ and $(\oplus b)$ both denote functions. Thus, if $\oplus$ has type $\oplus : A \to B \to C$, then we have

$$\begin{aligned}(a\oplus) &: B \to C \\ (\oplus b) &: A \to C\end{aligned}$$

for all $a \in A$ and $b \in B$. The definitions of these sections are:

$$\begin{aligned}(a\oplus)\, b &= a \oplus b \\ (\oplus b)\, a &= a \oplus b\end{aligned}$$

For example, $f*$ denotes a function which takes a list of values and maps f to each element of the list; but $(*xs)$ denotes a function which takes a function as input and applies it to each element of the list xs.

Function composition is denoted by $\circ$. This operator has lower precedence than all other operators. Thus, $f \circ g*$ denotes $f \circ (g*)$ and not $(f \circ g)*$.

2.5 Refinement to Processes

Function composition corresponds to functional parallelism and can be realized in a concurrency framework (for example **CSP**) by process piping ($\gg$). Careful checking must be done to ensure the correctness of this realization that the output of one process must match (have the same type as) the input of the next process in the pipe. If the common type is a stream, say [A], we will denote piping by $\gg$; but if it is a vector of length p, we will denote piping by the operator ($\gg_p$).

2.6 Algebraic Laws

One important asset of BMF is its richness in algebraic laws which allow the transformation of a program from one form to another while preserving its meaning. Here is a short list

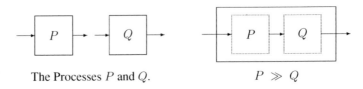

The Processes P and Q. $P \gg Q$

Figure 7: Stream Piping

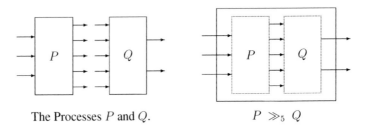

The Processes P and Q. $P \gg_5 Q$

Figure 8: Piping Generalized.

of frequently used algebraic rules which will be used in later examples. Historically, the "promotion rules" are intended to express the idea that an operation on a compound structure can be "promoted" into its components.

$$
\begin{aligned}
(f \circ g)* &= (f*) \circ (g*) &&\text{map distributivity} \\
f* \circ {+\!\!+}/ &= {+\!\!+}/ \circ (f*)* &&\text{map promotion} \\
\oplus/ \circ {+\!\!+}/ &= \oplus/ \circ (\oplus/)* &&\text{reduce promotion}
\end{aligned}
$$

3   Combinatorial List Generator Functions

3.1   *Segments*

A list s is a *segment* of t if there exist u and v such that $t = u +\!\!+ s +\!\!+ v$. If $u = []$, then s said to be an *initial segment* or a *prefix* of t. On the other hand, if $v = []$, then s is called a *final segment* or a *suffix* of t.

3.2   *Inits and Tails*

The function *inits* returns the list of initial segments of a list, in increasing order of length. The function *tails* returns the list of final segments of a list, in decreasing order of length. Thus, informally, we have

$$
\begin{aligned}
inits\,[a_1, a_2, \ldots, a_n] &= [[], [a_1], [a_1, a_2], \ldots, [a_1, a_2, \ldots, a_n]] \\
tails\,[a_1, a_2, \ldots, a_n] &= [[a_1, a_2, \ldots, a_n], [a_2, a_3, \ldots, a_n], \ldots, []]
\end{aligned}
$$

The functions $inits^+$ and $tails^+$ are similar, except that the empty list does not appear in the result.

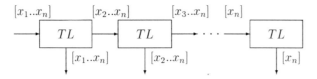

Figure 9: The process $TAILS$

We can define the functions $tails$ and $inits$ by explicit recursion equations (see [5]). For example, the suffixes of a list.

$$tails\,[] \quad = \quad [[]]$$
$$tails\,(x : xs) \quad = \quad (x : xs) : (tails\,xs)$$

For the examples given in this paper we use $tails^+$, rather than $tails$, so we will define a process corresponding to that function only for now. Here each item of the resulting list is produced on a separate channel- the output is modelled as a vector. The resulting network, $TAILS$, is depicted in Figure 9.

The function $inits$, which gives us the prefixes of a list can similarly be defined as follows (see [5]):

$$inits\,[] \quad = \quad [[]]$$
$$inits\,(x : xs) \quad = \quad [[]] \mathbin{+\!\!+} ((x :) * (inits\,xs))$$

This could be implemented with a similar network to that in Figure 9, except that the flow of data would come from the right instead of the left. This underlines the basic symmetry that exists between $inits$ and $tails$.

3.3   Segs

The functions $segs$ returns a list of all segments of a list, and $segs^+$ returns a list of all non-empty segments. A convenient definition is

$$segs \quad = \quad (+\!\!+)/ \; \circ \; (inits *) \; \circ \; tails$$
$$segs^+ \quad = \quad (+\!\!+)/ \; \circ \; (inits^+ *) \; \circ \; tails^+$$

For example,

$$segs\,[1,2,3] \quad = \quad [[],[1],[1,2],[1,2,3],[],[2],[2,3],[],[3],[]]$$
$$segs^+\,[1,2,3] \quad = \quad [[1],[1,2],[1,2,3],[2],[2,3],[3]]$$

Notice that the empty list $[]$ appears four times in $segs\,[1,2,3]$ (and not at all in $segs^+[1,2,3]$). The order in which the elements of $segs\,x$ appear is not important for our purposes and we shall make no use of it. In effect, we shall reduce over $segs$ with commutative operators only.

3.4   Splits

The function $splits$ returns the list of all possible ways of splitting a list into two parts such that the second part is non-empty. Informally, we have:

$$splits\,[a_1, a_2, \cdots, a_n] \quad = \quad [\; ([], [a_1, a_2, \cdots, a_n]), \; ([a_1], [a_2, \cdots, a_n]),$$
$$([a_1, a_2], [a_3, \cdots, a_n]), \; \cdots, \; ([a_1, a_2, \cdots, a_{n-1}], [a_n]) \;]$$

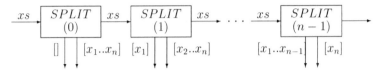

Figure 10: The process $SPLITS$

We can construct functional definition of $splits$ using the functions $take$ and $drop$ (see [5]):

$$splits\ s\ =\ [(take\ i\ s, drop\ i\ s) \mid i \leftarrow [0..\#s - 1]]$$

With this function we can associate the network $SPLITS$ which produces each item of the resulting list on a separate pair of channels. This is depicted in Figure 10.

3.5   Cartesian Product

The function cp returns a Cartesian product of its two input lists xs and ys, i.e. a list where every element of xs is paired with every element of ys. This can be defined quite simply as follows:

$$cp\ xs\ ys\ =\ [(x, y) \mid x \leftarrow xs; y \leftarrow ys]$$

Production of this list, as in the previous cases will require $O(n^2)$ steps. However, if we consider the result as a list of lists, each an element from xs paired with every element of ys, the result can then be produced in parallel in linear time. Thus we have a slight redefinition. We shall call this new function dcp for distributed Cartesian product.

$$dcp\ xs\ ys\ =\ [(pair\ x) * ys \mid x \leftarrow xs]$$

So, for example:

$$dcp\ [1, 2, 3]\ ['a','b','c']\ =\ [[(1,'a'), (1,'b'), (1,'c')],$$
$$[(2,'a'), (2,'b'), (2,'c')],$$
$$[(3,'a'), (3,'b'), (3,'c')]]$$

We can clearly define cp in terms of dcp to illustrate the relation between the two functions.

$$cp\ xs\ =\ (+\!\!+)/\ \circ\ dcp\ xs$$

This function can now be associated with the process CP, pictured in figure 11.

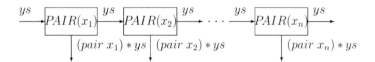

Figure 11: The process CP

3.6 Accumulations

The operator $-\!\!/\!\!\!/\!\!\rightarrow e$ (or *scanl*) takes a binary operator, say $\oplus$, on the left; a list of values on the right; and applies the function $(\oplus /\!\!\!\!\rightarrow e)$ to all the initial segments of the list. This function is often being refered to as "prefix sum" when the operator $\oplus$ is associative. We have

$$(\oplus -\!\!/\!\!\!/\!\!\rightarrow e)\, s \;=\; (\oplus /\!\!\!\!\rightarrow e) * (inits\ s)$$

For example:

$$(+ -\!\!/\!\!\!/\!\!\rightarrow 0)\,[1, 2, 3, 4, 5] \;=\; [0, 1, 3, 6, 10, 15]$$

In some cases we may not want to include the base value in the resulting list. For this purpose, in a similar manner to the $fold$ functions, we also introduce a function $scanl1$. This can be defined as follows:

$$scanl1\,(\oplus)\ e\ s \;=\; (\oplus /\!\!\!\!\rightarrow e) * (inits^+\ s)$$

For example:

$$scanl1\,(+)\ 0\,[1, 2, 3, 4, 5] \;=\; [1, 3, 6, 10, 15]$$

For each of these functions we are given two choices for implementation, in each case either using streams or vectors. The function $scanl1$ can be implemented with stream parallelism using the process $SCANL1$, as shown in Figure 12. This process will both input and output a stream. Alternatively, we have a vector implementation, and this is demonstrated by the process $VSCANL1$, shown in Figure 13. This process inputs a vector and outputs a vector.

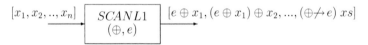

Figure 12: The Process $SCANL1(\oplus, e)$.

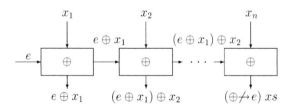

Figure 13: The process $VSCANL1(\oplus)$

4   Case Studies

4.1   The Maximum Segment Sum Problem

There is a famous problem, called the *maximum segment sum* (*mss*) problem, which is to compute the maximum of the sums of all segments of a given sequence of numbers, positive, negative or zero. For example, $mss\ [2, -3, 1, 2, -2, 3, -1] = 4$ which corresponds to the segment $[1, 2, -2, 3]$. For details see Bird's paper ... In symbols

$$mss = \max /\ \circ sum*\ \circ segs^+$$

Direct evaluation of the right-hand side of this equation requires $O(n^3)$ steps on a list of length n. There are $O(n^2)$ segments and each can be summed in $O(n)$ steps, giving $O(n^3)$ steps in all.

$$
\begin{aligned}
mss\ &=\quad \{\ \text{definition}\ \} \\
&\qquad \max /\ \circ sum*\ \circ segs^+ \\
&=\quad \{\ \text{definition of } segs^+\ \} \\
&\qquad \max /\ \circ sum*\ \circ +\!+\!/\ \circ inits^+ *\ \circ tails^+ \\
&=\quad \{\ \text{map promotion}\ \} \\
&\qquad \max /\ \circ +\!+\!/\ \circ sum* *\ \circ inits^+ *\ \circ tails^+ \\
&=\quad \{\ \text{map distributivity}\ \} \\
&\qquad \max /\ \circ +\!+\!/\ \circ (sum*\ \circ inits^+) *\ \circ tails^+ \\
&=\quad \{\ \text{definition of accumulation}\ \} \\
&\qquad \max /\ \circ +\!+\!/\ \circ (+\!\!-\!\!/\!\!\rightarrow) *\ \circ tails^+ \\
&=\quad \{\ \text{reduce promotion}\ \} \\
&\qquad \max /\ \circ \max /\ *\ \circ (+\!\!-\!\!/\!\!\rightarrow) *\ \circ tails^+
\end{aligned}
$$

Implementation is now an almost trivial matter of combining 'off the shelf' components that correspond with each stage of our algorithm. This gives us the following network:

$$TAILS \gg_n VMAP(SCANL(+)) \gg_n VMAP(FOLD(max)) \gg_n VFOLDR1(max)$$

where n is the length of the input list. The resulting network can be seen in Figure 14. This algorithm will now run in linear time.

4.2   Minimum Distance

Given two lists of points in three dimensional space, the minimum distance function, md compares every point from the first list with every point from the second list and returns the distance between the closest of these.

Here we need to make use of the Cartesian product function, cp. We simply need to map some function $dist$ to this list, and then find the minimum of this result.

$$md \qquad\qquad = \quad (min/)\ \circ (dist *)\ \circ cp$$

$$dist\ (x1, y1, z1)\ (x2, y2, z2)\ = \quad \sqrt{(x2 - x1)^2 + (y2 - y1)^2 + (z2 - z1)^2}$$

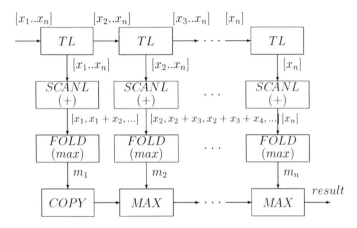

Figure 14: A network to solve the maximum segment sum problem for the list xs

However, given the nature of dcp, producing a list of lists, we need a little remodeling to achieve the actual definition.

$$
\begin{aligned}
md\ xs\ &=\quad \{\ \text{definition}\ \} \\
&\quad \min /\ \circ dist*\ \circ (cp\ xs) \\
&=\quad \{\ \text{definition of }cp\ \} \\
&\quad \min /\ \circ dist*\ \circ +\!\!+/\ \circ (dcp\ xs) \\
&=\quad \{\ \text{map promotion}\ \} \\
&\quad \min /\ \circ +\!\!+/\ \circ (dist*)*\ \circ (dcp\ xs) \\
&=\quad \{\ \text{reduce promotion}\ \} \\
&\quad \min /\ \circ \min /\ *\ \circ (dist*)*\ \circ (dcp\ xs)
\end{aligned}
$$

The implementation can now be constructed as before, giving us the network:

$$CP(xs) \gg_n VMAP(MAP(dist)) \gg_n$$
$$VMAP(FOLD(min)) \gg_n VFOLDL1(min)$$

Again n is the length of the input list. This is depicted in Figure 15.

4.3 Lists with Distinct Elements

Consider the problem of testing whether all the elements of a list are distinct. That is, no element of the list occurs more than once in the list.

Essentially we need to compare every element in the list with every other, see if they differ, and then *and* all these results together. This can be achieved with the following function:

$$distinct\ =\ (\wedge/)\ \circ noteq*\ \circ tails^{+}$$

Given a function $noteq$ which takes a list and dictates if the first item is different to all the others.

$$
\begin{aligned}
noteq\ &=\ (\wedge)/\ \circ diff \\
diff\ (x:xs)\ &=\ (\neq x)*xs
\end{aligned}
$$

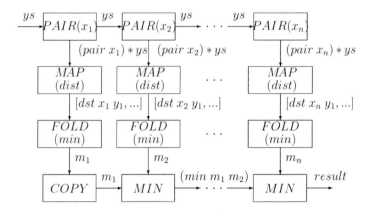

Figure 15: A network to solve the minimum distance problem for the lists xs and ys

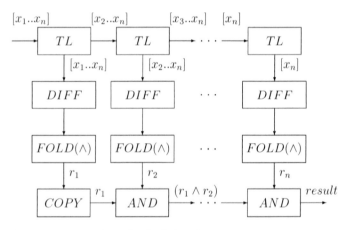

Figure 16: A network to solve the distinct elements problem for the list xs

This allows us to give a slight redefinition of $distinct$:

$$distinct \ = \ (\wedge/) \circ (\wedge/) * \circ diff * \circ tails^+$$

The above definition can then be transformed quite straightforwardly to the following network:

$$TAILS \gg_n VMAP(DIFF) \gg_n VMAP(FOLD(\wedge)) \gg_n VFOLDL1(\wedge)$$

where n is the length of the input list. The results can be seen in Figure 16.

4.4   Parallel Enumerate Sort

For each element in the input list $[a_1, a_2, \cdots, a_n]$, the *rank sort* algorithm aims at computing its final position (rank) in the sorted list. This is simply achieved by counting the number of elements in the list having smaller value ([9]). If j elements have smaller value than a_i then

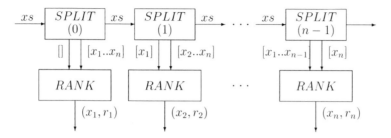

Figure 17: A network performing rank sort on the list *xs*

a_i is the $(j+1)^{th}$ element of the sorted list. If two or more elements have the same value, the algorithm must be slightly amended in order to produce a unique rank for each element in the unsorted list. This is achieved by counting the number of elements having smaller value or the same value and smaller index in the unsorted list. Formally, the rank of the ith element of the list $[a_1, a_2, \cdots, a_n]$ is captured as:

$$rank\ i\ [a_1, a_2, \cdots, a_n] = \#\{j \in \{1..n\} \mid a_j < a_i \vee (a_j = a_i \wedge j < i)\}$$

The functional specification of the *rank sorting* algorithm is:

$$rsort :: [a] \rightarrow [(\alpha, num)];\ rank :: ([a], [a]) \rightarrow (\alpha, num)$$
$$rsort \qquad\quad = \quad (rank *) \circ splits$$
$$rank\ (s, x: t) \quad = \quad (x, \#filter\ (< x)\ s + \#filter\ (\leq x)\ t)$$

The resulting implementation can be found in Figure 17.

5 Conclusion

In this paper we have presented a number of frequently used combinatorial list generator functions and showed how they can be efficiently implemented in parallel as networks of interacting processes. These list generator functions are the building blocks for many interesting algorithms and their proposed parallel implementations can be the basis for systematically parallelising such algorithms.

This paper attempts to combine both data parallelism and functional parallelism in one framework which is founded on concurrency. It also develops some real world algorithms which make use of this framework. Both the functions and algorithms which use them had at least quadratic (sequential) execution time and in every case we have successfully developed linear time parallel implementations.

The focus has been on these combinatorial functions, and how a mixture of data and functional parallelism can be used to remove the previous bottleneck of communicating their results (lists of lists). In the process we have introduced models for data parallelism into a transformational framework which previously concentrated solely on functional parallelism (see [1]).

We have presented an essentially skeletonic approach to implementation. Given a specification composed of several more commonly used functions, we can simply take each function in turn, find a pre-defined parallel implementation known to be efficient, and then link these all together to create our network. This approach has several advantages. The first and perhaps most obvious is speed of development. In addition, as already mentioned, our pre-defined 'off the shelf' components are already known to be efficient, and, whereas we cannot always guarantee that the resulting network will be optimal, we will in almost all cases see a substantial increase in execution time. Finally, this approach removes some of the burden of understanding the inherent parallelism from the programmer, which can allow them to concentrate more on what is actually required from an algorithm, rather than how is best to implement it. This highly systematic approach may then even lead to an entirely automatic tool for transformation from specification to parallel implementation. This is an area we are already investigating.

This work could be extended to include a larger class of combinatorial list generator functions, and a further study of the effects of higher order functions on vectors. We may then identify situations quite different to those encountered in this work where this combined parallelism could be used to great effect.

References

[1] A.E. Abdallah, Derivation of Parallel Algorithms from Functional Specifications to CSP Processes, in: Bernhard Möller, ed., *Mathematics of Program Construction*, LNCS 947, (Springer Verlag, 1995) 67-96

[2] A. E. Abdallah, Synthesis of Massively Pipelined Algorithms for List Manipulation, in L. Bouge and P. Fraigniaud and A. Mignotte and Y. Robert (eds), Proceedings of the *European Conference on Parallel Processing, EuroPar'96*, LNCS 1024, (Springer Verlag, 1996), pp 911-920.

[3] R. S. Bird, An Introduction to The Theory of Lists, in: M. Broy, ed., *Logic of Programming and Calculi of Discreet Design*, (Springer, Berlin, 1987) 3-42.

[4] R. S. Bird, Functional Algorithm Design, in: Bernhard Möller, ed., *Mathmeatics of Program Construction*, LNCS 947, (Springer Verlag, 1995) 2-17

[5] R. S. Bird and P. Wadler, *Introduction to Functional Programming*, (Prentice-Hall, 1988).

[6] M. I. Cole, *Algorithmic Skeletons: Structured Management of Parallel Computation*, in: Research Monographs in Parallel and Distributed Computing, (Pitman 1989).

[7] J. Darlington, A. Field and P.G. Harrison, *Parallel Programming Using Skeleton Functions*, in: A. Bode, M. Reeve and G. Wolf, eds., Parallel Architectures and Languages Europe (PARLE'93), LNCS 694.

[8] C. A. R. Hoare, *Communicating Sequential Processes*. (Prentice-Hall, 1985).

[9] Donald E. Knuth, *The Art of Computer Programming, Volume III: Sorting and Searching* Addison-Wesley 1973

Communicating Process Architectures 2004
Ian East, Jeremy Martin, Peter Welch, David Duce, and Mark Green (Eds.)
IOS Press, 2004

Reconfigurable Hardware Synthesis of the IDEA Cryptographic Algorithm

Ali E. ABDALLAH and Issam W. DAMAJ

Research Institute for Computing,
London South Bank University,
103 Borough Road,
London SE1 0AA,
United Kingdom.

A.Abdallah@lsbu.ac.uk, I.Damaj@lsbu.ac.uk

Abstract. The paper focuses on the synthesis of a highly parallel reconfigurable hardware implementation for the International Data Encryption Algorithm (*IDEA*). Currently, *IDEA* is well known to be a strong encryption algorithm. The use of such an algorithm within critical applications, such as military, requires efficient, highly reliable and correct hardware implementation. We will stress the affordability of such requirements by adopting a methodology that develops reconfigurable hardware circuits by following a transformational programming paradigm. The development starts from a formal functional specification stage. Then, by using function decomposition and provably correct data refinement techniques, powerful high-order functions are refined into parallel implementations described in Hoare's communicating sequential processes notation(*CSP*). The *CSP* descriptions are very closely associated with *Handle-C* hardware description language (*HDL*) program fragments. This description language is employed to target reconfigurable hardware as the final stage in the development. The targeted system in this case is the *RC-1000* reconfigurable computer. In this paper different designs for the *IDEA* corresponding to different levels of parallelism are presented. Moreover, implementation, realization, and performance analysis and evaluation are included.

1 Introduction

In the last few years, there has been dramatic advances in manufacturing Field Programmable Gate Arrays (*FPGAs*). It is now possible to make use of multi-million gates *FPGAs*. *FPGAs* offer much flexibility for the design of integrated circuits (ICs) chips for parallelism. Generally, parallelism and implementation in hardware provide us with two alternatives that can often deliver very dramatic improvements in efficiency. With the emergence of such reconfigurable hardware chips, the presence of a development environment for these scalable hardware circuits is very useful. Moreover, it would constitute the cornerstone solution for the ever-increasing need for more: efficiency, scalability and flexibility in realizing massively parallel algorithms for a wide area of applications.

The proposed rapid development model (RDM) adopts the transformational programming approach for deriving massively parallel algorithms from functional specifications [1, 2, 3]. The functional notation is used for specifying algorithms and for the reasoning about them. This is usually done by carefully combining small number of high order functions (like *map*, *zip* and *fold*) to serve as the basic building blocks for writing high-level programs. The systematic methods for massive parallelization of algorithms work by carefully composing "off the shelf" massively parallel implementation of each of the building blocks involved in the algorithm.

To describe parallelism we follow a step-wise provably correct refinement that maps the functional specification to a network of communicating processes. Hoare's *CSP* is used to describe the refined specification. This development step allows issues of immense practical importance (such as data distribution, network topology, and locality of communications) to be carefully reasoned about. Relating the Functional Programming and *CSP* fields gives the ability to exploit a well-established functional programming paradigms and transformation techniques in order to develop efficient *CSP* processes.

The final development stage follows the skeleton built by the previous stage, i.e. the refinement to *CSP* stage, to realize a corresponding reconfigurable hardware circuit. The reconfigurable hardware realization step is done using *Handel-C* an automated compilation development model [4]. *Handel-C* uses much of the syntax of conventional C with the addition of explicit parallelism. Handel-C relies on the parallel constructs in *CSP* to model concurrent hardware resources. Accordingly, algorithms described with *CSP* could be implemented with *Handle-C*. An overview of the transformational derivation and the hardware realization are shown in Figure 1.

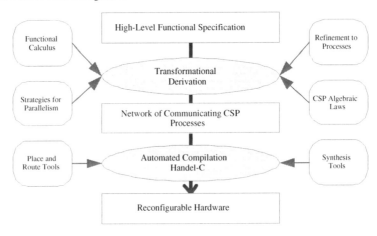

Figure 1: An overview of the transformational derivation and the hardware realization processes.

2 Background and Previous Work

Abdallah and Hawkins defined in [2] some constructs used in the development model. This looked in some depth at data refinement; the means of expressing structures in the specification as communication behavior in the implementation.

Firstly, streams are defined as a sequence of messages on a single channel, and correspond to a sequential method for communicating a list. Streams facilitate the communication of finite sequences and require some means of signalling the end of transmission (EOT). Secondly, vectors of items are a means of communicating a list on more than one channel. The assumption is that there are as many channels in the vector as there are items in the list, such that each item is communicated on its own channel. Thirdly, vectors of streams are the parallel composition of n streams, each communicating a sublist independently as a stream. Each stream has its own end-of-transmission signal (EOT), and they can finish transmitting at different times. Lastly, streams of vectors is defined where a complete sublist is communicated in a single step.

3   Data Refinement

In the following subsections, we present some data types used for refinement.

3.1   Stream of Values

The stream is a purely sequential method of communicating a group of values. It comprises a sequence of messages on a channel, with each message representing a value. Values are communicated one after the other. Assuming the stream is finite, after the last value has been communicated, the end of transmission (EOT) on a different channel will be signaled. Given some type A, a stream containing values of type A is denoted as $\langle A \rangle$.

3.2   Vector of n Values

Each item to be communicated by the vector will be dealt with independently in parallel. A vector refinement of a simple list of items will communicate the entire structure in a single. Given some type A, a vector of length n, containing values of type A, is denoted as $\lfloor A \rfloor_n$.

3.3   Refinement of a List of Lists

Whenever dealing with multi-dimensional data structures, for example, lists of lists, implementation options arise from differing compositions of our primitive data refinements - streams and vectors. Examples of the combined forms are the *Stream of Streams*, *Streams of Vectors*, *Vectors of Streams*, and *Vectors of Vectors*. These forms are denoted by:

$$\langle S_1, S_2, ..., S_n \rangle$$
$$\langle V_1, V_2, ..., V_n \rangle$$
$$\lfloor S_1, S_2, ..., S_n \rfloor$$
$$\lfloor V_1, V_2, ..., V_n \rfloor$$

4   High-Order Functions

Functional programming environments facilitate reusability through high-order-functions. Many algorithms can be built from components which are instances of some more general scheme. In this section we introduce the refinement of some high-order-functions detailed in [2].

Map applies a function to a list of items. Thus, in the functional setting, we have:

$$map\, f\, [x_1, x_2, ..., x_n] = [f(x_1), f(x_2), ..., f(x_n)]$$

Refining to *CSP* we have:

$$VMAP_n(F) = \|_{i=1}^{i=n} F[in_i/in, out_i/out]$$

where, F is the refinement of f. A data parallel processes visualization of map $VMAP_n(F)$ is shown in Figure 2.

The *fold* family of functions is used to *reduce* a list by inserting a binary operator between each neighboring pair of elements. The basic fold operator ($/$) has no concept of direction and as such requires an associative binary operator to be well defined.

$$f\, /\, [x_1, x_2, ..., x_n] = x_1 f x_2 ... f x_n$$

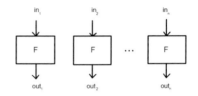

Figure 2: The Process $VMAP_n(F)$.

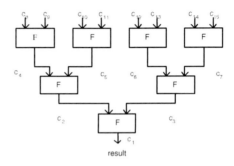

Figure 3: The Process $VFOLD_n(F)$.

Refining to *CSP* we have:

$$VFOLD_n(F) = \|_{i=1}^{i=n} F[c_i/out, c_{2i}/in_1, c_{2i+1}/in_2]$$

where, F is the refinement of the operator f. An instance of *VFOLD* is shown in Figure 3.

The high-order-function *zipWith* is used to zip two lists (taking one element from each list) with a certain operation.

$$zipWith\, f\, [x_1, x_2, ..., x_n][y_1, y_2, ..., y_n] = [x_1 f y_1, x_2 f y_2, ..., x_n f y_n]$$

Refining to *CSP* we have:

$$VZIP_n(F) = \|_{i=1}^{i=n} F[c_i/out, a/in_1, b/in_2]$$

5　The IDEA Algorithm

Cryptographic algorithms are an essential part in security. A well known cryptographic algorithm is the Data Encryption Standard (DES) [5, 6], widely adopted in security products. Another cryptographic algorithm is the International Data Encryption Algorithm, *IDEA* [7, 6]. Due to its high immunity to attacks [8, 6], *IDEA* is considered as one of the most important post-*DES* cryptographic algorithms.

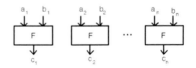

Figure 4: The Process $VZIP(F)$.

The *IDEA* algorithm is the evolution of an initial algorithm (the Proposed Encryption Standard, or *PES*) devised by Xuejia Lai and James Massey [7]. Some authors [6, 8] consider *IDEA* as one of the most secure cryptographic algorithms available at this time. In fact, there is no linear cryptanalytic attacks on *IDEA*, and there are no known algebraic weaknesses in *IDEA* other than the one discovered by Daemen [9]. Daemen discovered a weakness by using a class of 251 weak keys during encryption results in easy detection and recovery of the key. However, since there are a large number of possible keys this result has no impact on the practical security of the cipher for encryption provided, the encryption keys are chosen at random. *IDEA* is generally considered to be a very secure cipher; both the cipher development and its theoretical basis have been openly and widely discussed.

IDEA is a method to encrypt and decrypt data. A randomly secret key number is used to encrypt and decrypt the data. *IDEA* is a 64-bit iterative block cipher with a 128-bit key. The encryption process requires eight complex rounds. Decryption is carried out in the same manner as encryption once the decryption subkeys have been calculated from the encryption subkeys. The cipher structure was designed to be easily implemented in both software and hardware [10].

Hardware implementation of this cryptographic algorithm has been an active area of research. Davor and Mario presented an *FPGA* core implementation for the *IDEA*, which was addressed in [11]. They used a system with single core module to implement the *IDEA*. This module was implemented using a *Xilinx FPGA*. Cheung et al in [12] investigated a high-performance implementation of the *IDEA* using both bit-parallel and bit-serial architectures. They used a *Xilinx* Virtex XCV300-6 and XCV1000-6 *FPGAs* to evaluate and analyse the performance of the implementations. Beuchat et al in [13] presented a high-speed *FPGA* implementation of the *IDEA*. In [14] *IDEA* was addressed presenting hardware software tri-design of encryption for mobile communication units. A comparison was given between a *DSP* processor from Texas Instruments and the *Xilinx XC4000* series *FPGAs*. In [14] *VLSI* Implementation of the *IDEA* is presented. Allen et al in [15] presented an implementation comparison for the *IDEA* between the *SRC-6E* and *HC-36* general reconfigurable computers.

6 IDEA Formal Functional Specification

We view the *IDEA* algorithm as of three main blocks. A global view of these blocks would show the encryption (or decryption) as a block with 2 inputs, the private key and the plaintext (or ciphertext) and outputting the ciphertext (or plaintext). The two remaining blocks are for encryption and decryption subkeys generation. In the case of encryption subkeys generation, the block will take the private key as an input and outputs the desired subkeys. The decryption subkeys generator will input the generated encryption subkeys and output the decryption subkeys. As a first step, we define some types to be used in the following specification:

```
type Private    = [Bool]    type SubKey     = Int
type Plaintext  = [Int]     type Ciphertext = [Int]
modVal          = 65536
```

6.1 Basic Building Blocks

Three different key primitive building blocks are used within the *IDEA*:

* Bit-wise exclusive OR.

* Addition of 16-bit integers modulo $2^{16} (modulo\ 65536)$.

- Multiplication of 16-bit integers modulo $2^{16} + 1$ (*modulo* 65537), where an all zeros input block is considered as 2^{16}.

6.2   Encryption Subkeys Generation

As shown in Figure 5, 52 16-bit subkeys are generated from the 128-bit encryption key. The algorithm for generation is as follows:

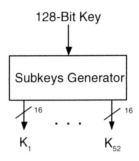

Figure 5: Subkeys Generator.

- The first eight subkeys are selected directly from the key by partitioning the key (128-bit list) into eight segments of equal length (16-bit).

- A circular shift of 25-bit positions is applied to the key of the previous step, and the eight subkeys are then extracted.

- This procedure is repeated until all 52 subkeys are generated i.e. 8-times and 4 subkeys are extracted in the final step.

In the following specification the subkeys generation is specified as the function *generateEncSubKeys*, this function takes the encryption key as input and outputs a list corresponding to the 52 16-bit subkeys. Tracing the steps of the function, it firstly takes the first eight rotations of the input key using the function *keyRotation* and generates accordingly the corresponding subkeys for each rotation through the function *generateSubKeys*. The generated subkeys are then concatenated in one list. The 52 subkeys are then extracted from the list and converted to integers equivalent to the 16-element list of *bool* representing each subkey. The conversion is done using the function *btoi*.

```
generateEncSubKeys :: Private -> [SubKey]
generateEncSubKeys key = map (btoi) (take 52
    (foldr1 (++) (map generateSubKeys (take 8 (keyRotation key)))))
```

All the rotated keys are determined by the function *keyRotation* which repeatedly generates the rotated keys. This function uses the polymorphic function *repeated* which takes a function f and a list xs and repeatedly applies the function f to xs. In this case, it repeatedly rotates the key in 25-bits steps. The rotation values would be $0, 25, 50, 75, 100, 125, 22, 47$ from the original key position.

```
keyRotation :: Private -> [[Bool]]
keyRotation key = take 8 (repeated (shift 25) key)

repeated :: (a -> a) -> a -> [a]
repeated f x = x: repeated f (f x)

shift :: Int -> [a] -> [a]
shift n key = (drop n key) ++ (take n key)
```

To generate the 16-bit subkeys from the rotated keys, the high-order function *map* is applied in the function *generateEncSubKeys* to the function *generateSubKeys* over the list of rotated keys. The function *generateSubKeys* employs *segs*, which selects *n* sublists from a list *xs*:

```
generateSubKeys :: Private -> [SubKey]
generateSubKeys key = segs 16 key

segs :: Int -> [a] -> [[a]]
segs n [] = []
segs n xs = (take n xs) : segs n (drop n xs)
```

We have the following assertion holding for all lists *xs*:

$$++/(segs\ n\ xs) = xs$$

Finally, the desired subkeys are packed in lists of 6 elements in one list of lists using the function *pack*.

```
pack :: [a] -> [[a]]
pack = segs 6
```

6.3   Decryption Subkeys Generation

After specifying the encryption subkeys generation, now we can introduce the decryption subkeys generation, where, every decryption subkey is a function of one of the encryption subkeys. The relation between the encryption and the decryption subkeys is as specified in the function *generateDecSubKeys*. This function is done by mapping a function *perform* to a prepared list of indices. The preparation of the indices list *indices* is done as shown in Figure 6. Furthermore, the function *perform* employs *addInv* and *mulInv*, which correspond to the additive and multiplicative inverse respectively. This function also uses the high-order function *mapWith* that takes a list of functions and a list of values and applies (using the function *apply*) each function in the first list to the corresponding value in the second list (using the high-order-function *zipWith*).

```
generateDecSubKeys :: [SubKey] -> [SubKey]
generateDecSubKeys eKeys = take 52 (foldr1 (++) (map perform indices))
   where
      indices = mapWith fs (map reverse (pack (reverse [1 | 1<-[0..51]])))
      f1(xs) = shift 2 xs
      f2(xs) = zipWith (+) (copy (xs!!2) 6) [0, 2, 1, 3, -2, -1]
      f3 = id
      fs = [f1, f2, f2, f2, f2, f2, f2, f2, f3]
      perform(as) = mapWith [mulInv , addInv, addInv, mulInv, id, id]
                            (zipWith (!!) (copy eKeys 6) as)
copy :: a -> Int -> [a]
copy x n = [x | i <- [1..n]]
```

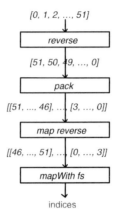

Figure 6: Indices permutation.

```
mapWith ::  [(a -> b)] -> [a] -> [b]
mapWith fs = zipWith (apply) fs

apply :: (a -> b) -> a -> b
apply f = f
```

Moving to the formal specification of modular arithmetic operations employed in the *IDEA* decryption. The additive inverse *(modulo 2^{16})* and the multiplicative inverse *(modulo $2^{16}+1$)*. We specify these operations as the functions *addInv* and *mulInv*. The function *addInv* is simply the input number subtracted from the modulus value:

```
addInv :: Int -> Int
addInv a = modVal - a
```

To calculate the multiplicative inverse, the Extended Euclidean algorithm [16] is used, The steps to calculate the multiplicative inverse are clarified in Figure 7. Accordingly, the functional specification is as follows:

```
mulInv :: Int -> Int
mulInv 0 = 0
mulInv b = if (y < 0) then ((modVal +1) + y) else (y)
   where
      y = (extendedEucA (modVal +1) b)!!2

extendedEucA :: Int -> Int -> [Int]
extendedEucA a b
| b == 0 = [a, 1, 0]
| otherwise = iterateSteps [a, b, 0, 1, 1, 0]

iterateSteps ls = if ((ls[1]) > 0)
                    then (iterateSteps s2)
                    else ([(ls[0]), (ls[3]), (ls[5])])
   where
      s1 = (step1 ls)
      s2 = (step2 [(ls[1]), (s1[1]), (ls[2]), (s1[2]), (ls[4]), (s1[3])])
```

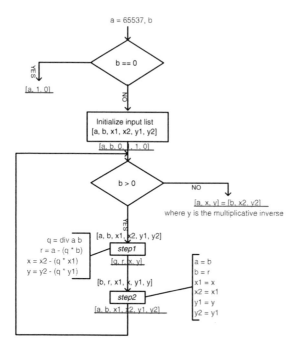

Figure 7: Extended Euclidean algorithm steps flow chart.

```
step1 :: [Int] -> [Int]
step1 ls1 = [q ,
              (ls1[0]) - (q * (ls1[1])),
              (ls1[3]) - (q * (ls1[2])),
              (ls1[5]) - (q * (ls1[4]))]
    where
      q = div (ls1[0]) (ls1[1])

step2 :: [Int] -> [Int]
step2 ls1 = [(ls1[0]), (ls1[1]), (ls1[3]), (ls1[2]), (ls1[5]), (ls1[4])]
```

6.4   IDEA Encryption and Decryption

The encryption (decryption) subkeys are made ready for the encryption (decryption) using the specified functions *generateEncSubKeys* and *generateDecSubKeys*. The encryption (decryption) works by taking a list of elements representing the plaintext (ciphertext) and the private key. Then, the list of plaintext (ciphertext) is segmented as segments of 4-elements each element representing a 16-bit word. These packed lists are then passed to encryption or decryption along with the input private key. A functional specification of *IDEA* encryption is formulated as a function *encryption*. The encryption function works by firstly segmenting the input list using the function *segs*. Secondly, it maps the function responsible for a single block encryption with the input private key to all segmented input list elements. The function responsible for encrypting a single 4-element list is called *encryptSegs*.

```
encryption :: Private -> Plaintext -> Ciphertext
encryption key ls = concat (map (encryptSegs key) (segs 4 ls))
```

A different specification that considers the input plaintext as an already segmented list *ls*:

```
encryption :: Private -> [Plaintext] -> [Ciphertext]
encryption key ls = map (encryptSegs key) ls
```

The decryption has a similar specification. Figure 8 shows the structure and the block diagram for the *IDEA*. A single 64-bit block from the plaintext segmented as a list of 4 elements each of 16-bit inputs to this structure. The output has a similar type, but it represents a block from the ciphertext.

We specify the encryption of one block as the function *encryptSegs*. This function firstly packs the encryption subkeys. Then, it folds (using the high-order-function *foldl*) with an initial list *xs* the function *singleRound* distributing the packed subkeys to each round. Note that the function *singleRound* is the formal specification of a round. The folded output is then passed to the function *outputTransformation* along with the last pack of subkeys, giving the final output. The function *outputTransformation* specifies the output transformation stage found as the final stage in *IDEA* encryption (decryption).

```
encryptSegs :: Private -> [Int] -> [Int]
encryptSegs key xs = [e, g, h, f]
   where
     kss = pack (generateEncSubKeys key)
     [a, b, c, d] = foldl singleRound xs (init kss)
     ([e, f], [g, h]) = outputTransformation [a, c, b, d] (last kss)
```

The decryption could be specified in a similar manner.

6.4.1   Single Round Specification

The main part of the *IDEA* algorithm consists of the application of 8 similar rounds to the input plaintext and the key as shown in Figure 8. In this section we introduce the round construct by introducing each of its building blocks.

A round is specified as a function *singleRound* with two input lists, one representing the input block from the plaintext and the other a pack of subkeys. A *singleRound* works by composing three different functions *firstSubRound*, *secondSubRound*, and *thirdSubRound* (See Figure 9).

```
singleRound :: [Int] -> [Int] -> [Int]
singleRound xs ks = thirdSubRound (secondSubRound (firstSubRound ks xs))
```

The function *firstSubRound* employs modular multiplication and addition to the first 4 elements of both input lists. This function also forwards the last two subkeys from input to output list.

```
firstSubRound  :: [Int] -> [Int] -> [Int]
firstSubRound  [k1, k2, k3, k4, k5, k6] [x1,x2,x3,x4] =
    [(mulMod x1 k1), (addMod x2 k2),
    (addMod x3 k3), (mulMod x4 k4), k5, k6]
```

In *IDEA*, each plaintext bit influence every ciphertext bit. The spreading out of a single plaintext bit over many ciphertext bits hides the statistical nature of the plaintext [10]. This diffusion is provided by the basic building block of the algorithm known as the multiplication/addition (*MA*) structure shown in Figure 9. The function that specifies this structure is called *mA*, and the multiplication/addition is done using the functions *mulMod/addMod*.

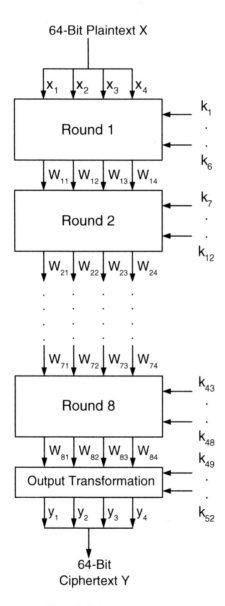

Figure 8: IDEA general structure.

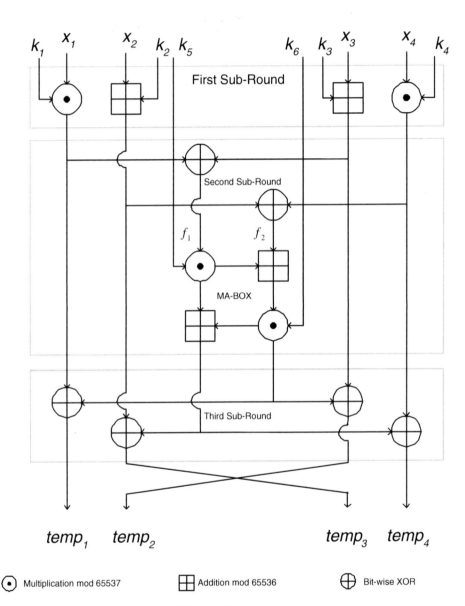

Figure 9: IDEA round.

```
mA :: [Int] -> (Int, Int)
mA [u, w, k5, k6] = (addMod a b, b)
  where
    a = mulMod u k5
    b = mulMod (addMod w a) k6
```

Thereby, the function *secondSubRound* employs the function *mA* over two subkeys and the result of XORing 4 elements from its own input.

```
secondSubRound  :: [Int] -> [Int]
secondSubRound [v1, v2, v3, v4, k5, k6] = [v1, v2, v3, v4, q1, q2]
  where
    (p1, p2) = ((fullexor v1 v3), (fullexor v2 v4))
    (q1, q2) = mA [p1, p2, k5, k6]
```

A third subround is specified to complete the scene of a whole round. This function, namely *thirdSubRound*, is responsible for XORing its inputs. For this sake the high-order-function *zipWith* is used.

```
thirdSubRound :: [Int] -> [Int]
thirdSubRound [y1, y2, y3, y4, p1, p2] =
    zipWith fullexor [y1, y3, y2, y4] [p2, p2, p1, p1]
```

As employed in specifying a single round's constructs, the modular addition *(modulo 65536)* is specified as a function *addMod* with two inputs and one output of type *Int*. The specification can use the modulo operation *mod* to calculate the modular addition as follows:

```
addMod :: Int -> Int -> Int
addMod i1 i2 = mod (i1 + i2) modVal
```

Escaping the cost of the parallel implementation of the operation *mod* as to be implemented by hardware the functional specification is done as follows:

```
addMod :: Int -> Int -> Int
addMod i1 i2 = fullAND (i1 + i2) (modVal - 1)
```

Where, the function *fullAND* is the bit-wise logic AND. It is worth to note at this step that an iterative addition/subtraction dependant version of the operation *mod* could be done as follows:

```
mymod :: Int -> Int -> Int
mymod a b
  | a < b = a
  | otherwise = mymod (a - b) b
```

However, The significance of different versions of these operations is to be more transparent at the realization step. The modular multiplication *(modulo 65537)* is considered one of the most expensive operations used in the *IDEA* from hardware usage and/or throughput points of evaluation.

Considerable research has been done trying to afford different economical and/or efficient implementations. In [16] different designs where addressed discussing the mathematical foundation of each and giving their reconfigurable hardware implementations. An efficient implementation is suggested in [17]. We specify this algorithm as follows:

```
mulMod ::   Int -> Int ->Int mulMod x y =
    if ((mulModEfficient x y) == modVal)
    then (0)
    else (mulModEfficient x y)

mulModEfficient ::   Int -> Int -> Int mulModEfficient x y
  | (x == 0) && (y == 0) = 1
  | (x == 0) && (y /= 0) = ((modVal+1) - y)
  | (x /= 0) && (y == 0) = ((modVal+1) - x)
  | otherwise = if (cL < cH)
                then (cL - cH + (modVal+1))
                else (cL - cH)
  where
    cL= b2i  (take 16 (i2b (x * y)))
    cH= b2i  (drop 16 (padWithFalse32BitR (i2b (x * y))))
```

6.4.2   Output Transformation Specification

This stage is designed to allow the decryption to have the same structure as encryption. The specification is the same as that for the function *firstSubRound*.

7   Refinement of the IDEA Formal Specification

Narrowing the distance from a specific hardware implementation, we apply the step-wise refinement suggested by the development methodology. Data and process refinements are executed with a main concern of demonstrating the design flexibility granted by the proposed methodology. Designs varying from data-parallel to pipelined are shown giving the *CSP* implementation of each.

7.1   Encryption Subkeys Generation

The following design is the refinement of the subkeys generating functions. Datatype refinement considers the input as a 128-bit integer *(Int128)* item to correspond to the 128-bit list of *bool*. An alternative implementation as a 128-element vector of *bool* items could be followed. The first implementation is chosen since, an integer as viewed in hardware is an array of individually manipulatable bits. This is nearly identical to the latter implementation, with a difference that the 128-bit integer item will be communicated on a single channel instead of a vector of channels. The output is refined to a vector of items thereat the 52 subkeys are to be taken. Generally, this design will fork a parallel computation aiming for an expectedly fast subkeys generation. This is done by executing 8 parallel instances of a subkey generator leading to a parallel production of all subkeys. The first step is done by refining the function *generateEncSubKeys* as the process *GENCSKEYS*, where:

$$generateEncSubKeys :: Int128 \rightarrow \lfloor Int16 \rfloor_{52}$$
$$generateEncSubKeys \sqsubseteq GENCSKEYS$$

The *CSP* implementation that corresponds to *generateEncSubKeys* is as follows:

$$GENCSKEYS =$$
$$(in?key \rightarrow SKIP); \; KEYROTATION(key) >>_8 VMAP_8(GSUBKEYS) >>_8 CONCAT$$

While, the following holds:

$$keyRotation \sqsubseteq KEYROTATION$$
$$generateSubKeys \sqsubseteq GSUBKEYS$$
$$concat \sqsubseteq CONCAT$$

Figure 10 is a visualization of the process *GENCSKEYS*.

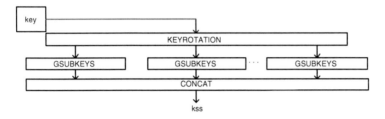

Figure 10: The process *GENCSKEYS*.

Moving to the sub-blocks of this generator, the functional specification for the function *keyRotation* is:

```
keyRotation :: Private -> [[Bool]]
keyRotation key = take 8 (repeated (shift 25) key)
```

Where, *take 8 (repeated (shift 25) key)* could be rewritten, depending on the specification of *repeated*, as:

```
take 8 (repeated (shift 25) key)=
    map (flip shift key) [0, 25, 50, 75, 100, 125, 22, 47]
```

The final specification would be:

```
keyRotation :: Private -> [[Bool]]
keyRotation key = map (btoi) (map (flip shift key) ls)
    where
    ls = [0, 25, 50, 75, 100, 125, 22, 47]
```

In this design we considered the refinement of the input key type to be an item, while the list *ls* and the output rotated keys as vectors of items.

$$keyRotation :: Int128 \rightarrow \lfloor Int128 \rfloor_8$$

The *CSP* implementation of the functional specification refines *keyRotation* to a process *KEYROTATION*.

The key could be passed as an argument to each of the processes *SHIFT(key)*, while distributing the list *ls* elements to the parallel processes as shown in Figure 11. The is described as follows:

$$KEYROTATION(key) = VMAP_8(PRD(key) \rhd SHIFT)$$

The key could be explicitly passed to the process *SHIFT*. The effect of applying this step to the previous design can be visualized as in Figure 12. In the above version the key is locally produced and fed to each process *SHIFT*. The effect of having 8 parallel copies of *PRD(key)* communicating with 8 instances of *SHIFT* can be eliminated by factorizing the

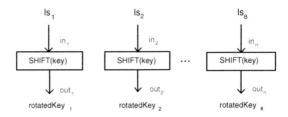

Figure 11: The process *KEYROTATION*.

process *PRD(key)* and broadcasting its output to the relevant processing elements in the network. Applying this rule will result in a semantically equivalent version of *KEYROTATION* which has a different layout. This is shown in Figure 13. The formal rule that justifies the above transformation is:

$$KEYROTATION(key) = BROADCAST_8(key)[d/out] \triangleright_8 VMAP_8(SHIFT)$$

where,

$$shift \sqsubseteq SHIFT$$

The refinement of the input n and the output rotated key realises them as items.

$$shift :: Int128 \rightarrow Int \rightarrow Int128$$

The *CSP* implementation of *shift* is the process *SHIFT*:

$$SHIFT = (in_1?key \rightarrow SKIP \;|||\; in_2?n \rightarrow SKIP); \; out!(key[n..127]{+}{+}key[0..n])$$

where, $key[n..127]{+}{+}key[0..n]$ is the integer equivalent of the concatenation of the upper $127 - n$ bits of the 128-bit key, and lower n bits. Figure 14 gives a general visualization of the process *GENCSKEYS*. The next step is presenting the refinement of *generateSubKeys*. The corresponding *CSP* process is *GSUBKEYS*.

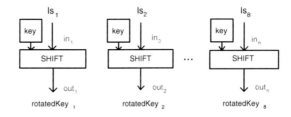

Figure 12: The process *KEYROTATION*, an alternative.

The *CSP* refinement realises the input as an item, and the output as a vector of items where each item is a list.

$$generateSubKeys :: Int128 \rightarrow \lfloor Int16 \rfloor_8$$
$$GSUBKEYS = (in?key \rightarrow SKIP); \; SEGS(key)$$

The recursion in *segs* is unrolled for n equals 16 in a similar way to that done for *keyRotation*.

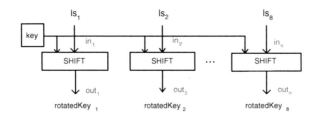

Figure 13: The process *KEYROTATION*, optimised implementation.

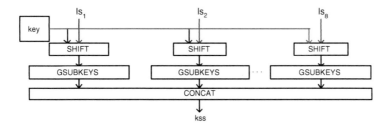

Figure 14: The Process *GENCSKEYS*.

```
segs 16 key =
    [(take 16 key), (take 16 (drop 16 key)),
    (take 16 (drop 32 key))), ..., (take 16
    (drop 112 key)))]
```

Then, the refinement to *CSP* is as follows:

$$SEGS = (in_1?n \rightarrow SKIP \,|||\, in_2?key \rightarrow SKIP);$$

$$|||_{i=0}^{i=\frac{length(key)}{n}-1} out[i]!(key[i*n..((i+1)*n)-1])$$

where $key[0..15], key[16..31], ...$ are the integers equivalent to each 16-bit word. The refinement of the function *pack* is the process *PACK*.

7.2 Decryption Subkeys Generation

The decryption subkeys generation is refined in two ways controlling the number of used processes. The first design replicates the use of the processes *MULINV* and *ADDINV* (the refinement of *addInv* and *mulInv*), where all subkeys are produced in parallel as a vector of vector of items. Each item is communicating on a different channel. The second design implements 4 parallel processes that are inputting the encryption subkeys as a stream of vectors and outputting the desired decryption subkeys as a stream of vectors. In the second design the replication of *MULINV* and *ADDINV* is restricted to 2 of each, thus an economical use of hardware resources is expected in the realization step.

7.2.1 Decryption Subkeys Generation - First Design

We firstly recall the part of the specification responsible for creating the permutation indices. The list *indices* is created as follows:

```
indices = mapWith fs (map reverse (pack (reverse [1 |1<-[0..51]])))
f1(xs) = shift 2 xs
f2(xs) = zipWith (+) (copy (xs!!2) 6) [0, 2, 1, 3, -2, -1]
f3 = id
fs = [f1, f2, f2, f2, f2, f2, f2, f2, f3]
```

The generated list indices has the following values:

```
indices = [[48,49,50,51,46,47],
           [42,44,43,45,40,41],
           [36,38,37,39,34,35],
           [30,32,31,33,28,29],
           [24,26,25,27,22,23],
           [18,20,19,21,16,17],
           [12,14,13,15,10,11],
           [6, 8, 7, 9, 4, 5 ],
           [0, 1, 2, 3]]
```

For simplicity in implementation we replace the computational constructs with a table of values containing the required indices. Accordingly, this permutation is applied to the input encryption subkeys. The modified specification is as follows:

```
generateDecSubKeys :: [SubKey] -> [[SubKey]]
generateDecSubKeys eKeys  = map perform eKeysPerm
  where
    indices =  [[48,49,50,51,46,47],
                [42,44,43,45,40,41],
                [36,38,37,39,34,35],
                [30,32,31,33,28,29],
                [24,26,25,27,22,23],
                [18,20,19,21,16,17],
                [12,14,13,15,10,11],
                [6, 8, 7, 9, 4, 5 ],
                [0, 1, 2, 3]]
    eKeysPerm = map (zipWith (!!) (copy eKeys 6)) indices
    perform(as) = mapWith [mulInv , addInv, addInv, mulInv, id,id] as
```

The input and output to and from the process *GDSKEYS*, the refinement of *generateDecSub-Keys*, are communicated as a vector and a vector of vectors:

$$generateDecSubKeys :: \lfloor Int16 \rfloor_{52} \rightarrow \lfloor \lfloor Int16 \rfloor_6 \rfloor_9$$

The input encryption subkeys are firstly permutated according to the given *indices*, and then produced to parallel instances of the process *PERFORM* the refinement of *perform*.

$$GDSKEYS = |||_{i=0}^{i=51} (in.elements[i]?skeys[i] \rightarrow SKIP);$$
$$(PRDp(skeys) \triangleright VMAP_9(PERFORM))$$

$$PERFORM = |||_{j=0}^{j=1} (ADDINV[in/in_j, out/out_j]$$
$$||| \ MULINV[in/in_j, out/out_j]$$
$$||| \ (Forward[in/in_j, out/out_j]))$$

$$PRDp(ls) = (|||_{i \in P, j=0}^{j=53} out.elements[j]!ls[i]) \rightarrow SKIP$$

$$P = \{48, 49, 50, 51, 46, 47, 42, 44, 43, 45, 40, 41,$$
$$36, 38, 37, 39, 34, 35, 30, 32, 31, 33, 28, 29, 24, 26,$$
$$25, 27, 22, 23, 18, 20, 19, 21, 16, 17, 12, 14, 13, 15,$$
$$10, 11, 6, 8, 7, 9, 4, 5, 0, 1, 2, 3, 0, 0\}$$

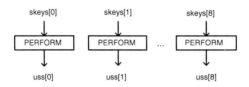

Figure 15: Decryption subkeys generation, first design.

7.2.2 Decryption Subkeys Generation - Second Design

In this design, the input and output are communicated as streams of vectors of 6 items. The input vector is ordered in the way needed for the process, where the first and the fourth elements are passed to the *MULINV* processes, the second and the third inputs are passed to the *ADDINV* processes. The last two input elements are forwarded to the output channels in their order. This process is visualized in Figure 16.

$$generateDecSubKeys :: \lfloor Int16 \rfloor_{52} \rightarrow \langle \lfloor Int16 \rfloor_6 \rangle$$

$$GDSKEYS = |||_{i=0}^{i=51} \, in.elements[i]?skeys[i] \rightarrow SKIP);$$
$$(SPRDp(skeys) \rhd SMAP(PERFORM)$$

$$SPRDp(ls) = ((; \,)_{i=0}^{i=8}(|||_{j\in P'[i],k=0}^{k=5} \, out.elements[k]!ls[j])) \rightarrow$$
$$out.eotChannel!eot \rightarrow SKIP$$

$$P' = \{\{48, 49, 50, 51, 46, 47\}, \{42, 44, 43, 45, 40, 41\},$$
$$\{36, 38, 37, 39, 34, 35\}, \{30, 32, 31, 33, 28, 29\},$$
$$\{24, 26, 25, 27, 22, 23\}, \{18, 20, 19, 21, 16, 17\},$$
$$\{12, 14, 13, 15, 10, 11\}, \{6, 8, 7, 9, 4, 5\}, \{0, 1, 2, 3, 0, 0\}\}$$

7.3 IDEA Encryption and Decryption

A parallel program for a block encryption (or decryption) could be viewed with different levels of parallelism. The first design is suggested to view the input subkeys as vector of vectors passed in parallel to the parallel rounds. This design replicates the process *SINGLEROUND* (which corresponds to the function *singleRound*) an 8-stage pipeline. The replication is done using a vector implementation off-the-shelf refined high-order-function *foldl*.

Another design considers input subkeys as stream of vectors using one instance of the process *SINGLEROUND*, thus a later minimal use of resources needed by *SINGLEROUND* processes. This is done using a sequential implementation of *foldl*.

A compromised design affording flexibility in controlling replication of the process *SINGLEROUND* is done by taking a part of the subkeys as vector of vectors while the remaining

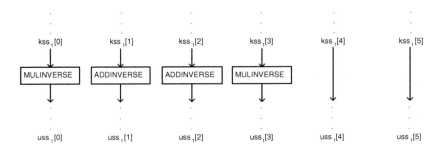

Figure 16: Decryption subkeys generation, second design.

subkeys as stream of vectors. This is a tradeoff between use of hardware resources and throughput of processing. These designs are elaborated in the following subsections.

The encryption for a whole set of plaintext also could be viewed in two levels of parallel execution. A first design could pass sequentially the plaintext blocks as a stream of vector of items. A second design could pass the blocks as streams of vector of vectors of items, replicating the whole *IDEA* block leading to a multi-way encryption. These two versions are presented for the encryption taking into consideration that the decryption is implemented similarly. Refining the input plaintext segmented blocks to a stream of vector of items, while the key is input once as an item, we get:

$$encryption :: \langle \lfloor Int16 \rfloor_4 \rangle \rightarrow \langle \lfloor Int16 \rfloor_4 \rangle$$

where:

$$ENCRYPTION(key) = SMAP(ENCRYPTSEGS(key))$$

The second version is implemented as follows, where n is limited to the available resources.

$$encryption :: \langle \lfloor \langle \lfloor Int16 \rfloor_4 \rangle \rfloor_n \rangle \rightarrow \langle \lfloor \langle \lfloor Int16 \rfloor_4 \rangle \rfloor_n \rangle$$
$$ENCRYPTION(key) = SMAP(VMAP_n(SMAP(ENCRYPTSEGS(key))))$$

7.3.1   IDEA First Design

The main point of the first design is to have a version of *IDEA* with all of its rounds working in parallel. This is apparent from the refinement of the input subkeys. The subkeys are refined as a vector of vectors of items and distributed to the parallel rounds. The refinement realises this function as the process *ENCRYPTSEGS* (See Figure 17), where the input and output segments are streams of vectors of items and the key is passed as an item. The key will be used to generate a vector of vectors of subkeys through *GENCSKEYS*.

$$encryptSegs :: Int128 \rightarrow \langle \lfloor Int16 \rfloor_4 \rangle \rightarrow \langle \lfloor Int16 \rfloor_4 \rangle$$
$$encryptSegs \sqsubseteq ENCRYPTSEGS$$
$$ENCRYPTSEGS = GENCSKEYS \gg_{52} PACK \gg_9$$
$$(VVFOLDL(SINGLEROUND)\|OTPTTRANS)$$

The process *VVFOLDL(SINGLEROUND)* is an off-the-shelf refinement for the high-order-function *foldl* over a vector of vectors of items.

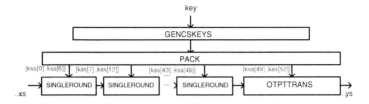

Figure 17: *IDEA* encryption block diagram, a fully-pipelined first design.

The refinement of a single round is a process *SINGLEROUND*. The data refinement realises the inputs and output of this function as vectors of items.

$$singleRound :: \lfloor Int16 \rfloor_4 \rightarrow \lfloor Int16 \rfloor_6 \rightarrow \lfloor Int16 \rfloor_4$$
$$singleRound \sqsubseteq SINGLEROUND$$
$$SINGLEROUND = FIRSTSUBROUND \ggg_6 SECONDSUBROUND$$
$$\ggg_6 THIRDSUBROUND$$

where:

$$firstSubRound \sqsubseteq FIRSTSUBROUND$$
$$secondSubRound \sqsubseteq SECONDSUBROUND$$
$$thirdSubRound \sqsubseteq THIRDSUBROUND$$

SINGLEROUND is depicted in Figure 18.

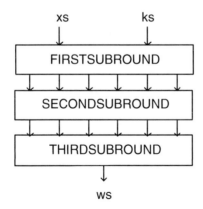

Figure 18: The process *SINGLEROUND* as the piping of the three subrounds.

The refinement of the function *firstSubRound* realises the inputs and output as vectors of items. The refinement of the functions *addMod* and *mulMod* (modular addition and multiplication) are the processes *AddMod* and *MulMod* respectively.

$$firstSubRound :: \lfloor Int16 \rfloor_4 \rightarrow \lfloor Int16 \rfloor_6 \rightarrow \lfloor Int16 \rfloor_6$$
$$FIRSTSUBROUND = |||_{j=0}^{j=1} (ADDINV[in/in_j, out/out_j] \ ||| \ MULINV[in/in_j, out/out_j]$$
$$||| \ (Forward[in/in_j, out/out_j]))$$

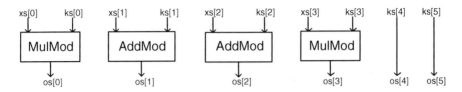

Figure 19: The process *FIRSTSUBROUND*.

Visualization of the process *FIRSTSUBROUND* is shown in Figure 19. The refinement of the function *secondSubRound* is *SECONDSUBROUND*. The *CSP* implementation consider the input and output as vectors of items:

$$secondSubRound :: \lfloor Int16 \rfloor_6 \rightarrow \lfloor Int16 \rfloor_6$$

$$SECONDSUBROUND = (VZIPWITH_2(EXOR)) \| MA$$
$$EXOR = (in_1?l1 \rightarrow SKIP \ ||| \ in_2?l2 \rightarrow SKIP); \ out!(l1 \oplus l2)$$
$$fullexor \sqsubseteq EXOR$$

where, $\oplus$ is the bit-wise execlusive-OR. This process is visualized in Figure 20.

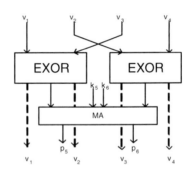

Figure 20: The processes *SECONDSUBROUND*.

The refined process *MA* satisfies the function *mA*. Accordingly, the *CSP* implementation is as follows:

$$mA :: \lfloor Int16 \rfloor_4 \rightarrow (Int16, Int16)$$

$$MA = (\|\|_{i=1}^{i=4} \ in_1?list.Elements[i] \rightarrow SKIP);$$
$$MULMOD \| IBROADCAST_2[d/out] \|$$
$$(ADDMOD \gg MULMOD) \| IBROADCAST_2[d/out] \| ADDMOD$$

The process *IBROADCAST_n* broadcasts a single input to an *n* independent channels. The Process *MA* is visualized in Figure 21.

Data refinement considers the input and output of the function *thirdSubRound* as vectors of vectors:

$$thirdSubRound :: \lfloor Int16 \rfloor_6 \rightarrow \lfloor Int16 \rfloor_4$$

$$THIRDSUBROUND = (\|\|_{i=0}^{i=5} \ in.elements[i]?[y1,y2,y3,y4,p1,p2] \rightarrow SKIP);$$
$$(PRD([y1,y3,y2,y4] \| PRD([p2,p2,p1,p1] \| VZIPWITH_4(EXOR))$$

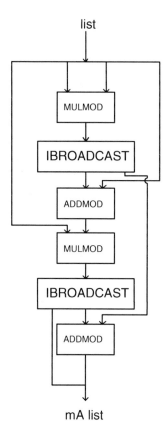

Figure 21: The process *MA*.

Visualization of the process *THIRDSUBROUND* is shown in Figure 22.

The refinement for the *outputTransformation* is done in a similar way to *FIRSTSUB-ROUND*.

7.3.2 IDEA Second Design

As indicated earlier, in this design the generated subkeys communicate with encryption (or decryption) process as a stream of vectors of items as depicted in Figure 23. The refinement for this design is as follows:

$ENCRYPTSEGS =$
$$GENCSKEYS \gg_{52} PACK \gg_9 (SVFOLDL(SINGLEROUND) \| OTPTTRANS)$$

The process *SVFOLDL(SINGLEROUND)* uses an off-the-shelf refinement for the high-order-function *foldl* over a stream of vectors of items.

7.3.3 IDEA Third Design

This design is a compromised solution between the first and the second design. The *CSP* implementation of this design allows the passing of the subkeys in two ways. Some of the

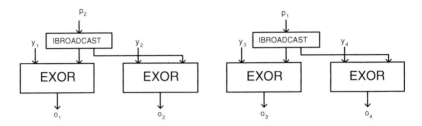

Figure 22: The process *THIRDSUBROUND*.

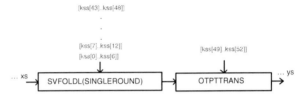

Figure 23: *IDEA* encryption block diagram in its second design with streamed input and output.

subkeys elements are passed as a vector of vectors, while the remaining subkeys are communicated as a stream of vectors. This design is shown in Figure 24.

$$ENCRYPTSEGS(n) = GENCSKEYS \gg_{52} PACK \gg_9$$
$$((n \rhd VVFOLDL(SINGLEROUND))$$
$$\| SVFOLDL(SINGLEROUND)$$
$$\| OTPTTRANS)$$

The processes *VVFOLDL(SINGLEROUND)* and *SVFOLDL(SINGLEROUND)* are running in parallel synchronising on the output of *VVFOLDL(SINGLEROUND)* to be the input to *SVFOLDL(SINGLEROUND)*. The number of folded processes is produced for each where n is the number of folded processes having subkeys as vector of vectors.

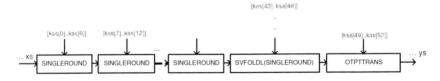

Figure 24: *IDEA* encryption block diagram, partially pipelined third design.

8 Reconfigurable Hardware Realization

In this section we discuss only some pieces of the code implementing the presented designs. The whole implementations were tested and the practical evaluation and analysis is presented in the next section. Coding with *Handel-C*, the structure of the implementation is based on the network of communicating processes given by the refinement. A part of the code implementing the macro *GenerateEncSubKeys* is as follows:

```
par {
    KeyRotation (Key1, Vlst, VoVOut1);
    VMap (VoVOut1, VoVOut2, Size, GenerateSubKeys);
    // The output is concatenated in one vector of vectors VoVOut2
}
```

The used datatypes were declared as:

```
Item (key1, Int128);  // The Key
VectorOfVectorsOfItems (voVOut1, 8, 8, Int16);  // Intermediate
VectorOfVectorsOfItems (voVOut2, 8, 8,Int16);  // Result
```

Another example is the hardware implementation of the second design for decryption sub-keys generation. In this code the encryption subkeys are loaded from the memory bank produced as a stream of vectors of 6 elements to a macro *Perform* that performs the required computation based on the *CSP* refinement.

The macro that performs the computation and the main program that uses it are as shown in the following listing.

```
StreamOfVectorsOfItems (sKssIn, 6, Int16);
StreamOfVectorsOfItems (sUssOut, 6, Int16);
 .
 .
 .
par{
    ProduceStreamOfVectorsOfItems (sKssIn, 9, 6, P');
    Map (sKssIn, sUssOut, Perform);
    StoreStreamOfVectorsOfItems (sUssOut, 6, decSubKeyss);
}

macro proc Perform (sKIn, sUOut) {
    par {
        MulInv (sKIn.elements[0], sUOut.elements[0]);
        AddInv (sKIn.elements[1], sUOut.elements[1]);
        AddInv (sKIn.elements[2], sUOut.elements[2]);
        MulInv (sKIn.elements[3], sUOut.elements[3]);
        ForwardItem (sKIn.elements[4], sUOut.elements[4]);
        ForwardItem (sKIn.elements[5], sUOut.elements[5]);
    }
}
```

The implementation for a single round is done by implementing each sub-round as a macro. The macro that corresponds for the process *FIRSTSUBROUND* is:

```
macro proc FirstSubRound (xs, ks, ts) {
    par {
        AddMod (xs.elements[1], ks.elements[1], ts.elements[1]);
        MulMod (xs.elements[0], ks.elements[0], ts.elements[0]);
        AddMod (xs.elements[2], ks.elements[2], ts.elements[2]);
        MulMod (xs.elements[3], ks.elements[3], ts.elements[3]);
        ForwardItem (ks.elements[4], ts.elements[4]);
        ForwardItem (ks.elements[5], ts.elements[5]);
    }
}
```

Thus for a single round:

```
macro proc Round (xsIn, ksIn, wsOut) {
    .
    .
    .
    par {
        FirstSubRound (xsIn, ksIn, one);
        SecondSubRound (one, two);
        ThirdSubRound (two, wsOut);
    }
}
```

Turning our attention to another example, we choose the implementation of the encryption third design. Whereby, a combination of parallel and sequential fold are employed. Comments on the functionality are included near each statement.

```
void main (void) {
    .
    .
    .
    par {
        // Get plaintext.
        ProduceStreamOfVectorsOfItemsFromBank0 (xsSOV, 4);

        // Produce subkeys for VVFoldL
        ProduceVectorOfVectorsOfItems (vVSubKeys, pRnds, 6, subKeyss);
        VVFoldL (vVSubKeys, 6, xsSoVector, 4, pRnds, Round, xsSOV);

        // Produce the remaining subkeys for SVFoldL
        ProduceStreamOfVectorsOfItems (sVSubKeys, sRnds, 6, subKeyss1);
        SVFoldL (sVSubKeys, 6, sWs, Round, xsSoVector, 4, sRnds);

        // Produce subkeys for the output transformation
        ProduceVectorOfItems (ks9, 4, subKeys9);
        OutputTransformation (sWs, ks9, xsSoVector1);

        // Store the ciphertext
        StoreStreamOfVectorsOfItemsInBank1 (xsSoVector1, 4);
    }
}
```

9 Performance Analysis and Evaluation

Generally, the suggested algorithms inherit all the advantages from the development method applied. Key issues are granted, like the production of reusable, scalable, and correct solutions by construction as opposed to trial and testing. Correctness, which is an important aspect in security algorithms, is ensured by construction through the functional specification step. Recall that according to this specification, the implementation under *HUGs98 Haskell* compiler is tested at the unit, component and integration levels.

Table 1 shows the results for the encryption and decryption subkeys generation. Note that the test key used for the generation is the key whose 16-bit segments are: $\{1, 2, 3, 4, 5, 6, 7, 8\}$. We also recall that the execution time of doing only the handshaking between the host and the *RC-1000* system with no computations costs approximately $132\,\mu\,Sec$. Some of decryption first design's results are marked as not available as the design was too large for the compiled device. The encryption keys are expanded with a throughput of 4.089 Gbps occupying an area of 5846 Slices, i.e. 12% of the area of the available *FPGA*. The speed dramatically goes down with the decryption subkeys expansion using the second stream-based design (6.68 Mbps and an area of 9032 Slices).

Table 1: Results for encryption and decryption subkeys generation.

Metrics Designs	Encryption Subkeys Generation	Decryption Subkeys Generation First Design	Decryption Subkeys Generation Second Design
Number of Gates	64906 NANDs	4094334 NANDs	162923 NANDs
Number of Occupied Slices	5846 Slices (12%)	92091 Slices (321% Overmapped)	9032 Slices (47%)
Total equivalent gate count	80784 Gates	1012481 Gates	132128 Gates
Number of Cycles	14 Cycles	88 Cycles	588 Cycles
Maximum Frequency of Design	68.81MHz	NA	4.72 MHz
Throughput	4.089 Gbps	NA	6.68 Mbps
Measured Execution Time	167 Micro sec.	NA	299 Micro sec.
Measured Throughput	23.77 Mbps	NA	4.98 Mbps

Table 2 presents the results for the different designs of encryption (decryption). The findings reflect the change of performance with respect to the change of design. The first design, as intended, is the fastest with a max throughput of 21.33 Gbps (average throughput of 21.5 Mbps) noted from testing random input test vectors with a key $= \{1, 2, 3, 4, 5, 6, 7, 8\}$. The second design, which correspond to a sequential execution of the rounds has an expected slowest throughput (maximum throughput of 5.82 Gbps and average throughput of 19.53 Mbps), but the minimum circuit area 5650 Slices (29% of the area of the used *FPGA*). The third design trades the throughput for the used area, thus it has a compromised performance as compared to the first and second designs. Many tests are run using random test vectors and keys to measure the average throughput shown in Table 2. Table 3 shows different ratios relative to a suggested design. For instance, This table shows the Gates Saving Ratio with respect to the second design. This ratio is an indicator for how many times more (or less) a design would use gates taking the second design result as a reference value.

Table 2: Results for encryption (or decryption) for different test vectors.

Metrics Designs	1st Fully-Pipelined Design	2 nd Stream-Based Design	3 rd Partially-Pipelined (2 Parallel and 6 Sequential)
Number of Gates	394526 NANDs	88651 NANDs	176583 NANDs
Number of Occupied Slices	19198 Slices (99%)	5650 Slices (29%)	10147 Slices (52%)
Total equivalent gate count	363682 Gates	93659 Gates	172719 Gates
Number of Cycles / Key ={1,2,3,4,5,6,7,8}	88 Cycles	415 Cycles	382 Cycles
Maximum Frequency of Design	34.975 MHz	44.72 MHz	36.42 MHz
Throughput	25.4 Mbps	6.89 Mbps	6.1 Mbps
Best Measured Execution Time	0.036 Micro Sec.	0.04475 Micro Sec.	0.0425 Micro Sec.
Average Measured Execution Time	2.98 Micro sec.	3.276 Micro sec.	3.086 Micro sec.
Best Measured Throughput	1.777 Gbps	1.430 Gbps	1.505 Gbps
Average Measured Throughput	21.5 Mbps	19.53 Mbps	20.73 Mbps

Different implementations of modular arithmetic operations dramatically affect the performance of the *IDEA*. Three implementations for the modular multiplication are being investigated. The first implementation uses a fast and expensive version of the modulo operator *mod*. A second implementation corresponds to an iterative version of the operation *mod*. The third implementation is for the efficient implementation shown in the specification section,

Table 3: Comparisons among suggested designs.

Metrics Designs	First Design	Second Design	Third Design (2 parallel and 6 sequential)
Gates Saving Ration wrt Second Design	3.88 (288% more gates)	N_1 = T E No. Gates (No Comm.) N_2 = T E No Gates (No Comm.) of 2nd Design N_1/N_2 ((N$_1$ - N$_2$) / N$_2$ %)	1.84 (84% more gates)
Number of Cycles Ratio wrt First Design	C_1 = No. Cycles C_2 = No cycles of 1st Design C_1/C_2 (C$_1$ - C$_2$) / C$_2$ %)	4.7159 (371.59% more cycles)	4.3409 (340.9% more cycles)
Best Time Ratio wrt First Design	E_1 = Exec. Time E_2 = Exec. Time of 1st Design E_1/E_2 (E$_1$ - E$_2$) / E$_2$ %)	1.24 (24% more time)	1.18 (18% more time)
Average Time Ratio wrt First Design		1.099 (9.9% more time)	1.035 (3.5% more time)
Best Measured Speedup Ratio wrt First Design	S_1 = Speed of 1st Design S_2 = Speed	1.24 (24% faster)	1.18 (18% faster)
Average Measured Speedup Ratio wrt First Design	S_1/S_2 (S$_1$ - S$_2$) / S$_2$ %)	1.1 (10% faster)	1.037 (3.7% more time)
Occupied Area (Slices) Ratio wrt Second Design	3.39 (239% larger area)	A_1 = Area (No Comm.) A_2 = Area (No Comm.) of 2nd Design A_1/A_2 (A$_1$ - A$_2$) / A$_2$ %)	1.77 (77% larger area)

which eliminates the use of the operation *mod*. Table 4 shows comparisons among the suggested implementations of the modular multiplication as used in the second design. This table shows that the efficient implementation of the modular multiplication has affected the performance of the *IDEA* positively. This is shown in the reduced cycle count taken by this implementation as compared to the two other implementations. It also reduced the used area to 5650 Slices after being 6263 and 10739 Slices in the other implementations.

Table 4: Results for encryption second design for different versions of 'mod', for different test vectors.

Second Design Modular Multiplication Implemented using: (Key Used = {1,2,3,4,5,6,7,8})	'mod' Operator	Iterative 'mod'	Efficient Implementation Eliminating 'mod'
Number of Gates	172164 NAND Gates	95226 NAND Gates	93659 NAND Gates
Number of Cycles	988 Cycles	106060 Cycles	415 Cycles
Best Measured Execution Time	0.04475 Micro Sec.	0.15075 Micro Sec.	0.011 Micro sec.
Best Measured Speed	1.430 Gbps	424.54 Mbps	5.82 Gbps
Number of Occupied Slices	10739 (55%)	6263 (32%)	5650 (29%)
Total equivalent gate count	168889	103057	93659

To present some results from the literature for hardware implementations of the *IDEA* algorithm, A summary of findings is shown in Table 5. In [12, 13, 11, 18], the authors present different ad hoc hardware implementations of the *IDEA* algorithm. The *IDEA* block cipher has been implemented at throughput ranging from 8.5 Gbps [13] to 177 Mbps [18] on *FPGAs*. Note that while a 528 Mbps throughput was achieved [14], with a fully pipelined architecture, the implementation required four *Xilinx XC4020 FPGAs*.

Table 5: Comparison among different hardware implementations of the IDEA.

System Metrics	Speed (Mbps)	Clock Frequency (MHz)	Area
PCI Pamette - 4 Xilinx XC4020 FPGAs (Zimmermann et al)	528	33	3200 CLBs
UNICORN Architecture; Xilinx FPGA (Runje et al)	2.8	NA	NA
XCV1000-6 Xilinx FPGA (2 Cores) (Cheung et al)	5250	82	11602 Slices
XCV1000-6 Xilinx FPGA (Beuchat et al)	8000	NA	4845 Slices
XCV2000e-6 Xilinx FPGA (Beuchat et al)	8500	NA	18164 Slices
XC2V4000-6 Xilinx FPGA (Beuchat et al)	7900	NA	18537 Slices

10 Conclusion

We investigated in this paper the synthesis of highly parallel reconfigurable hardware implementation for the *IDEA*. Important aspects for hardware implementations of cryptographic algorithms like correctness, reliability along with efficiency are stressed through the application of the proposed development model. The development for the *IDEA* started by formally specifying the algorithm in a functional setting. At that point, provably correct refinement rules are applied transforming the specification to different proposed designs. Thereby, implementations with different levels of parallelism are studied. The refined designs include the blocks from *IDEA* responsible for encryption and decryption in addition to their subkeys generators. The reconfigurable circuits' realization using *Handel-C* is done based on the refined *CSP* networks. The first design requires 88 computing cycles yielding an average throughput of 25.4 Mbps. The maximum throughput achieved with random test vectors was 21.33 Gbps. The second design occupied the minimum area among the different designs with 5650 slices. Currently, our research is concentrating on widening the area of application of the development model, besides, automating the development process.

References

[1] A. E. Abdallah. Derivation of Parallel Algorithms from Functional Specifications to CSP Processes. *Mathematics of Program Construction, LNCS 947, (Springer Verlag, 1995)*, pages 67–96, 1995.

[2] J. Hawkins and A. E. Abdallah. Functional process modelling. *Proceedings of the 7th IEEE International Conference on Electronics, Circuits and Systems*, December 2000.

[3] I. Damaj, J. Hawkins, and A. Abdallah. Mapping high level algorithms onto massively parallel reconfigurable hardware. *ACS/IEEE International Conference on Computer Systems and Applications*, pages 14–22, July 2003.

[4] Celoxica. Handel-c documentation. *http://www.celoxica.com/*, 2003.

[5] National Bureau of Standards, U.S. Department of Commerce. *Data encryption standard*, January 1977.

[6] B. Schneier. *Applied Cryptography*. John Wiley and Sons, New York, 1996.

[7] X. Lai and J. Massey. A proposal for a new block encryption standard. In *Proceedings of the EUROCRYPT 90 Conference*, pages 389–904, 1990.

[8] A. Tanenbaum. *Computer Networks*. Prentice Hall, Upper Saddle River, NJ, third edition, 1997.

[9] J. Daemen, R. Govaerts, and J. Vandewalle. Weak keys for IDEA. *Springer-Verlag*, pages 224–231, 1994.

[10] William Stallings. *Network Security Essentials*. Prentice Hall, third edition, November 2002.

[11] D. Runje and M. Kovac. Universal strong encryption FPGA core implementation. In *Proceedings of Design, Automation and Test in Europe*, pages 923–924, 1998.

[12] O. Y. H. Cheung, K. H. Tsoi, P. H. W. Leong, and M. P. Leong. Tradeoffs in parallel and serial implementations of the international data encryption algorithm IDEA. *Lecture Notes in Computer Science*, 2162:333, 2001.

[13] Jean-Luc Beuchat and Jean-Michel Muller. Modulo *m* multiplication-addition: Algorithms and FPGA implementation. *Electronics Letters*, 40(11):654–655, May 2004.

[14] O. Mencer, M. Morf, and M.J. Flynn. Hardware software tri-design of encryption for mobile communication units. In *Proceedings of the 1998 IEEE International Conference on Acoustics, Speech and Signal Processing*, volume 5, pages 3045–3048, 1998.

[15] Allen Michalski, Kris Gaj, and Tarek El-Ghazawi. An Implementation Comparison of an IDEA Encryption Cryptosystem on Two General-Purpose Reconfigurable Computers. In *Field-Programmable Logic and Applications: 13th International Conference, FPL*, Lecture Notes in Computer Science, pages 204 – 219, Lisbon - Portugal, 2003. Springer.

[16] Jean-Luc Beuchat. Modular multiplication for FPGA implementation of the IDEA block cipher. In Ed Deprettere, Shuvra Bhattacharyya, Joseph Cavallaro, Alain Darte, and Lothar Thiele, editors, *Proceedings of the 14th IEEE International Conference on Application-Specific Systems, Architectures, and Processors*, pages 412–422. IEEE Computer Society, 2003.

[17] Alfred J. Menezes, Paul van Oorschot, and Scott A. Vanston. *Handbook of Applied Cryptography*. CRC Press, fifth edition, August 2001.

[18] R. Zimmermann, A. Curiger, H. Bonnenberg, H. Kaeslin, N. Felber, and W. Fichtner. A 177 MBps VLSI implementation of the International Data Encryption Algorithm. *IEEE Journal of Solid State Circuits*, 29(3):303–307, March 1994.

Author Index